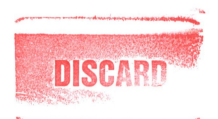

Prosthetics and Patient Management

A Comprehensive Clinical Approach

Prosthetics and Patient Management

A Comprehensive Clinical Approach

Kevin Carroll, MS, CP, FAAOP
Hanger Prosthetics
Orlando, Florida

Joan E. Edelstein, MA, PT, FISPO
Columbia University
College of Physicians and Surgeons
New York, New York

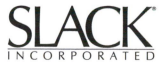

SLACK®
INCORPORATED

Delivering the best in health care information and education worldwide

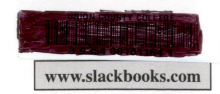

ISBN 10: 1-55642-671-2
ISBN 13: 978-1-55642-671-1

Published by: SLACK Incorporated
                  6900 Grove Road
                  Thorofare, NJ 08086 USA
                  Telephone: 856-848-1000
                  Fax: 856-853-5991
                  www.slackbooks.com

Contact SLACK Incorporated for more information about other books in this field or about the availability of our books from distributors outside the United States.

Library of Congress Cataloging-in-Publication Data

Prosthetics and patient management : a comprehensive clinical approach / [edited by] Kevin Carroll, Joan E. Edelstein.
    p. ; cm.
  Includes index.
  ISBN-13: 978-1-55642-671-1 (hardcover : alk. paper)
  ISBN-10: 1-55642-671-2 (hardcover : alk. paper)
  1. Amputees--Rehabilitation. 2. Prosthesis.
  [DNLM: 1. Amputation--rehabilitation. 2. Amputation--adverse effects. 3. Amputees--rehabilitation. 4. Artificial Limbs.
  5. Joint Prosthesis. WE 170 P966 2006] I. Carroll, Kevin. II. Edelstein, Joan E.

RD553.P76 2006
617.5'8--dc22

                                        2006007679

Printed in the United States of America

Last digit is print number: 10   9   8   7   6   5   4   3   2   1

DEDICATION

To my wife, Mary Carroll, PT, in appreciation for her help and support on this project. To Michael and Aoife, whose encouragement was enormous throughout this endeavor. To Carol Wade, for many weekends of hard work coordinating this project, and to Sherri Edge, for her invaluable advice and contributions.

—KC

For David, Benjamin, and, most of all, for Haskell.

—JEE

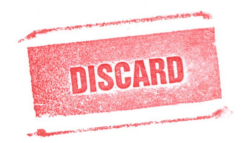

CONTENTS

Section I: Early Management

Section II: Rehabilitation of Adults With Lower-Limb Amputations

Section III: Rehabilitation of Adults With Upper-Limb Amputations

Section IV: Beyond the Basics

ACKNOWLEDGMENTS

We acknowledge the contribution of our patients and colleagues, who shape our professional insights, and our students, who challenge us to harmonize the theoretical with the practical aspects of clinical practice. We sincerely thank John Bond, Carrie Kotlar, Robert Smentek, and Michelle Gatt from SLACK Incorporated, for their confidence in us and their patience, enthusiasm, and guidance that helped bring this book into existence.

ABOUT THE EDITORS

Kevin M Carroll, MS, CP, FAAOP has a simple guiding philosophy: people first. This has served him well in his clinical consultations with thousands of prosthetic consumers across the World. By listening to each person's thoughts and concerns, and understanding their unique situations, Kevin has found a sure path to assisting people in their rehabilitation. He specializes in the care of older adults and also has a degree in gerontology, enhancing his expertise in this area.

Kevin's practice began in his native country of Ireland in 1978 at the National Medical Rehabilitation Center in Dublin. In 1984, he moved to the United States and continued his education, earning degrees in Family Studies, Gerontology, and Counseling Psychology. He serves as Vice President of Prosthetics for Hanger Prosthetics & Orthotics, the largest provider of prosthetic care in the World. Kevin's commitment to improving prosthetics has placed him at the forefront of numerous prosthetic breakthroughs.

His professional background encompasses the roles of researcher, educator, international speaker, and clinician. Kevin travels extensively throughout North America and various parts of the World presenting continuing education courses at professional conferences, and conducting Patient Evaluation Clinics. He is certified by the American Board for Certification as a Certified Prosthetist and has been named a Fellow of the American Academy of Orthotics and Prosthetics, one of the highest honors of the profession. Professional contributions include Practitioner Advisory Council for *O&P Business News*; Editorial Advisory Board for *Orthopedic Technology Review*; Editorial Board for Jointe Centre for Research in Prosthetics & Orthotics and Rehabilitation Programs, Kingdom of Saudi Arabia; Professional Advisory Board for *O&P Edge*; and Editorial Board of *O&P Business World*. Kevin has written on all aspects of prosthetics for publications such as *Physical Medicine and Rehabilitation Clinics of North America, American Academy of Orthopaedic Surgeons, Foot and Ankle Clinics of North America, Amputee Coalition of America*, and various magazine articles.

He is a member of the International Society for Prosthetics and Orthotics, and is a professional advisor for the Amputee Coalition of America, and a member of the National Association of Professional Geriatric Care Managers; Kevin is also a member of the British Association of Prosthetics and Orthotics (BAPO).

Kevin's hobbies include playing music and building sport prosthetic systems, and watching athletes put them to the test at track and field events and the Paralympics.

Joan E. Edelstein, MA, PT, FISPO, is a world-renowned authority in prosthetics and orthotics. After graduating from New York University, NY, magna cum laude, she entered clinical practice in the Children's Division of the Institute of Physical Medicine and Rehabilitation, subsequently renamed the Rusk Institute of New York University, where she became chief physical therapist. When invited to join the faculty of the University of Wisconsin, Madison, she began the academic phase of her career. Returning to New York, she became a senior research scientist at New York University's Prosthetics and Orthotics Program, originally part of the College of Engineering, later a division of the Department of Orthopedic Surgery and the School of Education. She conducted laboratory and field-testing of a wide variety of prostheses and orthoses for the upper and lower limbs, as well as trunk orthoses. She is highly regarded for her enthusiastic instruction in the postgraduate courses offered to physicians, prosthetists, therapists, and other members of the rehabilitation team. Professor Edelstein pioneered the establishment of the first undergraduate curriculum leading to the baccalaureate in prosthetics and orthotics. Upon the closing of the New York University program, she became an associate professor of clinical physical therapy at the College of Physicians and Surgeons, Columbia University, New York, NY, and served as Director of the Program in Physical Therapy. She continues as Special Lecturer at Columbia University and adjunct faculty at New York University; George Washington University, Washington, DC; Touro College, Bay Shore, NY; and Husson College, Bangor, ME.

Professional contributions beyond the university include presenting post-graduate and continuing education courses throughout North America, Europe, Africa, Asia, and the Middle East. She has been a keynote speaker at professional conferences and congresses. Her numerous publications pertaining to all phases of prosthetics and orthotics include journal articles, book chapters, monographs, and books, particularly *Orthotics: A Comprehensive Clinical Approach* (published by SLACK Incorporated).

Professor Edelstein has been editor or member of the editorial boards of *Archives of Physical Medicine and Rehabilitation, Journal of the Association of Children's Prosthetic-Orthotic Clinics, Journal of Rehabilitation Research and Development, Physical and Occupational Therapy in Geriatrics,* and *Topics in Geriatric Rehabilitation.* She was honored by being named a Fellow of the International Society for Prosthetics and Orthotics.

Contributing Authors

Randall D. Alley, CP
Upper-Limb Prosthetics Society
Thousand Oaks, California

Diane Atkins, OTR, FISPO
The Woodlands, Texas

James C. Baird, CPO
Hanger Prosthetics & Orthotics
Frazer, Pennsylvania

Katherine Binder, CP
Hoboken, New Jersey

Dawn M. Ehde, PhD
Department of Rehabilitation Medicine
University of Washington School of Medicine
Seattle, Washington

Elizabeth Smith Cole, PT
Department of Physical Therapy
Amputee Services of Austin
Austin, Texas

Janos P. Ertl, MD
Assistant Clinical Professor
Department of Orthopaedic Surgery
University of California, Davis
Sacramento, California

William J. J. Ertl, MD
Assistant Professor
Department of Orthopaedic Surgery
University of Oklahoma Health Science Center
Oklahoma City, Oklahoma

Troy Farnsworth, CP
Hanger Prosthetics & Orthotics
Salt Lake City, Utah

Pamela G. Forducey, PhD, ABPP
Integris Neuroscience Institute and Telehealth
Oklahoma City, Oklahoma

Mark Geil, PhD
Department of Kinesiology and Health
Georgia State University
Atlanta, Georgia

Marisol A. Hanley, PhD
Department of Rehabilitation Medicine
University of Washington
Seattle, Washington

Kawaljeet Kaur, MD
Brookfield, Wisconsin

Clay M. Kelly, MD
Chief of Amputee Rehabilitation
Assistant Professor of Physical Medicine and
    Rehabilitation
Case Western Reserve University
MetroHealth Medical Center
Cleveland, Ohio

Lawrence R. Lange, CPO, FAAOP
Scottsdale, Arizona

Stephen Mandacina, CP, FAAOP
Hanger Prosthetics & Orthotics
Lees Summit, Missouri

Matthew A. Parente, PT, CPO
Newington Certificate Program in Orthotics and
    Prosthetics
Newington, Connecticut

John Rheinstein, CP, FAAOP
Hanger Prosthetics & Orthotics
Bronx, New York

William D. Ruwe, PhD, PsyD
Integris Neuroscience Institute and Telehealth
Oklahoma City, Oklahoma

Randy Richardson, RPA
Hanger Prosthetics & Orthotics
Oklahoma City, Oklahoma

Christina Skoski, MD
HP/HD HELP
Santa Ana, California

Douglas G. Smith, MD
Associate Professor of Orthopaedic Surgery
Director, Prosthetics Research Study
Medical Director, Amputee Coalition of America
University of Washington
Harborview Medical Center
Seattle, Washington

Elaine N. Uellendahl, CP
Hanger Prosthetics
Phoenix, Arizona

Jack E. Uellendahl, CPO
Hanger Prosthetics
Phoenix, Arizona

Mary Witt, PT
Eagle, Colorado

Melissa Wolff-Burke, PT, EdD, ATC
Shenandoah University
Winchester, Virginia

Christopher Kevin Wong, MS, PT
Touro College
School of Health Sciences
Bay Shore, New York

PREFACE

Patients with amputation deserve optimal management which involves coordinated interaction of many members of the rehabilitation team. The interdisciplinary authorship of this book reflects this belief. We are proud of our colleagues' breadth of clinical experience. Variety is not limited to the contributors to *Prosthetics and Patient Management: A Comprehensive Clinical Approach*; amputation affects many facets of humanity, from the infant born with limb absence to the octogenarian who sustained amputation because of vascular disease, from the adolescent coping with cancer to the athlete eager to return to the playing field.

While the popular media may devote a headline or a sound bite to the latest prosthetic or surgical technology, in this book we are able to detail the attributes of computerized knee units, externally powered upper-limb components, and the newest biomaterials. These developments are based on established principles. Because most patients are fitted with less dramatic prostheses, we offer clinicians firm grounding in contemporary practice.

Prosthetic fitting is part of the continuum of rehabilitation. Care often begins prior to surgery or when the infant is born or as part of management of sarcoma. Consequently, issues in early management, pain control, and patient and family psychology strongly influence prosthetic effectiveness. After fitting, a structured, comprehensive training program enables the patient to obtain the maximum benefit from the prosthesis.

This book mirrors scope of prosthetics, beginning with Section I: Early Management, encompassing professional roles within the clinic team are described; amputation surgery, postoperative care, and management of pain, skin disorders, and psychological consequences of amputation. Section II: Rehabilitation of Adults With Lower-Limb Amputations considers the anatomic and prosthetic implications of amputations from a single toe to removal of the pelvis, as well as basic training for these patients. Section III: Rehabilitation of Adults With Upper-Limb Amputations includes both body- and externally-powered prostheses, and the training required to enable patients to use their prostheses most effectively. *Prosthetics and Patient Management: A Comprehensive Clinical Approach* concludes with Section IV: Beyond the Basics, intended to equip readers with the special considerations pertaining to children, plus evidence-based rehabilitation outcomes, and many ways people with amputations engage in recreation and other avocational activities. Finally, we polish the crystal ball to glimpse prosthetic, surgical, and educational advances and challenges.

It is our sincere hope that the prosthetists, therapists, physicians, nurses, and other current and aspiring clinicians who read this book will be inspired to foster greater achievement and better life satisfaction on the part of their patients and clients who have sustained amputation.

Section

I

Early Management

Chapter 1

Clinic Team Approach to Rehabilitation

Joan E. Edelstein, MA, PT, FISPO

OBJECTIVES

1. Explore the roles of each member of the rehabilitation clinic team
2. Name the organizations responsible for conferring professional credentials on each member of the team
3. Identify interdisciplinary organizations concerned with prosthetic rehabilitation

INTRODUCTION

Individuals and families who must confront congenital or acquired limb loss can draw upon a wide network of health care providers. Ideally, the patient will be treated by a smoothly functioning clinic team. The rehabilitation team concept gained popularity after World War II with the need to care for a large number of injured veterans, particularly those with amputations. Because contemporary medical care is often fragmented with insufficient communication among clinicians, it is especially worthwhile to describe a model of excellent care in which all parties work cooperatively.

Ideally, the adult who is about to undergo elective lower-limb amputation or who has sustained traumatic limb loss will interact with a core prosthetic clinic team composed of a physician, prosthetist, and physical therapist. Initially, medical care will be rendered by a surgeon; subsequently, either the surgeon will continue to care for the patient or may transfer responsibility to a physiatrist. Regardless of specialty, the physician bears the ultimate legal responsibility for the patient's welfare. If the patient faces upper-limb amputation, an occupational therapist should be a member of the core team. In the case of a child, a pediatrician is a central participant. People who have foot amputation may be treated by a pedorthist.

The clinic team should meet on a regular basis, depending on the volume of patients. Each team member brings specific insights to influence the treatment plan based on particular evaluation procedures. Once the patient has been assessed the team meets to formulate a coordinated treatment plan. Depending on the patient's medical condition, the plan may include prosthetic prescription. When the completed prosthesis is delivered, the clinic team determines the adequacy of its fit and function. Implementing the treatment plan calls for each clinician's special clinical skills. The clinic team is an excellent forum for sharing new technical data. Often during rehabilitation two or more team members may confer, in addition to plenary discussions. Frequently, the prosthetist and therapist will meet with the patient during treatment sessions. Throughout the rehabilitation process, the patient and family should be in close contact with the team, engaging in cooperative interaction. In such fashion, problems can be raised openly and readily resolved.

In addition to the core team, the patient and family may benefit from interventions provided by a social worker, psychologist or psychiatrist, a vocational counselor, or any combination of these specialists. The core team may call upon other clinicians, such as a dermatologist or plastic surgeon. During the patient's initial hospitalization, nurses are integral to recovery. A patient who transfers to a rehabilitation center will probably work with a rehabilitation nurse.

Each team member has particular qualifications that enable the clinician to provide the best care to enable the patient to achieve optimal rehabilitation success. In addition to initial qualification, all professions promote ongoing education so that practitioners may be informed about new developments in the field. In some instances, continuing education is mandated by licensing or professional agencies.

PHYSICIANS AND SURGEONS

Most amputations in the United States are elective procedures performed on adults who have peripheral vascular disease. Consequently, the surgery is usually performed by a general surgeon or a vascular surgeon. Amputations necessitated by trauma or skeletal disease are often carried out by an orthopedic surgeon. Subsequent care is likely to be provided by a physiatrist or pediatrician. Any of these physicians may serve as chief of the clinic team. Other physicians who may participate in treatment include a dermatologist, plastic surgeon, and psychiatrist.

General surgeons are licensed physicians who become members of the American Board of Surgery (1617 John F. Kennedy Boulevard, Suite 860, Philadelphia, PA 19103) upon completion of 5 years of specialty training plus written examination, according to the Accreditation Counsel for Graduate Medical Education (515 North State Street, Suite 2000, Chicago, IL 60610).

Vascular surgeons may belong to the Peripheral Vascular Surgery Society (c/o DMC Companies, 824 Munras Avenue, Suite C, Monterey, CA 93940).

Orthopedic surgeons are eligible for membership in the American Board of Orthopaedic Surgery (400 Silver Cedar Court, Chapel Hill, NC 27514) after licensure, 5 years of specialty training, 2 years of clinical experience, in addition to passing written examination. The American Academy of Orthopaedic Surgeons (6300 North River Road, Rosemont, IL 60018) sponsors educational programs and publications. An orthopedic technician may work closely with the orthopedist if a rigid plaster dressing is applied at the time of amputation.

Some patients have scars that are adherent, invaginated, or otherwise unsatisfactory. Plastic surgeons can revise the faulty scar to facilitate prosthetic fitting. They earn recognition from the American Board of Plastic Surgery (7 Penn Center, Suite 400, 1635 Market Street, Philadelphia, PA 19103) after 3 years of prerequisite training, 2 years of specialty training, and examination.

Physiatrists are specialists in physical medicine and rehabilitation who focus on restoring function, caring for patients with acute and chronic pain and musculoskeletal problems, as well as those who have various neuropathies. These physicians receive credentials from the American Board of Physician Medicine and Rehabilitation (3015 Allegro Park Lane SW, Rochester, MN 55902) after licensure, 1 year of prerequisite training, 3 years of specialty training, 1 year of clinical experience, and written examination. The American Academy of Physical Medicine and Rehabilitation (One IBM Plaza, Suite 2500, Chicago, IL 60611) is the national medical society representing physiatrists.

If the patient is a child, a pediatrician is an important member of the clinic team and may be its leader. Pediatricians are certified by the American Board of Pediatrics (111 Silver Cedar Court, Chapel Hill, NC 27514) after 3 years of specialty training and examination.

When dermatitis, verrucuous hyperplasia, or other skin disorders disrupt rehabilitation, the team may call upon the services of a dermatologist. Dermatologists are members of the American Board of Dermatology (Henry Ford Hospital, 1 Ford Place, Detroit, MI 48202) who have completed 1 year of prerequisite training, 3 years of specialty training, and an examination.

Severe emotional problems, perhaps pertaining to the circumstances of the amputation or phantom pain, may require the intervention of a psychiatrist. These clinicians are accredited by the American Board of Psychiatry and Neurology (500 Lake Cook Road, Suite 335, Deerfield, IL 60015), which requires 4 years of specialty training and examination.

PROSTHETIST (CP OR CPO)

A prosthetist fabricates and fits prostheses, formerly known as artificial limbs. A certified prosthetist is known as CP, whereas those who are certified in both prosthetics and orthotics add CPO to their names. The American Board for Certification in Orthotics and Prosthetics requires a baccalaureate degree, plus 1 year of postgraduate education provided by any of the eight accredited programs, plus 1 year of internship and passing written and practical exams: California State University—Dominquez Hills (Carson City, Calif), Los Amigos Research and Education Institute (Downey, Calif), Hanger Prosthetics Orthotics Inc—Certificate Program (Newington, Conn), Georgia Institute of Technology (Atlanta, Ga), Northwestern University (Chicago, Ill), Century Community and Technical College (White Bear Lake, Minn), University of Texas Southwestern Medical Center (Dallas, Tex), and University of Washington (Seattle, Wash). Eight states (Alabama, Florida, Illinois, New Jersey, Ohio, Oklahoma, Texas, and Washington) now license prosthetists. A CP may join The American Academy of Orthotists and Prosthetists (526 King Street, Suite 201, Alexandria, VA 22314), which furthers the scientific and educational attainments of professional practitioners. The American Orthotic and Prosthetic Association (330 John Carlyle Street, Suite 200, Alexandria, VA 22314) is the trade association serving the interests of orthotic and prosthetic facilities, manufacturers, and suppliers.

ORTHOTIST (CO OR CPO)

An orthotist fabricates and fits orthoses, also known as braces. Orthoses may be fitted to patients with partial foot amputations. A certified orthotist is known as CO, whereas those who are certified in both prosthetics and orthotics add CPO to their names. The educational and legal requirements and professional organizations noted for prosthetists also pertain to orthotists.

PEDORTHIST (CPED)

The patient with foot anomaly, whether congenital or acquired, may be referred to a pedorthist. The profession of pedorthics encompasses the design, manufacture, modification, and/or fit of footwear, including shoes, orthoses, and foot devices, to prevent or alleviate foot problems caused by disease, congenital defect, overuse, or injury. The Board for Certification in Pedorthics (2517 Eastlake Avenue East, Suite 200, Seattle, WA 98102) specifies that the practitioner complete 120 hours of pedorthic education and pass an examination. The Board accepts a reduced number of hours of education if the applicant is an accredited athletic trainer, prosthetist, orthotist, chiropractor, osteopath, podiatrist, physician, or physical therapist. Florida, Illinois, Ohio, and Oklahoma license pedorthists. The professional organization is the Pedorthic Footwear Association (9861 Broken Land Parkway, Columbia, MD 21046).

PHYSICAL THERAPISTS

Physical therapists (PT) provide services that help restore function, improve mobility, relieve pain, and prevent or limit permanent physical disabilities, as well as restoring, maintaining, and promoting overall fitness and health. All physical therapy education is at the post baccalaureate level. Graduation from a master's or doctoral curriculum that combines didactic and laboratory studies and clinical affiliations entitles the individual to take the national licensure examination. Physical therapists are licensed by all states. Some PTs are also certified by the American Board of Physical Therapy Specialties. Members of the prosthetic clinic team are most apt to be either Orthopaedic Certified Specialists or Geriatric Certified Specialists. Certification requires advanced knowledge, clinical experience, and examination

Physical therapist assistants (PTA) work under the supervision of PTs. Although PTs, rather than PTAs, evaluate the patient, PTAs may conduct exercise programs and gait training. Physical therapist assistants are graduates of associate degree programs. The American Physical Therapy Association (1111 North Fairfax Street, Alexandria, VA 22314) represents PTs and PTAs, sponsoring instructional courses, national conferences, and scholarly publications.

OCCUPATIONAL THERAPISTS

Patients with upper-limb amputation will receive much of their treatment from an occupational therapist (OT), particularly instruction in the control and use of the prosthesis. Occupational therapy is skilled treatment that helps individuals achieve independence in all facets of their lives, giving people the skills for living independent and satisfying lives. Occupational therapists enter the field with a bachelor's, master's, or doctoral degree, which includes classroom and fieldwork experience; they must also pass a national examination. Most states regulate occupational therapy practice.

Certified Occupational Therapy Assistants (COTA) complete an associate's degree. The professional organization for OTs and COTAs is The American Occupational Therapy Association, Inc. (4720 Montgomery Lane, Bethesda, MD 20824)

NURSE (RN)

Nurses promote health, prevent disease, and help patients cope with illness. When providing direct patient care, they observe, assess, and record symptoms, reactions, and progress in patients; assist physicians during surgery, treatments, and examination; administer medications; and assist in convalescence and rehabilitation.

Nurse specialists who are likely to be part of the clinic team are rehabilitation nurses who usually work in rehabilitation departments and nurse practitioners who provide basic, primary health care, diagnosing and treating common acute illnesses and injuries and prescribing medications. State laws govern the tasks that nurses may perform. The National League for Nursing (61 Broadway, New York, NY 10006) and the American Nurses Association (600 Maryland Avenue SW, Washington, DC 20024) are the principal professional organizations.

SOCIAL WORKER (MSW)

Psychosocial problems complicate rehabilitation. Social workers help people function the best way they can in their environment, deal with their relationships, and solve personal and family problems. Of particular relevance to people with amputations, social workers address problems of housing and employment. Although a bachelor's degree is the minimum entry requirement, most positions require a master's degree or doctorate. Accredited educational programs require at least 400 hours of supervised field experience at the baccalaureate level and 900 hours at the master's level. All states have licensing, certification, or registration requirements. The National Association of Social Workers (750 First Street, NE, Washington, DC 20002) offers voluntary credentials.

PSYCHOLOGIST (PHD OR PSYD)

Psychologists study the human mind and behavior. Those in health service provide mental health care. Clinical psychologists help mentally and emotionally disturbed clients adjust to life and may assist medical and surgical patients in dealing with illnesses or injuries. They may interview patients and administer diagnostic tests, then provide individual, family, or group psychotherapy and design and implement behavior modification programs. A doctoral degree, most often PhD or PsyD, is usually required for employment. The American Psychological Association (750 First Street NE, Washington, DC 20002) accredits doctoral training programs. The American Board of Professional Psychology, Inc (514 East Capitol Avenue, Jefferson City, MO 65101) recognizes professional achievement by awarding specialty certification to those who have a doctorate in psychology, postdoctoral specialty training, 5 years of experience, and a passing grade on an examination.

REHABILITATION COUNSELOR

Rehabilitation counselors help people deal with the personal, social, and vocational effects of disabilities. They evaluate the strengths and limitations of individuals, provide personal and vocational counseling, and arrange for medical care, vocational training, and job placement. A master's degree is often required to be licensed or certified. Education encompasses 48 to 60 semester hours of graduate study and supervised clinical experience. Forty-seven states require some form of licensure or certification for practice outside of schools. Many counselors choose to be nationally certified by the National Board for Certified Counselors, Inc (3 Terrace Way, Suite D, Greensboro, NC 27403). The Commission on Rehabilitation Counselor Certification (1835 Rohlwing Road, Suite E, Rolling Meadows, IL 60008) requires passing a written examination. The American Counseling Association (5999 Stevenson Avenue, Alexandria, VA 22304) is a prominent professional organization for rehabilitation counselors.

INTERDISCIPLINARY RESOURCES

Whether or not the clinician works within a clinic team, interdisciplinary organization enables exchange of information through local and national meetings, publications, and, increasingly, Internet sites. The International Society for Prosthetics and Orthotics is an international organization (Borgervaenget 5, 2100 Copenhagen Ø, Denmark) composed of national member societies. The United States National Member Society (5613 Stockton Way, Dublin, OH 43016) attracts physicians, surgeons, prosthetists, physical therapists, orthotists, occupational therapists, and engineers. The Association of Children's Prosthetic-Orthotic Clinics (6300 North River Road, Suite 727, Rosemont, IL 60018) has both individual and clinic members who are concerned with habilitation and rehabilitation of children with amputations or limb loss. The American Congress of Rehabilitation Medicine (6801 Lake Plaza Drive, Suite B-205, Indianapolis, IN 46220) is an organization fostering interdisciplinary collaboration and cooperation in research. The Amputee Coalition of America (900 East Hill Avenue, Suite 285, Knoxville, TN 37915) is an advocacy organization composed of consumers and clinicians. It operates the National Limb Loss Information Center (NLLIC), which provides comprehensive resources for lay and professional users, including the NLLIC comprehensive limb loss catalogue on the Internet.

CONTEMPORARY CLINICAL PRACTICE

The foregoing discussion presents a model for patient management, which may not be feasible if the team members are not employed by the same clinical facility or are not participants in the patient's health insurance plan. The prosthetist or pedorthist often works for a private company, which may not be a contracted vendor with the medical institution. In such circumstances, it is incumbent on each clinician to make every effort to communicate with colleagues, as well as to be attuned to new research and technical developments. Rehabilitation can be successful whether the patient is treated by a formal clinic team or by dedicated clinicians working on an individual basis who communicate with one another.

Chapter 2

Amputation Surgery: Osteomyoplastic Reconstructive Technique

Janos P. Ertl, MD and William J. J. Ertl, MD

OBJECTIVES

1. Identify the indications for amputation surgery
2. Trace the history of osteomyoplastic reconstruction
3. Indicate the indications for osteomyoplastic reconstruction
4. Describe preoperative clinical and instrumented evaluation procedures
5. Outline the osteomyoplastic procedure for transtibial, transfemoral, transmetatarsal, and transhumeral amputations
6. Present the results of osteomyoplastic reconstruction for various amputation levels

Editors' note: Although not widely practiced, the osteomyoplastic amputation procedure continues to hold great promise as a means of maximizing the patient's function. The following discussion responds to the increase in interest in this procedure.

INTRODUCTION

Lower-limb amputation is a surgical procedure that dates to prehistory. Neolithic man survived traumatic, ritualistic, punitive, and therapeutic amputation. Plato and Hippocrates described therapeutic amputation techniques.

Surgical treatment of severe lower-limb trauma and peripheral vascular disease has greatly advanced, especially revascularization, internal fixation of fractures, and microvascular and free tissue procedures, which have favorably enhanced patients' outcomes. Amputation may be necessary when efforts to salvage the extremity fail and may be the only alternative to return the patient to a more satisfactory lifestyle. Often after significant time, funds, and emotion have been invested into salvage of the limb with both the patient and surgeon feeling defeated, amputation is then viewed as a failure. The patient may picture himself as incomplete by societal standards.

In some regions of the world advanced surgical limb salvage techniques are unavailable, or are too costly, making amputation the primary form of treatment for damaged limbs.

When compared to the prosthetic industry, amputation techniques have changed relatively little and are usually performed by the most junior member of the surgical team. Even if the amputation is well performed and the prosthesis well fitted, some patients have persistent symptoms of residual limb pain, swelling, sense of instability, and decreased prosthetic wear. They pose a challenging situation from a surgical reconstructive perspective. The effects of previous surgery, altered anatomy, muscle and bone atrophy, aerobic deconditioning, and the attempt to retain maximum residual limb length create difficulties when surgical reconstruction is considered.

The osteomyoplastic lower extremity amputation procedure described by Professor Janos V. Ertl, MD, in 1939 originated as reconstructive surgery. Ertl's experience was developed by operating on an estimated 13,000 amputees.[1,2] The principles of osteomyoplasty are based on amputation, reconstructive surgery, and physiology and anatomy. The procedure arose from the observation that in bony injuries the periosteum might regenerate. Ertl first applied this principle to procedures using osteoperiosteal grafts to the mandible and the skull during World War I[1,2] when many soldiers survived trench warfare with maiming injuries to their face and cranium. He reconstructed osseous defects with flexible, osteoperiosteal grafts harvested from the tibia. Subsequently, he applied the same principle to the spine, long bones, and amputations. With osseous reconstruction in amputations, particular attention was applied to the handling of the soft tissues. Neuromuscular isolation, high ligation of the nerves, myoplasty, and smooth skin closure provided the patient with a cylindrical residual extremity with end-bearing capabilities. Ertl believed that this returned the residual extremity to as well-balanced an anatomic and physiologic state as possible. The Ertl procedure is now applied to both primary and secondary diaphyseal amputations of the femur, tibia, humerus, metatarsals, and digits. Our positive experience with this procedure makes it an option when dealing with difficult primary and reconstructive amputations.

INDICATIONS

Amputation is performed in the presence of peripheral vascular disease (PVD), trauma, tumor, infection, and congenital anomalies. The leading indication for limb amputation in the United States is PVD. Persons with diabetes mellitus account for half of those with PVD, with an estimated 65,000 lower extremity amputations performed for this group annually. Peripheral vascular disease necessitates amputation when the patient presents with uncontrollable soft tissue or bony infection or unrelenting rest pain due to muscle ischemia. These patients usually have had extensive vascular studies and attempts at revascularization. Progressive small vessel occlusion and neuropathy cause the toes to become gangrenous. Pressure points develop trophic ulcers, allowing bacteria to invade the bone. The patient has often undergone multiple foot amputations and numerous debridements and may have to use a wheelchair to relieve pressure on the extremity. Ascending cellulitis due to venostasis may be present.

Traumatic limb loss occurs primarily because of industrial and motor vehicle accidents even though equipment safety is legislatively mandated. Accidents usually involve high-grade open fractures with associated nerve injury, soft tissue loss, and ischemia and unreconstructable neurovascular injury. Modern limb salvage is often successful. If, however, salvage fails, the result is an infected painful extremity that sabotages the patient's daily activities and work. Limb salvage with less-than-favorable results leaves the patient with a painful limb that is less functional than a prosthesis, resulting in lost workdays and high medical expense.

Osteomyelitis may result from systemic disease or open fracture. Cultures or biopsy can identify the infecting organism. Gas gangrene is a very serious infection due to *Clostridium* species. *Clostridial myonecrosis* develops rapidly. Patients present with symptoms of pain, sepsis, and delirium. Examination often reveals a brownish discharge and crepitation within the soft tissues on palpation. Streptococcal myonecrosis develops more slowly than clostridial infections. Persons with diabetes mellitus often have polymicrobial infections that involve anaerobic gas-forming gram-negative organisms.

Malignancies often manifest pain initially. The patient may be referred for amputation following a work-up for a tumor, after limb salvage is excluded as an option.

Limb salvage surgery remains the primary treatment for bone tumors when the risk of local recurrence equals that of amputation, and the salvaged limb is expected to be functional. Whether the patient has limb salvage or amputation, the goal in treating malignant bone tumors is to remove the lesion at the site having the lowest risk of recurrence.

Congenital limb deficiencies and malformations are evident at birth and account for a small percentage of amputations. With growth, functional difficulties may develop to limit the child's mobility. Each situation is evaluated on an individual basis because anomalous limbs are often functional and amenable to orthotic management or limb reconstruction. Amputation is indicated when a functional level greater than the patient's current level is anticipated.

The decision to perform an amputation often comes after all other options have been exhausted. It is a final decision that cannot be reversed once initiated. The only contraindication to amputation is poor health impairing the patient's ability to tolerate anesthesia and surgery. However, the diseased limb often is at the center of the patient's illness, leading to a compromised medical status. The removal of the diseased limb segment is necessary to eliminate systemic toxins and save the patient's life.

Whatever the indication for amputation, the goal remains creating the most functional limb possible so that the patient may enjoy the greatest lifestyle satisfaction.

PREOPERATIVE EVALUATION

Although a diseased limb can be removed readily resolving the local problem of the extremity, care does not end there. The patient must learn to apply and remove the prosthesis, monitor the skin, care for the prosthesis, and walk on various terrain. Because of the complexity of these issues, a multidisciplinary approach should be taken. The preoperative treatment team should include the surgeon, primary care physician or physiatrist, a physical therapist, a prosthetist, and a social worker. Patients undergoing amputation should be evaluated for cognitive and physical abilities. In some instances, consultation with a psychiatrist may be useful to determine the ambulatory potential. Patients with PVD should have an evaluation by a vascular surgeon to determine the feasibility of vascular reconstruction. Consultation with an internal medicine specialist is also recommended to manage general health, cardiovascular disease, and, where present, diabetes mellitus. Many patients with PVD are often malnourished and may have cardiac and cerebral ischemic disease. They can develop polymicrobial infections, which usually can be managed with broad-spectrum antibiotics and wide debridement.

The extent and location of the disease, trauma, or malformation determine the level of amputation. Surgery must be performed so that the patient will be able to wear a prosthesis comfortably. Knee joint salvage enhances rehabilitation, decreasing the energy expenditure required for ambulation.

Allowing the patient to talk with someone who has undergone an amputation successfully can also prepare the patient and address issues the patient may not have considered. The input of each team member and peer counseling will lead to a prepared and involved patient with the understanding needed to achieve a positive postoperative, rehabilitative, and life-long result.

Laboratory Studies

Amputation wound healing is a concern because most amputations are performed for compromised circulation. Standard laboratory studies are recommended, as are elective laboratory studies depending on the patient's medical condition. Laboratory studies relative to wound healing are as follows:

- C-reactive protein: This is an indicator of infection. Less than 1.0 indicates no infection; above 8 indicates significant infection.
- Hemoglobin: More than 10 g/dL is required. Oxygenated blood is necessary for wound healing.
- Absolute lymphocyte count: Less than 1500 μ/L indicates immune deficiency and increases the possibility of infection.
- Serum albumin level: Less than 3.5 g/dL indicates malnutrition and diminished ability of wound healing.

In patients with nonprogressive gangrene, physiologic inadequacy as determined by these laboratory studies should be optimized (eg, by oral or intravenous hyperalimentation prior to amputation for malnutrition). When progressive infection or intractable ischemic pain is present, an open amputation can be performed and the soft tissue closure established later.

Imaging Studies

Anteroposterior and lateral radiography of the involved extremity is essential.

Computed tomography (CT) scanning and magnetic resonance imaging (MRI) are performed for tumor work-up or osteomyelitis to ensure that the surgical margins are appropriate.

Technetium Tc-99m pyrophosphate bone scanning is used to predict the need for amputation in individuals with electrical burns and frostbite. A 94% sensitivity rate and a 100% specificity rate have been reported in demarcating viable from nonviable tissues.

Other Studies

Doppler Ultrasonography

This is used to measure arterial pressure; the area under the waveform is a measure of flow. In approximately 15% of patients with PVD, the results are falsely elevated because of the noncompressibility of calcified arteries. Doppler ultrasonography has also been used to predict wound healing. A minimum measurement of 70 mm Hg is believed to be necessary for wound healing.

Ischemic Index

This index is the ratio of the Doppler pressure at the level being tested to the brachial systolic pressure. An ischemic index of 0.5 or greater at the surgical level is necessary to support wound healing.

Ankle-Brachial Index

The ischemic index at the ankle is probably the best indicator for assessing adequate inflow to the ischemic limb. An index lower than 0.45 indicates that incisions distal to the ankle will not heal.

Transcutaneous Oxygen Pressure Measurement

This noninvasive test assesses the partial pressure of oxygen diffusing through the skin. It can be applied to any area of intact skin and records the oxygen-delivering capacity of the vascular system. It is believed to be the most reliable and sensitive test for wound healing. Values greater than 40 mm Hg indicate acceptable wound-healing potential. Values less than 20 mm Hg indicate poor healing potential. Studies have reported an 88% sensitivity rate and an 84% specificity rate. Pressure may be falsely low in areas of edema, cellulitis, and venous stasis changes.

TRANSTIBIAL RECONSTRUCTIVE OSTEOMYOPLASTIC PROCEDURE

Informed consent is obtained from all patients. For those who are candidates for very short residual extremities, knee disarticulation, and transfemoral amputation are discussed. Nevertheless, every attempt is made to maintain the knee and maximize residual extremity length.

The patient is positioned supine. A bumper under the hip may be used to control rotation of the limb. A tourniquet may be applied, although its use in vascular patients is discretionary. After preparing and draping the extremity, any previous incisions are identified and used. Wound healing does not differ whether the incision is anteroposterior, oblique, or mediolateral. Following incision, dissection is carried down to the muscular layer. Frequently, the residual extremity has no distal bony muscular coverage because the musculature was either poorly secured or allowed to retract. Dissection is then carried more proximal with the anterior, lateral, and posterior compartments being identified and isolated. If a long posterior muscle flap was used for anterior coverage in the primary amputation, care should be taken to preserve the length of this posterior muscle compartment. During isolation of the muscular compartments, care should also be taken to maintain fascial attachments to the musculature for later myoplastic reconstruction. The main neurovascular structures are identified, including the tibial nerve, artery, and vein; superficial and deep peroneal nerves; peroneal artery and vein; sural nerve; and the saphenous nerve and vein. They are released from scar tissue and separated. Palpation of neuromas may aid in localizing neurovascular bundles; in the original amputation, they are commonly ligated in unison. Once separated, each identified nerve should be transected as high as possible and allowed to retract into the soft tissue bed. The artery and nerve are separated and ligated in a separate fashion.

After soft tissue dissection is completed, osseous structures are managed. The periosteum is incised from anterior to posterior on the fibula and tibia. Using a 45-degree angled chisel, an osteoperiosteal flap is elevated medially and laterally, maintaining the proximal attachment. Small cortical fragments are left attached to the periosteum to create a flexible bone graft. Any exposed cortical bone that remains is resected to the same level, facilitating the suturing of the osteoperiosteal flaps. This requires no more than 1.5 to 2.0 cm of bone to be resected. The medial tibial flap is sutured to the lateral fibular flap and the lateral tibial flap is sutured to the medial fibular flap, resulting in a tubular structure. Occasionally, it is necessary to split the fibula or lateral tibia longitudinally to create medial and lateral periosteal-cortical flaps, which are secured in the same fashion as noted above. Care should be taken not to abduct the fibula too much as this will place undue stress on the proximal tibiofibular joint.

In short or very short residual extremities, the lateral tibia periosteal-cortical flap or free osteoperiosteal grafts are harvested from the proximal tibia, contralateral extremity, or iliac crest to maintain bony length. This may also be performed on any length of residual extremity. We have used free osteoperiosteal grafts in primary amputations harvested from the removed limb without difficulty and obtained complete synostosis formation.

Some short transtibial extremities exhibit fibular abduction secondary to the pull of the biceps femoris muscle. This may lead to a distolateral pressure point and subsequent prosthetic difficulties. In such instances, the fibula is reduced in an adducted position and a lag screw placed into the proximal tibiofibular joint, stabilizing the realignment with or without arthrodesis of this joint.

The mobilized musculature is then brought distally to cover the osteoperiosteal bridge. Myoplasty is completed with the posterior musculature sutured to the anterior and lateral musculature. The goal is to provide soft tissue coverage to the distal aspect of the residual extremity. The anterior musculature is frequently rotated over the prominent distal tibia and sutured to the posterior lateral gastroc-soleus fascia. After completion of the myoplasty, the skin is mobilized over the myoplasty. Care is given to reapproximate the skin symmetrically, leaving neither dog-ears nor crevices. Drains are placed for hematoma decompression. After sterile dressings are applied, the extremity is placed in a plaster splint in knee extension. The splint is removed between 2 and 7 days postoperatively. A temporary total contact end bearing prosthesis is provided in 5 to 8 weeks. Physical therapy focuses on education on transfers, desensitization of the residual extremity, aerobic conditioning, and upper body strengthening.

Primary amputations are approached in a similar fashion, with care given to ensure that sufficient skin is maintained for coverage of the greater muscle bulk.

Results

Between January 1980 and January 1995 three surgeons performed transtibial osteomyoplastic lower extremity amputation reconstructions in 164 patients. Seven patients with bilateral amputations were treated in stages. Twelve patients died from unrelated causes and nine patients were lost to follow-up. Consequently, 143 patients with 150 osteomyoplastic reconstructions with a minimum of 2-year follow-up were available for review. The average follow-up was 9 years with a range of 2 to 15 years. The group included 102 men and 41 women, with an average age at the time of reconstruction of 48.5 years (range: 12 to 88 years). The initial causes of amputation were trauma in 63.3% (95), PVD in 27.3% (41), infection in 7.3% (11), and tumor in 2% (3). The average time to surgical reconstruction after primary amputation was 9.5 years (range: 2 months to 47 years).

Table 2-1

THE 30-POINT RATING SYSTEM

Pain	Points
a) No pain	5
b) Slight pain/no compromise with activities	4
c) Mild pain with normal activity	3
d) Pain with standing in prosthesis	2
e) Pain without prosthesis	1

Function	
a) Unlimited walking ability	5
b) 6 to 12 blocks	4
c) 2 to 5 blocks	3
d) 1 to 2 blocks	2
e) Indoors only or wheelchair assistance	1

Stability	
a) No weakness/no limitations	5
b) Difficulty with uneven terrain	4
c) Difficulty with stairs/inclines	3
d) Extremity weakness	2
e) Thigh lacer/walking aids	1

Swelling	
a) None/minimal/no socket compromise	5
b) With walking 6 to 12 blocks	4
c) With walking 2 to 5 blocks	3
d) With walking 1 to 2 blocks	2
e) With indoor walking	1

Hours of Prosthetic Wear	
a) 14 to 18 hours	5
b) 10 to 13 hours	4
c) 6 to 9 hours	3
d) 3 to 5 hours	2
e) 1 to 2 hours	1

Radiographs	
a) Full synostosis	5
b) Up to 75%	4
c) Up to 50%	3
d) Up to 25%	2
e) No synostosis	1

Total	30

Grading System	
Excellent:	25 to 30
Good:	20 to 24
Fair:	15 to 19
Poor:	<15

The overall results when using the 30-point scale shown in Table 2-1 were 73.3% (110) excellent, 18.7% (28) good, 5.3% (8) fair, and 2.7% (4) poor. The poor results were in dysvascular patients who had continued pain despite improvements in all other functional categories. When questioned about overall satisfaction, 97.3% of all patients stated their final result improved the residual extremity function and their quality of life.

TRANSFEMORAL RECONSTRUCTIVE OSTEOMYOPLASTIC PROCEDURE

The patient is informed of the surgical risks and complications. All attempts are made to maintain maximum residual extremity length to reduce energy expenditure. A diagram of the transverse section at the appropriate transfemoral level is helpful during surgery. In secondary reconstruction, the previous operative report should be reviewed and attention directed toward the original treatment of the muscles and nerves, which may assist in the exposure and dissection during osteomyoplasty.

The extremity is prepared in standard fashion. A sterile tourniquet may not always be feasible. A bumper is placed under the hip of the involved extremity to assist with rotational control. The previous incisions are identified and used.

Dissection is carried to the muscular layer. The muscles are often retracted and atrophic, necessitating proximal dissection. Adductors, abductors, quadriceps, and hamstrings are isolated in their respective groups. The fascial envelope, or more often scar tissue attachments, are maintained for subsequent myoplasty. The neurovascular structures are identified, released from scar, and separately isolated. The nerve must be separated from the artery to avoid pulsatile irritation of the nerve. Often the neurovascular structures have been ligated together. The sciatic nerve may be identified by palpation of its neuroma, which may be as large as 4 cm in circumference. The nerve trunk is mobilized by blunt dissection, distracted, and transected at a higher level, allowing retraction into soft tissue surroundings. If a tourniquet has been used, it may be released to evaluate bleeding. The vascular structures are often friable and need to be handled carefully to avoid proximal retraction. The artery and associated veins are separately ligated to avoid arteriovenous connections.

Attention is directed towards the distal femur. Any exostoses are removed and the periosteum incised anterior to posterior. Using a 45-degree angled chisel, medial and lateral osteoperiosteal flaps are elevated maintaining their proximal attachments. Elevation of the flaps is aided by rotating the chisel 180 degrees. The femur is transected at the level of the osteoperiosteal flaps, with minimal femur necessitating removal. The medial and lateral flaps are sutured together and circumferential periosteal sutures are placed occluding the end of the open medullary canal. An alternative method is to prepare a longer medially or laterally based osteoperiosteal flap, securing it to the opposing and circumferential periosteum, achieving medullary coverage.

Myoplasty is performed by suturing the antagonistic muscle groups to each other and anchoring them into the periosteum, covering the osteoplasty. The adductors are sutured first to the abductor group or anchored to the lateral femoral periosteum. The abductors are imbricated over the adductor attachment and additionally secured to the periosteum anterior and posterior. The flexors are sutured to the extensor group and the underlying adductor/abductor groups, centralizing the distal femur in a muscular envelope.

The skin is fashioned to the underlying myoplasty symmetrically, avoiding dog-ears and invaginations of the incision. A smooth contour is the goal, allowing for a better residual limb-prosthetic interface. Penrose drains are placed prior to completion of the closure.

Postoperatively, the residual extremity is placed in an elastic bandage hip spica or a plaster splint, depending on length. Sutures are removed at 2 to 3 weeks depending on wound healing. Temporary total contact end-bearing prosthetic fitting is coordinated with the prosthetist, between 5 and 8 weeks postoperatively. Physical therapy is initiated for transfers, desensitization, range of motion, aerobic conditioning, and upper body strengthening.

Primary amputations are approached in a similar fashion with care given to ensure sufficient skin coverage for the greater muscle bulk.

Results

Between January 1980 and January 1995 three surgeons performed transfemoral osteomyoplastic lower extremity amputation reconstructions in 91 patients, including two patients with bilateral amputations. Thirteen patients died from unrelated causes and six patients were lost to follow-up. A total of 72 patients (40 men and 32 women) with 74 transfemoral osteomyoplastic amputation reconstructions with minimum 2-year follow-up were available for review. The average postoperative follow-up was 9.8 years (range: 2 to 5 years). Average patient age at operation was 57.4 years (range: 29 to 79 years). Causes of amputation were trauma in 60% (43), PVD in 30% (22), infection in 4% (3), and tumor in 6% (4). The average time to surgical reconstruction after primary amputation was 13.3 years (range: 10 months to 40 years).

The final overall results using the 30-point rating system (see Table 2-1) demonstrated 70% (52) excellent, 20% (15) good, 4% (3) fair, and 6% (4) poor. The poor results occurred in three patients with unilateral amputation and one patient with bilateral amputation, all of whom had PVD. They had continued pain despite improvements in other responses. When questioned about overall satisfaction, 95.8% of patients reported that their final result improved the residual extremity function and their quality of life.

TRANSMETATARSAL PROCEDURE

Use of a tourniquet in vascular patients is discretionary. The extremity is prepared in standard fashion. The skin incision is made as distal as possible, and dorsal and plantar flaps created. The flexor and extensor muscle groups are elevated as one musculofascial flap.

The vessels are isolated and ligated. Digital nerves are separated, distracted, and ligated at a more proximal level.

Osteoperiosteal flaps are elevated from the first and fifth metatarsals as described above. The metatarsals are equally transected at the level of the osteoperiosteal elevation. The osteoperiosteal flaps are sutured end-to-end and to each metatarsal, covering the exposed diaphysis. The flexor and extensor groups are sutured to each other through the fascial attachments, forming the myoplasty.

If used, the tourniquet is released and bleeding controlled. The skin is contoured to the underlying myoplasty, achieving a smooth transition. Penrose drains are placed for hematoma decompression. Sterile dressings and a well-padded posterior splint are applied.

The splint is removed between 2 and 7 days. Physical therapy is instituted for education on transfers, desensitization of the residual extremity, aerobic conditioning, and upper body strengthening. Full weight-bearing begins between 4 and 6 weeks or pending wound healing.

TRANSHUMERAL PROCEDURE

Sterile upper extremity preparation is completed in standard fashion. A sterile tourniquet may be used on a discretionary basis. Previous incisions are used and anteroposterior or mediolateral flaps elevated. The muscles are separated into anterior and posterior groups. Depending on the amputation level, the median, ulnar, and radial nerve, and their extensions are isolated, distracted, and proximally ligated. The brachial artery is separated from its veins and separately ligated. Similar to the transfemoral amputation, osteoperiosteal flaps are created and sutured over the exposed medullary canal. If used, the tourniquet is released and bleeding controlled. The myoplasty is fashioned by suturing the flexor and extensor myofascial groups together and into the underlying periosteum. The skin is contoured to the myoplasty in similar fashion as above. A bulky soft-tissue dressing is applied. A prosthesis is fitted between 4 and 6 weeks postoperatively.

DISCUSSION

Conventional amputations can create multiple difficulties. Loon[3,4] described two problem categories. The first concerns the amputation and includes pain, circulatory disturbance, local osteopenia, and muscle atrophy. The second category consists of problems caused by the attachment of a prosthesis; the extremity is a passive, inactive participant in function. The constellation of symptoms is known as the inactive residual extremity syndrome.

Animal and human studies demonstrate numerous pathophysiologic effects of conventional amputation contributing to the inactive residual extremity syndrome. Conventional amputation leaves the intramedullary canal open. Nontraumatized bone exhibits an intramedullary pressure gradient of approximately 65 mm Hg.[5] The increased venous pressure is necessary to maintain a centrifugal venous drainage in a rigid tubular bone. Medullary pressure appears to be important in venous drainage[6] and in osteocyte nutrition.[7] An open medullary canal causes loss of the normal venous pressure, which has been measured as 0 mm Hg. Slowing of dye material on contrast venogram and dilated, tortuous intramedullary sinuses are also observed.[3,4] Closure of the canal with osteoperiosteal flaps allows these conditions to reverse themselves as shown on postoperative venograms. The transtibial bone bridge also stabilizes the fibula and creates a broader surface to load during prosthetic wear[3,4,8-12] with complete end weight-bearing possible on a mature bone bridge. Animal studies have shown improvement in regional blood flow with osteoplasty, myoplasty, and an even greater sustained synergistic effect when performed together.

Muscle and soft tissue blood flow is essential for primary healing and future function. Many conventional amputations are performed without restoring the length–tension relationship of the musculature. Subsequently, the muscle atrophies, fatty degeneration occurs, circulation slows, venous stasis arises as the muscles do not aid in pumping venous blood, and the result can be chronic edema. Soon after amputation vessels become more numerous and tortuous.[13] Hypervascularity decreases within 1 to 2 weeks following the amputation. The soft tissue then becomes hypovascular but the tortuous vessels remain.[8-11] Similar angiographic findings are seen in patients with vessel occlusion and PVD, indicating pathologic circulation.[13-16] Arteriovenous malformations can also be seen at the distal portion of the residual extremity creating a shunt in the extremity.

Myoplasty with muscles secured to bone via the periosteum restores muscle tension and provides soft tissue covering over the distal osseous structures, resulting in a well-balanced residual extremity. Angiographic studies after myoplasty have shown an improvement in arterial supply and venous drainage.[8] Vascular changes seen with inactivity and immobilization are reversed with myoplasty.[11] Terminal circulation in PVD patients is improved with myoplasty.[17] Animal studies show improvement in regional blood flow with osteoplasty, myoplasty, and an even greater sustained synergistic effect when performed together.[8-11] The residual extremity demonstrates a more rhythmic and phasic activity on electromyography as opposed to an irregular pattern without myoplasty.[18]

Another adverse effect of conventional amputation is edema, which alters the size and shape of the residual extremity.[3,4] This may result from the relative inactivity of the extremity when myoplasty is not performed. Volume changes hinder fitting into the prosthetic socket, limiting ambulation, and can result in chronic skin disorders. Continuing the cascade of changes, inactivity and the inability to load the bone will lead to atrophy of the muscle and local osteopenia/osteoporosis, poor venous return, loss of the pumping action of muscle, and fatty degeneration. Osteomyoplastic reconstruction, in contrast, maintains the size and shape of the residual extremity.

Pain is the most frequent and often the most disabling symptom, and usually is the reason for seeking medical intervention. The genesis of pain may be phantom sensations, circulatory disturbances, local skin changes, exostosis, bone necrosis, and neuroma formation. Medullary closure, high neuroma resection, myoplasty, and meticulous skin closure decreases pain in the majority of patients treated. Eight PVD patients in our study group continued to experience pain. Although experiencing improvement in all other categories rated on the 30-point scale, including length of prosthetic wear, they exhibited symptoms that were most likely due to continued vascular claudication.

Stability of the residual extremity is difficult to measure objectively. The clinician usually relies on the patient's ability to function with the prosthesis. Functional gains experienced by our patients were related not only to decrease of pain, but also the patients' ability to remain stable within the socket. As function improved, patients appeared to become more confident in late stance, increasing their overall walking distance.

Osteomyoplastic procedure, whether applied to primary or secondary amputations, is intended to create a functional, active residual extremity based on reestablishing a physiologic, well-balanced environment. The resultant residual extremity is stronger and more durable with improved stability and proprioception. We have used free osteoperiosteal grafts to form our bone bridge in short residual limbs to maintain length and achieve good results. In longer residual limbs, minimal length is removed, in contrast to what has been described in conventional amputation surgery.[19-21] The myoplasty contributes to the length of the extremity.

Difficulty assessing the long-term result of osteomyoplasty relates to the fact that many variables affect the results. Socket design and fit, prosthetic components, and interaction with different prosthetists with varying experience all influence function and satisfaction.

Osteomyoplastic amputation reconstruction is technically challenging with a somewhat greater operative time than conventional techniques. Nevertheless, it is suitable for traumatic and vascular amputations and offers the surgical community a dynamic procedure for both primary and secondary reconstructions in upper- and lower-limb amputation surgery.

REFERENCES

1. Ertl J. *Regeneration: Ihre Anwedung in der Chirurgie*. Leipzig, Germany: Verlag von Johann Ambrosius Barth; 1939.

2. Ertl JP, Barrack R, Alexander AH, VanBuecken K. Triplane fracture of the distal tibial epiphysis. Long-term follow-up. *J Bone Joint Surg Am*. 1988;70:967-976.

3. Loon HE. Biological and biomechanical principles in amputation surgery. Proceedings of the Second International Prosthetics Course. Copenhagen, Switzerland: Prosthetics International; 1962.

4. Loon HE. Below the knee amputations. *Artificial Limbs: National Academy of the Sciences-National Research Council*. 1963;6:86.

5. Ascenzi A. Physiologic relationship and pathological interferences between bone tissue and marrow. In: Bourne GH, ed. *The Biochemistry and Physiology of Bone*. New York, NY: Academic Press; 1956:403-444.

6. Lopez-Curto JA, Bassingthwaighte JB, Kelly PJ. Anatomy of the microvasculature of the tibia diaphysis of the adult dog. *J Bone Joint Surg Am*. 1980;62:1362-1369.

7. Sturmer KM. Measurement of intramedullary pressure in an animal experiment and propositions to reduce pressure increase. *Injury*. 1993;24:S7-S27.

8. Hansen-Leth C, Reimann I. Amputations with and without myoplasty in rabbits with special reference to the vascularization. *Acta Orthop Scand*. 1972;43:68-77.

9. Hansen-Leth C. Muscle blood flow after amputations with special reference to the influence of osseous plugging of the medullary cavity. *Acta Orthop Scand*. 1976;47:613-618.

10. Hansen-Leth C. Muscle blood flow after amputations with special reference to the amputation level. *Acta Orthop Scand*. 1977;48:10-14.

11. Hansen-Leth C. The vascularization in the amputation stumps of rabbits. A microangiographic study. *Acta Orthop Scand*. 1979;50:399-406.

12. Langhagel J. *Angiographische Untersuchung der Stumpfdurchblutung bei Beinamputierten*. Stuttgart, Germany: Arbeit und Gesundheit, Georg Thieme Verlag; 1968.

13. Leriche R. Traitement de certaines ulcerations spontanees des moignons par la sympathectomie priarterielle. *Press Med*. 1950.

14. Erikson U, Hulth A. Circulation of amputations stumps. Arteriographic and temperature studies. *Acta Orthop Scand*. 1962;32:159-170.

15. Erikson U. Circulation in traumatic amputation stumps. An angiographic and physiologic investigation. *Acta Radiol*. 1965;238(Suppl).

16. Erikson U, Olerud S. Healing of amputation stumps, with special reference to vascularity and bone. *Acta Orthop Scand*. 1966;37:20-28.

17. Medhat MA. Rehabilitation of the vascular amputee. *Orthopaedics Review*. 1983;12.

18. Condie DN. Electromyography of the lower limb amputee. *Medicine and Sport, Biomechanics*. 1973;8:482-488.

19. Bowker JH, Goldberg B, Poonekar PD. Transtibial amputation. In Bowker JH, Michael JW, eds. *Atlas of Limb Prosthetics: Surgical, Prosthetic, and Rehabilitation Principles*. 2nd ed. St Louis, Mo: Mosby; 1992:429-452.

20. Smith D. Amputations and prosthetics. *OKU*. 1993;4,23,267.

21. Smith DG, Fergason JR. Transtibial amputations. *Clin Orthop*. 1999;361:108-115.

Chapter 3

Postoperative Management

John Rheinstein, CP, FAAOP; Christopher Kevin Wong, MS, PT;
Joan E. Edelstein, MA, PT, FISPO

OBJECTIVES

1. Establish the goals of postoperative management
2. Detail the elements of postoperative assessment, including history, and physical and psychological assessments
3. Compare the techniques for postoperative care of the amputation limb, including soft, semi-rigid, and rigid dressings
4. Explain interventions intended to maintain or increase joint excursion and muscular strength
5. Describe procedures addressed at improving the health status of the patient as a whole person, including foot care, functional mobility, general conditioning, and emotional adjustment
6. Provide criteria to determine the patient's readiness for prosthetic fitting

Rehabilitation of people recovering from amputation surgery has three phases: 1) *Healing*, from surgery to first fitting of a temporary prosthesis, usually 4 to 8 weeks; 2) *Maturation*, temporary prosthesis to provision and use of definitive prosthesis, average time 4 to 6 months; and 3) *Definitive*, the remainder of the person's life. This chapter focuses on the healing phase.

Most patients with recent amputations are treated as in-patients in an acute care hospital. The amputated limb is likely to be edematous, painful, hypersensitive to touch, and weakened by muscle imbalance. Elderly adults are often debilitated and subject to orthostatic hypotension because of months or years of reduced physical activity, previous operative procedures, comorbidities, and numerous medications. Others may present with trauma, cognitive deficits, or may be coping with chemotherapy with or without radiation for treatment of malignancy. Psychologically, patients may be embroiled in denial, grief, anger, or depression regarding the loss of a limb. Almost all struggle with uncertainty about their future functional, social, and vocational capabilities.

After hospital discharge, patients are transferred to an in-patient rehabilitation department or are sent home and directed to an out-patient rehabilitation facility. Generally, surgical wounds heal and pain subsides so prosthetic use can begin. Without proper postoperative care, however, complications may develop, which can increase the time needed for rehabilitation and compromise long-term function. A critical determinant of rehabilitation success is the quality and amount of attention devoted to the patient. Frequent, conscientious follow-up is essential. The ultimate objective of rehabilitation is for each person to return to daily life functioning at the highest level possible based on the individual's capabilities and goals.

Written protocols for postoperative care and regular staff training are needed, especially in settings where turnover of personnel is frequent. Protocol documents should be distributed to all staff having any contact with patients who have amputations. Specific instructions should also be entered in the patient's chart and posted at the bedside. Results are best when one individual is responsible for supervising and coordinating all postoperative care.

GOALS

Management during the postoperative period is crucial to the patient's future functional abilities. Physical and psychological issues not addressed during this critical time can hinder a person's recovery and quality of life. Effective care requires the focused attention of each member of the rehabilitation team (surgeon, physiatrist, physical therapist, prosthetist, social worker, mental health professional, nurse, case manager, and payers) to plan and implement treatment protocols that take into account the unique needs of each patient. Many postoperative techniques have proven effective, yet no single procedure can be used in all cases.[1] Because the patient's response during the postoperative period is dynamic, health care professionals should be vigilant in monitoring progress and be willing to change treatment methods as needed. Understanding the various treatment options, their benefits and risks, will allow the most appropriate techniques to be applied as healing progresses.

All postoperative protocols have similar goals to: 1) heal the surgical wound, 2) minimize pain, 3) protect the amputated limb from trauma, 4) preserve and improve range of motion and strength of the entire body, 5) reduce swelling and begin shaping the amputated limb, 6) enable the patient to learn to use appropriate mobility aids, 7) begin controlled weight bearing, 8) accomplish functional activities, and 9) facilitate psychological adjustment to limb loss. Even if future prosthetic use is unlikely, patients need sufficient muscle strength and cardiopulmonary reserve to meet their daily functional needs. Emphasis on the goals needs to be balanced. For example, wound healing is a primary goal but it should not be overemphasized at the expense of other objectives such as limb shaping and joint mobilization.

ASSESSMENT

Postoperative treatment should be based on a thorough history and physical and psychological assessment. Clinical judgments are guided by the patient's healing and ambulation potential as well as the individual's ability and willingness to follow instructions (see Figure 3-4). The rehabilitation team should review the assessment periodically as the individual progresses through rehabilitation.

History
1. Age
2. Gender
3. Weight
4. Date of amputation(s)
5. Date of revision(s)
6. Etiology of amputation(s)
7. Complications pertaining to the amputation(s)
8. Previous prosthetic use
9. Current prosthetic concerns
10. Comorbidities
11. History of smoking
12. Family medical history
13. Home environment
14. Family and other social support
15. Access to physical therapy
16. Access to prosthetic care
17. Current and future work plans
18. Current and future hobbies
19. Economic considerations
20. Cultural considerations

Physical Assessment
For each amputated limb:
1. Level and length
2. Overall condition and girth
3. Condition of the wound
4. Strength
5. Range of motion
6. Pain: Local, phantom

Other Assessments
1. Strength in the other limbs and trunk
2. Range of motion in the other limbs and trunk
3. Manual dexterity
4. Cardiopulmonary function
5. Nutritional status
6. Vision
7. Ability to stand on the remaining leg
8. Days since patient last stood
9. Functional level assessment[2]

Psychological Assessment
1. Orientation
2. Cognition, particularly memory
3. Motivation
4. Other emotional considerations

AMPUTATION LIMB

Surgery

The quality of the amputation surgery sets the course of the patient's rehabilitation. Although consensus does not exist regarding the best surgical technique, there is general agreement that the condition of the amputation limb has a profound effect on the patient's future.

Optimally, the surgeon should approach the amputation as a reconstructive procedure. Prudent selection of the amputation level is critical to wound healing. The ideal level balances the need for wound healing with the functional benefits of maximum amputation limb length. Prosthetic component requirements also should be considered when deciding on limb length. For example, a knee unit adds length to the thigh; consequently, a long transfemoral amputation may be slightly shortened so that the patient will have equal thigh length when sitting.

The shape of the residuum is determined by the way the surgeon sections and shapes the musculature and bone. An excessively bulbous limb is difficult to fit into a prosthesis; however, a limb with insufficient distal soft tissue is also troublesome. Healing is facilitated by meticulous skin closure with the muscle flap under correct tension. Range of motion of the adjacent joint is optimized by surgical closure in full knee extension for the transtibial amputation and neutral hip extension and adduction for a transfemoral amputation. Otherwise the adjacent joint is apt to develop a flexion contracture. Unbalanced tension of opposing muscles during closure can also produce contractures. Patients are well served when physicians, therapists, and prosthetists provide feedback to surgeons as to the effect of particular surgical procedures on rehabilitation outcomes.

If the incision is left open, the amputation is termed an open amputation. This procedure is indicated in emergencies when there is risk or presence of infection. Wound closure is planned for a later date. Once closure has been achieved, the amputation limb is eligible for the dressing techniques described below.

Wound Healing

Amputation limb dressings influence wound healing. The dressings are intended to be applied to a closed amputation wound, namely one in which staples or sutures secure the edges of the skin.

The major purposes of a postoperative dressing are to reduce postoperative pain and edema, foster healing, and promote a well-shaped amputation limb. Edema develops quickly after tissue disruption. Dressings reduce edema by applying extravascular hydrostatic pressure to increase venous flow velocity.[2] For the individual with peripheral vascular disease, edema control is particularly important because impaired circulation delays healing.

Some people have difficulty achieving primary wound healing. Factors affecting healing include diabetes, vascular disease with or without surgery, smoking, nutrition,[3] abnormal blood composition, preoperative gangrene, antibiotic use, amputation level, surgical technique, post surgical drain, and postoperative dress-ing.[4] Consequently, the rehabilitation team should have an array of techniques available to meet the needs of each patient. Chapter 5 describes skin care.

Postoperative dressing techniques are broadly classified as soft, semirigid, and rigid. Each type has variations, with advantages and disadvantages. All are applied over a sutured amputation wound. The suture line is covered by one or more of the following: nonadherent impregnated gauze, sterile gauze, absorbent pads, semiocclusive, or colloid wound dressings. Selection among postoperative treatment protocols is usually based on clinical experience.[5] The challenge is to select the method most appropriate for the given patient and to recognize when another method becomes preferable. (see Figure 3-4) Until surgical wound healing and residual limb volume stabilization, one of the available dressings should be left in place 24 hours per day. Although these techniques are focused on lower limb amputees they can be applied to upper limb patients as well.[6]

Soft Dressings

The most common techniques for postoperative care involve use of elastic fabric, either in the form of a bandage or a shrinker sock.

Elastic Bandage

A 4- or 6-inch wide elastic bandage is applied to the amputation limb in a series of off-setting figure-of-eight turns. Circular turns tend to create hourglass constriction in the mid portion of the amputation limb. Elastic bandage should be applied with greater pressure distally. A dog ear (ie, redundant tissue at the distal medial and lateral portions of the limb) should be pulled into a broad conical shape. The bandage is secured with adhesive tape. Metal clasps may damage fragile skin if the clasp rubs on the contralateral limb.

Bandaging of the transtibial limb may begin either on the anterior or posterior surface. The latter application is preferable because it enables the bandage to be pulled anteriorly, thereby approximating the superior and inferior aspects of the incision. The posterior to anterior pull of soft tissue draws tissues under the terminal bone. Bandaging terminates at the distal thigh. When bandaging the transfemoral amputation limb, one should attempt to contain the proximal medial tissues to prevent formation of an adductor roll, which would chafe when the patient walks. The bandage should be secured around the lower torso.[7]

Elastic Bandage Advantages

Elastic bandaging is the oldest amputation limb dressing. Bandages are inexpensive and readily available in all hospitals. They can be applied by virtually anyone, including medical staff, family members, and, in the case of the transtibial limb, the patient.

Elastic Bandage Disadvantages

The bandage must be reapplied several times a day because it loosens as the patient moves about in bed or transfers from one seat to another. Self-bandaging requires that the patient have trunk flexibility, hand strength and dexterity, visual acuity, and endurance.[8,9] When the bandage is applied by different people, variation in pressure occurs.[10] If applied incorrectly, in extreme circumstances, the bandage can produce areas of high pressure that lead to tissue breakdown or even a tourniquet effect. Leaving the amputated limb exposed for as little as 10 minutes can result in edema formation, making the many reapplications of elastic bandage a detriment to patient care. The training required for the patient to learn to self-bandage skillfully, in addition to reapplications after the dressing loosens, becomes soiled, or is removed for wound inspection, results in the amputation limb being uncovered part of each day. Edema control is poor, as indicated by patients requiring more analgesics than those who have rigid dressings.[11] Elastic bandages are associated with misshapen limbs as well as poor edema control and skin breakdown.[8,9,12] Elastic bandages offer minimal protection from accidental trauma to the residual limb, especially if the patient falls.

Shrinker Socks

Elastic shrinker socks are manufactured in various lengths and widths, with the distal end intended to accommodate either a conical or cylindrical shape. The transtibial sock is knitted uniformly, whereas the transfemoral sock has a loosely knitted top. Shrinkers are sometimes applied over elastic bandage or after other modalities are removed. One alternative is elasticized fabric tubing, which is applied to the amputated limb, twisted, and reflected back over the limb. Tubing is sold in rolls in 1-inch width increments and is cut to the length needed. Another alternative is the use of elastic fabric shorts.[13]

Shrinker Sock Advantages

Shrinker socks are more effective than elastic bandage in reducing limb volume.[14]

Shrinker Sock Disadvantages

Care must be taken when applying the shrinker sock not to displace any staples or sutures that may be present. The sock is apt to roll down the transfemoral amputated limb unless garter belt suspension is worn. Socks eventually stretch and must be replaced by fresh ones. Replacement is also necessary when the amputation limb reduces volume. Consequently, different sizes must be stocked or specially ordered for each patient. Two or more shrinker socks of the same size should be supplied to allow for drying time between washings.

Resources for Soft Dressings

Elastic bandage is manufactured by Johnson & Johnson (New Brunswick, NJ) and many other companies. Shrinkers are available through prosthetists. Compressogrip elasticized tubing is sold by Knit-Rite Company (Kansas City, Kan).

Semi-Rigid Dressings

Unna dressings, air splints, and silicone liners encase the amputation limb in a semirigid dressing.

Unna Dressing

The Unna dressing is made of gauze bandage infiltrated with zinc oxide and calamine, with gelatin and glycerin as moisture retention agents. After the surgical incision is protected with a thin wound dressing, the bandage is applied in strips directly to the skin of the amputated limb.[15] The Unna dressing can be applied in the operating room[15-17] or later in the rehabilitation process.[18,19] It is usually left in place for 7 days, but can be removed for inspection or significant atrophy occurs, as indicated by loosening of the distal portion of the dressing. It is removed with bandage scissors. The Unna bandage can be used as a protective interface with an air splint or temporary prosthesis for early ambulation.

Unna Dressing Advantages

The inextensible dressing remains on the limb continually, promoting faster edema reduction and wound healing as compared to soft dressings.[19] Tension applied to the distal aspect of the amputation limb helps avoid dog ears. The lightness, slimness, and self-suspending qualities of Unna dressing facilitate functional mobility without limiting hip or knee motion. Its streamlined contour makes it especially suitable for transfemoral amputated limbs.[19] The Unna dressing is readily available and can be applied by the rehabilitation professional with minimal special instruction. Because the dressing does not have to be reapplied frequently, the risks associated with inappropriate reapplication are minimized.[8] The Unna dressing can be used in an outpatient setting because ordinarily it does not need to be reapplied for at least 1 week. Patients managed with the Unna dressing were ready for prosthetic fitting after surgery in half the time required for those with elastic bandage; the outcome was similar whether the Unna dressing was applied in the operating room[16] or in the rehabilitation department.[19] Functional outcome after rehabilitation is also better with the Unna dressing, particularly in patients with transfemoral amputations who are more likely to walk with a prosthesis.[19] For the transtibial amputated limb, Unna dressing resists substantial knee flexion, thus preventing contracture without completely immobilizing the knee.

Unna Dressing Disadvantages

A few patients have inserted a pencil beneath the Unna dressing to scratch the skin. In usual practice, the Unna dressing does not permit daily wound inspection. Unna bandage is somewhat more expensive than elastic

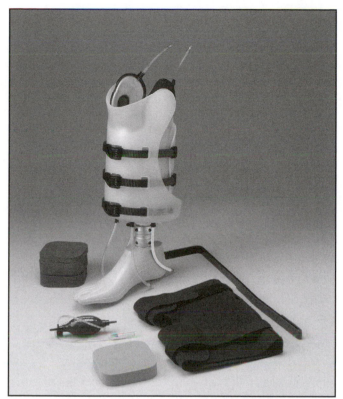

Figure 3-1. Air-Limb IPOP temporary prosthesis with inflatable lining.

bandage or plaster. The Unna bandage does not protect the residual limb from high impact trauma.

Unna Dressing Resources

Unna bandage is available from most medical supply companies. It is manufactured by Glenwood Inc (Tenafly, NJ) and Beiersdorf-Jobst (Charlotte, NC), among other suppliers.

Air Splint

The air splint is an inflatable plastic splint. The amputated limb, encased in stockinet, is placed in the splint, which is then closed and inflated to 25 mm Hg to promote edema reduction and wound healing.[20] For a transtibial amputated limb, the air splint extends to the mid thigh. The proximal edge of the air splint for a transfemoral amputation limb should be at the groin. The air splint may be applied either in the operating room or in the rehabilitation department.[21,22] An aluminum frame may be added to the outside of the air splint to enable limited weight bearing.[23,24] Another version of air splint is a temporary prosthesis with an inflatable lining (Figure 3-1).

Air Splint Advantages

Air splint is suitable for patients with transtibial, knee disarticulation and long transfemoral amputated limbs. It promotes edema reduction and wound healing.[21,22]

It compresses the amputated limb uniformly. It is easy to apply and take off. The air splint accommodates changes in limb volume because it is reinflated with each application. It protects the amputated limb from trauma and, for the transtibial amputated limb, resists knee flexion. The plastic does not absorb bacteria and is easily cleaned and sterilized. Compared to the soft dressing, the air splint decreases the time to prosthetic fitting.[25] With an aluminum frame, the Pneumatic Post Amputation Mobility Aid (Hosmer Dorrance Company, Campbell, Calif) can be worn for early ambulation. Although it can be reused for successive patients if the plastic is sterilized,[25,26] it is preferable to use fresh splints.

Air Splint Disadvantages

The plastic creates a humid environment for the limb. The patient who intends to apply it needs moderate manual dexterity and mobility. If the plastic is not cleaned regularly with alcohol, infection may occur.[23,26] The air splint is designed for partial weight bearing only. One manufacturer recommends using it only after the fifth postoperative day.

Air Splint Resources

The basic air splint is sold by Sammons Preston Rolyan (Bolingbrook, Ill). The Pneumatic Post Amputation Mobility Aid PPAM Mark 11 is available through the Hosmer Dorrance Company.

Silicone Liners

A roll-on silicone liner can be applied directly to the amputated limb, either in the operating room or later during the healing period. Liner size is determined by limb circumference 4 cm proximal to the distal end. If the exact size cannot be matched, the next smaller size is selected. The surgical incision is covered with a standard or hydrocolloid wound dressing. The liner is then inverted and rolled on the limb. Wearing time is based on individual circumstances. The wound should be inspected and aired at least once daily as well as following weight-bearing activity. Silicone can be sterilized using heat autoclaving.

Silicone Liner Advantages

The silicon liner provides compression to reduce postoperative edema. It tends to smooth scar tissue. The liner also provides the patient with an early opportunity to learn to use a silicone liner, which may also be used with the definitive prosthesis.

Silicone Liner Disadvantages

The liner traps sweat, which may create skin disorders if the liner is not cleaned at least daily. The liner only provides minimal protection against trauma. Contraindications to the silicone liner include skin grafts, poor blood flow, necrosis, infection, allergy to perspiration, contracture, lack of hand strength or dexterity, poor cognition, and noncompliance.

Silicone Liner Resources

Silicone liners are available from a number of manufacturers including: MediPro distributed by Southern Prosthetic Supply (Alpharetta, Ga), Ossur Inc (Aliso Viejo, Calif) and Alps South Corp. (St. Petersburg, Fla).

Rigid Dressings

A rigid dressing is a plaster or fiberglass cast intended to be applied in the operating room immediately after surgery by a specially trained surgeon, prosthetist, cast technician, or physical therapist. A sterile dressing is placed over the wound, and then the limb is covered with a sterile sock. For the transtibial limb, felt pads are situated over bony prominences. The limb is then wrapped with a layer of elastic plaster and the cast is reinforced with regular plaster. The plaster dries into a rigid cast. The transtibial rigid dressing extends over the knee; it may have a circular opening over the patella to prevent breakdown of fragile skin. The transfemoral rigid dressing reaches the groin. One or more straps are incorporated into the cast to be buckled to a waist belt or harness for suspension.[27,28] The patient and the health care staff must monitor the straps, keeping them taut to prevent cast slippage. Manual pressure against the distal end of the rigid dressing may be introduced to simulate weight bearing stress. The rigid dressing remains in place for 7 to 15 days until the time of suture removal.[27] It is removed sooner if it fits loosely because the limb has atrophied, or if infection is evident. Nursing and other rehabilitation staff must be trained to recognize infection, bleeding, ischemia, or excessive pain. A qualified person needs to be available at all times to remove the rigid dressing if such problems arise. Sometimes the rigid dressing is applied as the first postoperative dressing after which the patient receives a removable rigid dressing at the time of the first cast change.

Rigid Dressing Advantages

Rigid dressings apply mild pressure to the amputated limb to control edema, foster healing, and shape the limb. Healing occurs faster than with an elastic bandaging, facilitating earlier prosthetic fitting.[28,29] The rigid dressing protects the wound from trauma, eg, if the patient strikes the amputated limb against the bedrails or other hard surface or if the person should fall.[28,30,31] Controlling edema reduces the need for analgesics.[11] The transtibial rigid dressing limits knee motion thereby preventing flexion contracture.[27,29]

Rigid Dressing Disadvantages

Patients with infection or excessive drainage are not candidates for rigid dressings. A member of the rehabilitation team must be on call to apply a rigid dressing or to remove it if any problem arises or if it slips because limb volume markedly reduces. An improperly applied rigid dressing may cause local skin breakdown or ischemia. If a good fit is not maintained, movement inside the cast can cause blisters and abrasions.[33] An unmotivated or disoriented patient may attempt to remove the rigid dressing or may not maintain the suspension straps adequately taut. Postoperative pain can be mistakenly attributed to the rigid dressing if the amputated limb swells against the plaster. When the rigid dressing is removed, pain may increase with rapid increase of edema. In one study, investigators found no difference in infection rate or time to prosthetic fitting when comparing patients fitted with a rigid dressing as compared with soft dressings. Although most surgeons (64%) and all physiotherapists and nurses in the group felt that the rigid dressing was an improvement on their normal regime.[32]

Rigid Dressing Resources

Regular and elastic plaster or fiberglass bandage and sterile socks are readily available.

Removable Rigid Dressing

A removable rigid dressing is a custom-made plaster or fiberglass shell that is sectioned to form an anterior and a posterior portion that allow minor circumferential adjustments.[34] Recent innovations include the Hanger Kiwi Comfort Protector which combines a custom formed removable rigid dressing with a silicone liner (Figure 3-2) and the Hanger Nuttmegger (Figure 3-3) a custom plastic device made from a laser scan of the patient's residual limb (both Hanger Prosthetics & Orthotics, Bethesda, Md). A prefabricated alternative is the plastic removable rigid dressing known as the FLO-TECH-TOR (Flo-Tech Inc, Trumansburg, NY).

A removable rigid dressing is appropriate if the patient's balance or strength is such that restricted or nonweight bearing is indicated. Limited weight bearing can be introduced by having the patient pull with a strap wrapped around the distal end of the removable rigid dressing or by standing with the distal end of the removable rigid dressing on a stool, the sound foot on the floor, and the hands on a walker. The removable rigid dressing is ordinarily worn 24 hours a day with daily wound inspection followed by range of motion of the proximal joints. If the removable rigid dressing is removed, another dressing should be substituted immediately to prevent edema. Prosthetic socks may be added to compensate for volume reduction.

Removable Rigid Dressing Advantages

The removable rigid dressing reduces hospital stays and increases the likelihood that the patient will be ambulatory at discharge.[5,9,34,35] It protects and compresses the amputated limb, yet it can be removed for limb inspection. Upon removing this dressing, the patient should move the knee. The removable rigid

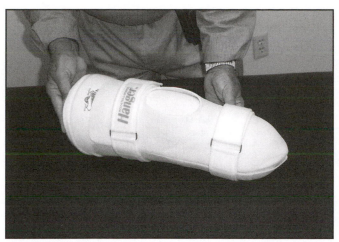

Figure 3-2. Hanger Kiwi Comfort Protector with straps fastened.

dressing should be reapplied before the amputated limb swells. If significant volume loss has occurred, a new removable rigid dressing needs to be applied. Plastic removable rigid dressings can be washed and adjusted as the limb atrophies.

Removable Rigid Dressing Disadvantages

The removable rigid dressing is ineffective if the patient removes it without authorization. With prefabricated devices, the residual limb may lose so much volume that a smaller size needs to be obtained. The removable rigid dressing is not designed for ambulation.

Immediate Postoperative Prosthesis

The technique used to form the socket for the immediate postoperative prosthesis is the same as for the plaster or fiberglass rigid dressing.[27,28] The clinician secures a pylon and foot to the rigid device to allow limited weight bearing. The physical therapy and nursing staff must be trained to instruct patients to restrict weight bearing to less than 25 pounds on the immediate postoperative prosthesis. In the first few postoperative weeks, standing and walking should be closely supervised by a physical therapist. If there is any doubt about the patient's ability or willingness to comply with weight-bearing restrictions, the pylon should be detached when the patient is not supervised in the rehabilitation department. This allows the patient to benefit from early ambulation while minimizing risk to the surgical wound. Patients should be reminded to pause before standing to control weight bearing and to recognize whether they are wearing the prosthesis. If difficulties with wound healing develop, weight bearing should be discontinued until the problem is resolved. Following suture removal and complete wound healing, weight bearing can be increased gradually as tolerated over 1 to 3 weeks until full single-leg

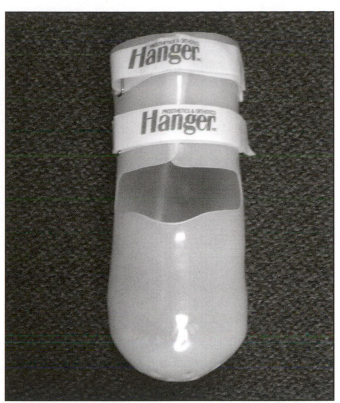

Figure 3-3. Hanger Nutmegger custom rigid dressing.

standing on the immediate postoperative prosthesis is achieved. Once full weight bearing is established, the custom-molded prosthesis should be prescribed. Immediate postoperative prostheses are generally kept on 24 hours a day with the pylon removed except for wound inspection and range of motion exercises. If the prosthesis is removed, another dressing should be substituted immediately to prevent edema.

Immediate Postoperative Prosthesis Advantages

An immediate postoperative prosthesis offers the benefits of the rigid dressing or removable rigid dressing, plus allowing three-point standing and ambulation. Early activity may reduce some comorbidities associated with prolonged bed rest, such as weakness, general deconditioning, and joint stiffness.[33] Falling and injuring the amputation limb while transferring or walking is less likely with an immediate postoperative prosthesis.[30] No significant difference in revision rates between patients fitted with immediate postoperative prostheses and other dressings have been reported.[13,29,35] Psychologically, the immediate postoperative prosthesis replaces the appearance of the amputated leg, which the patient can see soon after recovering from anesthesia, potentially easing the adaptation to a new body image.[11,27,31,33] Anecdotal evidence suggests that individuals fitted with immediate postoperative prostheses become more involved in their rehabilitation and have less uncertainty about prosthetic use. The immediate postoperative prosthesis acts as a bridge from surgery to the definitive prosthesis. Allowing people with amputation to stand and gradually begin using both legs improves overall function. Immediate postoperative prostheses help patients make the transition to a temporary or definitive prosthesis with greater ease than if they were to sit in a wheelchair, waiting for wound healing. The transtibial version discourages formation of a knee flexion contracture (see Figure 3-1).

Immediate Postoperative Prosthesis Disadvantages

The patient may put excessive weight on the immediate postoperative prosthesis, thus risking opening of the surgical wound. For this reason, a person who is disoriented or noncompliant should not be fitted with an IPOP. The patient may injure the contralateral leg by inadvertently striking it with the pylon of the immediate postoperative prosthesis. The other disadvantages described for the rigid dressing also apply to the immediate postoperative prosthesis.

Immediate Postoperative Prosthesis Resources

The detachable pylon is available from Seattle Systems (Poulsbo, Wash). Prefabricated immediate postoperative prostheses are manufactured by Aircast (Summit, NJ), Flo-Tech Inc (Trumansburg, NY), Otto Bock Health Care (Minneapolis, Minn), and Fillauer (Chattanooga, Tenn).

Pain

Control of postoperative local pain and phantom pain is an essential part of early management. Phantom sensations are the nonpainful sensations perceived to emanate from the missing portion of the amputation limb. Chapter 4 delineates the management of pain.

Joint Excursion

Adequate motion of the adjacent proximal joint is necessary to use a prosthesis effectively. Full joint excursion is optimized by surgical closure in full knee extension for a transtibial amputation and full hip extension and adduction for a transfemoral amputation. Otherwise the adjacent joint is apt to develop a flexion contracture. Unbalanced muscle tension during operative closure can produce a contracture. Hamstring hyperactivity inhibits the quadriceps muscle[36] and contributes to knee flexion contracture.[37] Postoperative edema and pain inhibit muscles from normal function.[38] For the patient with transtibial amputation, edema at the knee inhibits the quadriceps. Knee flexion contracture is even more likely if the amputation limb is allowed to dangle from the wheelchair seat. Hip flexion, abduction, and external rotation contracture are common after transtibial or transfemoral amputation due to prolonged sitting. Many people have hamstring and

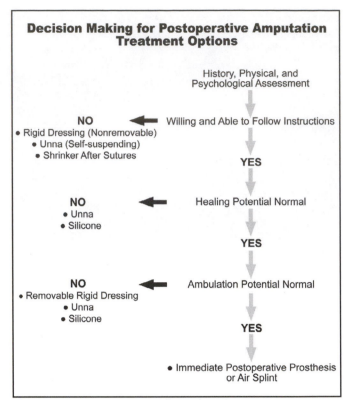

Figure 3-4. Postoperative clinical pathway.

iliopsoas tightness prior to amputation. Older or sedentary individuals, including those who had delayed amputation and spent prolonged time in a wheelchair, are particularly susceptible to developing contractures. A knee flexion contracture of 5 degrees or a hip flexion contracture of 15 degrees is not usually a problem because alignment of the prosthesis can accommodates slight contractures. However, a moderate contracture complicates prosthetic alignment and may compromise ambulation.

Optimal range of motion (ROM) can be obtained and maintained using different methods of positioning, immobilization, manual therapy, and exercise. ROM exercises should be introduced on the first postoperative day. The person with transtibial amputation should have a wheelchair with a horizontal support on which the amputated limb rests. If a contracture has developed, an adjustable stretching orthosis is usually effective. Once a patient uses a prosthesis on a regular basis, extension forces help reduce a contracture. Setting the prosthetic alignment so it does not fully accommodate the contracture creates a dynamic stretching force with each step. A prosthesis with adjustable components can be realigned as the contracture resolves.

Positioning

Static positioning is an important intervention for maintaining muscle length and joint range after lower-limb amputation. Positioning to emphasize hip extension, adduction, and knee extension should be introduced immediately after surgery and should be encouraged by all team members for consistent care during the patient's rehabilitation. Even in the absence of contractures, positioning is an important means of preventing contractures from occurring.

When the patient is in bed the hips should be kept adducted. Pillows can be used to support the lateral aspect of the thighs to maintain adduction. The knee should be kept extended. If tolerated, the patient should lie prone for at least 20 minutes a day to enable gravity to maintain hip flexor length and hip extension excursion.

When the patient sits the amputated limb should be adducted. A towel roll on each side of the wheelchair seat can be used to maintain the adducted position. Alternately, sitting in a bucket seat design cushion decreases iliotibial band contracture 30% over a 6-week period.[39] The knee should be kept extended with the distal end of the amputated limb elevated to the horizontal to stretch the hamstrings and prevent dependent edema. As noted, a specialized leg rest attached to the wheelchair seat can be used. If the hamstrings are exceptionally tight, a reclining wheelchair is beneficial; however, these cumbersome wheelchairs may limit independent mobility.

Immobilization

A benefit of the rigid dressing, Unna dressing, and air splint is that the knee is kept extended. Alternatively, orthoses can be used to maintain knee extension after transtibial amputation. A knee splint can be used to immobilize the knee when the patient is resting yet be removed for exercise. Additionally, an orthosis can protect the limb from trauma during transfers and wheelchair use. A posterior shell knee orthosis is an inexpensive, mass-produced option. The shell has straps over the anterior knee to maintain extension. Because the straps are adjustable, full extension may be difficult to maintain if the patient loosens them. Straps can press into the thigh or leg, subjecting the patient to the risk of skin breakdown.

Manual Therapy

Soft tissue interventions may be required to restore full ROM and muscle length. This is particularly true for the iliopsoas, the primary hip flexor.

Skin grafts following trauma or surgical harvesting present a special problem due to the large area of scar tissue usually present. Once healing has occurred, mobilization of the soft tissues around the borders of the graft and harvest site are imperative for restoring tissue flexibility and increasing pressure tolerance. Skin mobilization of the suture line should be taught to all patients.

Case Study

A patient who was a Vietnam War veteran of multiple combat tours, returned to the United States unscathed, only to be struck by a car while walking on the sidewalk. He sustained multiple surgical procedures, including split-thickness grafts to close the wounds. Repeated grafts harvested from the thigh and abdomen were unsuccessful. For 7 years he used crutches and a wheelchair while his leg remained painful and dysfunctional. He finally underwent a transtibial amputation with a graft from the plantar surface of his foot transferred to the anterior distal surface of the amputated limb. The graft was positioned with the thick skin of the heel over the end of the tibia to protect the severed bone. An adherent scar formed over the tibia just inferior to the patella, causing pain. The borders of the graft were mobilized using soft-tissue mobilization and myofascial release techniques. A prosthesis was eventually fitted, the pain receded, and the patient returned to full community ambulation without an assistive device.

Strengthening

Developing strength is also a priority because the strength loss before and after amputation is considerable. Most people who undergo amputation are elderly with peripheral vascular disease. Amputation occurs after a period of decreased activity and muscular atrophy. Postoperative edema and pain inhibit muscles from normal function.[36] Isometric, concentric, and eccentric muscular contractions are significantly weakened in the quadriceps (35% to 51% of sound limb strength) and hamstrings (42% to 60% of the contralateral limb) following transtibial amputation. Notably, individuals who had amputation within 7 years of measurement were not significantly stronger or weaker than those who had amputation more than 7 years ago,[37] suggesting that weakness occurs in the first few years of amputation and that exercise may forestall subsequent weakness.

Strengthening is best achieved with exercises aimed first at minimizing atrophy and loss of neuromuscular control, then progressing to increasing strength, and finally preparing the amputation limb for the forces involved in gait and functional activities with a prosthesis.

Exercises should be progressed from simple to more demanding. For example, separate quadriceps and gluteus maximus isometric exercises can be progressed to co-contractions. Simple isotonic exercise can be made more challenging with weights. Open-chain exercises are progressed to closed-chain exercises. Non-weight-bearing exercises performed in recumbency are advanced to weight-bearing exercises in the upright position. Similarly, lateral weight shifts can start with iliotibial band stretching to isometric exercise and isotonic hip abduction. Isolated leg-to-abdominal motion is first performed in the frontal and sagittal planes, then diagonally. If tolerated, strengthening exercises are best performed while the patient wears the prosthesis. This adds resistance and helps develop the patient's proprioceptive awareness of the prosthesis.

Isometric Exercise

Isometric exercise requires muscles to contract against resistance without joint motion. It is a convenient form of exercise that requires no equipment and can be performed in bed and in the wheelchair. It is useful when limb movement is painful.[40] Force is controlled by the individual within tolerance because no external load is used. Isometric exercise is most appropriate for low levels of strength. Most gains are made within the first few weeks of training[40] attributed to neural adaptations and recruitment of muscle.[41] Isometric exercise is highly appropriate for initial exercise of the amputated limb to minimize atrophy and maintain neuromuscular control. It develops angle-specific strength. To develop strength throughout the full joint excursion, isometric exercises need to be performed at varying angles.[40] When the new patient is able to move the leg into different angles, the person is ready to advance to active range of motion exercises.

Simple muscle setting should be initiated immediately following surgery to maintain neuromuscular activity and slow postoperative atrophy. Gluteus maximus isometric exercise performed in supine and iliopsoas isometric exercise performed prone use the bed for stability. Isometric iliopsoas contractions may be done supine with a pillow on the anterior portion of the leg providing counter-pressure. Isometric gluteus medius exercise can be performed against the bed rail or wheelchair side. A pillow can be squeezed for hip adductor isometric contraction. The individual with transtibial amputation should perform quadriceps and hamstrings isometric contraction. Isometric contractions should be held for 6 seconds to obtain peak tension in the muscle.[42]

Isometric exercise is associated with a rapid increase in blood pressure due to the Valsalva maneuver during the contraction.[42] Because many patients have cardiovascular disease, it is especially important to teach them to inhale and exhale during isometric contractions.

Active Range of Motion

Active joint excursion indicates individual's willingness to move the amputated limb. Once the person has sufficient strength, motivation, and pain tolerance to move the limb, simple active exercises can be initiated to build strength throughout the joint's excursion. Active exercises can be performed in a gravity-elimi-nated position if necessary and progressed to the anti-gravity position. For instance, hip abduction can be performed in supine with the leg sliding across the bed to eliminate the effect of gravity on the gluteus medius. Progression to gravitational resistance is achieved by abducting the hip while side-lying. Active hip exercise uses straight-leg raises for hip extension, flexion, abduction, and adduction, with the patient changing position from prone to side-lying to supine. Heel slides exercise hip and knee flexors, whereas long- and short-arc knee extension exercises the quadriceps. Active ROM exercises do not involve resistance that can be altered. Consequently, the individual who is able to perform three sets of 10 exercises should progress to resisted exercises.

Resistance Exercises

Resistance is provided manually or with cuff weights applied to the distal limb during straight plane hip exercises such as straight-leg raising in four directions. One set of six repetitions at full resistance increases strength.[43,44] More repetitions at lower resistance levels, however, builds endurance.[40]

Progressive resistance can also be provided by elastic ribbons or tubing. Elastic creates greater resistance at greater tension, thus more resistance is delivered at the end of the range of motion. Elastic ribbon and tubing are color coded for different resistances. Tubing length can also be altered to change the resistance.

Isokinetic exercise machines can also be used for strength training after amputation. Machines insure equal resistance throughout the joint excursion. In addition, machines can be adjusted to elicit concentric and eccentric contractions, with varying speeds of movement.

Isotonic exercise, whether using the therapist's hands, cuff weights, elastic ribbons or tubing, or isokinetic machines, has limited application in the postoperative period. Resistance is typically applied at the distal end of the limb. The short lever arm of the amputation limb demands less torque production from the muscle than if the limb were intact; consequently, greater resistance is required to create substantial torque. In the postoperative stage, the unhealed surgical incision is sensitive. Excessive resistance can create deleterious force on the limb. Cuff weights and elastic tubing can slide, imposing dangerous shear forces. Once the incision is healed, isotonic exercise can be an effective method for strengthening.

Closed Kinetic Chain Exercise

When the patient can perform repetitive active exercises, tolerate weight bearing, and protect the incision with an appropriate dressing, closed chain exercises can be initiated. These exercises stimulate co-contractions and dynamic stabilization in weight-bearing positions that more closely resemble muscular forces experienced in upright activities as compared with isotonic exercises.[40] For instance, when ascending a step, the quadriceps and gluteus maximus contract together to raise the body to the next step. Specificity of training produces greater function and strength increases.[40] In addition, closed-chain exercises are usually performed in the upright position, which allows meaningful upper-limb activity. Closed-chain exercise allows the patient to develop strength throughout the joint excursion while exposing the amputated limb to weight-bearing forces that prepare it for the forces applied by the socket during prosthetic gait.[45] Pictures and videos can be purchased from Advanced Rehabilitation Therapy (7641 SW 126 Street, Miami, FL 33156).

Recumbent Closed-Chain Exercises: Hip Extension

- *Position*: Supine. The amputated limb rests on a towel roll with the hip slightly flexed.
- *Exercise*: The patient presses the amputated limb into the towel with sufficient force to lift the lower torso off the mat. The patient with transtibial amputation achieves quadriceps and hamstring/gluteus maximus co-contraction. Performed at first with the sound leg resting on the mat, the level of difficulty can be progressed by lifting the sound limb and upper limbs off the mat.
- *Clinical notes*: Hip extension strength is adversely affected by hip flexor tightness, common in sedentary individuals. Joint or soft-tissue mobilization and stretching to the hip flexors to restore full hip extension augments hip extension strengthening. Patients should be instructed to stretch daily to maintain joint range. This is especially important for the person with transfemoral amputation who needs to maintain flexibility of the hip flexors for optimal gait with the prosthesis.

Recumbent Closed-Chain Exercises: Hip Abduction

- *Position*: Side-lying on the amputated side against the mat. A bolster is placed under the residual limb; the intact limb rests on another bolster or pillow in front.
- *Exercise*: The patient performs hip abduction by pressing the residual limb into the bolster and lifting the lower torso off the mat. Hip extension should be maintained to target the gluteus medius. This exercise facilitates co-contraction of the ipsilateral quadratus lumborum and the gluteus medius. Performed initially with the sound limb supported, the exercise is progressed by elevating the sound limb to eliminate the assistance of contralateral hip adductors when lifting the pelvis off the mat.

- *Clinical notes*: A flexed hip position emphasizes tensor fascia lata contraction, which plays a less significant role in maintaining frontal plane pelvic stability during gait. In contrast, emphasis on the gluteus medius is critical because ipsilateral gluteus medius strength (hip abduction with hip extension) correlates positively with prosthetic weight bearing. Further, greater gluteus medius strength enables a longer step, faster walking speed, and decreased sound-limb stance:swing phase ratio.[46] If neutral hip extension position can not be obtained, the patient should first restore hip extension range.

Recumbent Closed-Chain Exercises: Hip Adduction

- *Position*: Side-lying on the sound limb against the mat in hip and knee flexion. The amputated limb is positioned in hip abduction with a bolster under the medial aspect of the limb.
- *Exercise*: The patient performs hip adduction by pressing the amputated limb into the bolster and lifting the lower torso off the mat. This exercise facilitates co-contraction of the contralateral quadratus lumborum and the hip adductor muscles. The exercise can be made more difficult by eliminating contact between the sound limb and the mat to reduce the assistance of contralateral hip abductors.
- *Clinical notes*: Hip extension biases this exercise to the adductor magnus, which is particularly active in the first half of stance phase.[47] Hip flexion causes the adductor longus and brevis to become more active, which is typical in the latter half of stance phase.[48]

Recumbent Closed-Chain Exercises: Hip Flexion

- *Position*: Prone. A bolster is under the anterior aspect of the amputated limb. The intact limb lies extended on the mat.
- *Exercise*: The patient performs hip flexion by pressing the amputated limb into the bolster and lifting the lower torso off the mat. This exercise is best performed with co-contraction of the abdominals in a posterior pelvic tilt to maintain pelvic stability. If the knee is intact, the bolster can be positioned under the anterior aspect of the distal portion of the amputated limb to create a quadriceps and iliopsoas co-contraction as the pelvis is lifted. As the body is lowered to the mat, iliopsoas works eccentrically while the quadriceps maintain the knee in extension, similar to the functions of these muscles after midstance. The exercise can be made more difficult by reducing the support of the sound limb.

- *Clinical notes*: The quadriceps should be exercised in isolation and in conjunction with other muscles. The importance of the quadriceps is demonstrated in prosthetic gait. Electromyographic activity of the quadriceps during the second half of swing phase is more than double that of the sound limb[49] to maintain knee extension. The resting position may be also used as a stretch for the iliopsoas. Contract-relax principles can be applied by the patient by maintaining this position after contracting the iliopsoas during the exercise.

Once the patient has demonstrated weight-bearing tolerance in the recumbent position and the incision is healed with no more than a 2-cm opening, closed-chain exercises can be performed in other weight-bearing positions. For people with transtibial amputation, the quadruped position is excellent for increasing weight bearing. Four-limb support can be reduced to three-, then two-limb support for increased weight bearing. Resisted isometric holding in quadruped, active hip motion exercises, and trunk stability exercises using the upper and/or lower limbs are examples of exercises in quadruped position.

When two-limb support is tolerated, the patient with transtibial amputation can perform upright closed-chain exercises in tall kneeling on a padded surface. Tall kneeling requires co-contraction of the quadriceps and gluteus maximus to maintain stability. The abdominal muscles must contract to prevent excessive anterior pelvic tilt; they are stimulated when the weight line falls behind the hips. After transfemoral amputation, tall kneeling is achieved by straddling a bolster or by end-bearing on a height-adjusted padded surface. Maintaining tall kneeling can be made more difficult with visual tasks such as counting the men and women in the gym or reading a sign; upper-limb tasks such as folding laundry or using a tool; and activities that demand hand-eye coordination such as playing catch with a ball.

Proprioceptive Neuromuscular Facilitation

In general, the isometric, isotonic, and recumbent closed-chain exercises are performed in the straight planes. Because most functional activities occur diagonally, integrating the trunk into the movement of the extremities is important. Proprioceptive neuromuscular facilitation (PNF) uses diagonal movement with specific manual contacts to facilitate the retraining of coordinated movements.[40] Patterns can be used to facilitate anterior and posterior elevation and anterior and posterior depression of the pelvis once the patient can tolerate side-lying. Selecting the patterns to be practiced is based on the part of the gait cycle on which to focus (eg, anterior elevation to initiate swing phase). Pelvic patterns prepare the patient for coordinated pelvic and extremity movements in bed mobility and transfer training immediately after surgery and eventually, walking with a prosthesis.

Strengthening exercises should be progressed from simple to more demanding. For example, quadriceps and gluteus maximus co-contraction can be presented first as a separate isometrics exercise, then isotonic exercise, from open- to closed-chain, from lying to upright, from non-weight bearing to weight bearing. Similarly, lateral weight shifts might start with iliotibial band stretching, isometric exercise, to isotonic hip abduction, isolated leg to abdominals, and movement in straight frontal and sagittal planes to diagonal motion. If tolerated, strengthening exercises are best performed while wearing the prosthesis. This adds resistance and helps develop the proprioceptive sense of the prosthesis.

PATIENT AS A WHOLE PERSON

Concurrent with attention to the amputated limb, the rehabilitation team should address the care of the patient as a whole person, with emphasis on promoting psychosocial adjustment, protecting the intact limb from trauma, and fostering functional mobility. Commonly, patients undergoing amputation have comorbidities including hypertension, cardiac disease, and vascular surgery prior to the amputation, such as endarterectomy, angioplasty, and bypass graft, leaving the patient debilitated. People with diabetes may have retinopathy, nephropathy, and hypertension.[50] Older people are more susceptible to the complications of bed rest, such as pneumonia, pressure sores, urinary tract infection, as well as embolism, myocardial infarct, and cerebrovascular accident.

Facilitating the patient's emotional adjustment to limb loss is inherent throughout the rehabilitation process, beginning with the patient's first contact with the rehabilitation team. Chapter 6 addresses key psychosocial issues confronting the patient and family.

The patient's economic circumstances have to be taken into account when developing a rehabilitation plan. For example, if there are insurance limitations on the number of therapy sessions, it may be wise to ration them in the postoperative period so that some reimbursement remains for prosthetic training. Additionally, if the number of prostheses is limited, devices that provide the most long-term benefit should be prescribed.

Foot Care

To minimize the risk of contralateral amputation, especially for those with diabetes, regular foot hygiene with fastidious skin drying can help avoid skin maceration and infection. The toe nails should be trimmed by a nurse or podiatrist. The agile patient can inspect the plantar surface of the foot with a hand mirror; otherwise, a family member or a foot clinic must become involved. A wound can also be detected if the patient wears white socks, which would show any drainage stain. Routine screening with a 10-g monofilament applied to the mid dorsum and on the plantar surface at the heel, medial and lateral aspects of the mid foot, and beneath the first, third, and fifth metatarsal heads will indicate tactile acuity or its lack. Vibration perception threshold is correlated with vulnerability to amputation in those unable to detect vibration having a 14:5 odds ratio.[51]

Visual and tactile inspection of the shoe interior before donning can help the patient avoid injury caused by debris in the shoe. The upper portion of the shoe should have a sufficiently high toe box to accommodate any toe deformity and be of supple material. Whenever standing or walking, the patient should wear a sock and shoe to prevent minor trauma such as splinters and stubbed toes. The insole should be of a material and design that distributes weight-bearing forces over a broad area, especially over boney or callused areas. The insole should be replaced regularly whenever the cushioning compresses.

Functional Mobility

Once wound healing has begun, the patient should be guided to regain the ability to turn in bed, transfer from bed to chair, manage a wheelchair, and for most people, to achieve nonprosthetic ambulation. Even the person who is not a candidate for a prosthesis should be able to move to reduce the lifting burden that caregivers would otherwise have to provide. Those who will be fitted with a prosthesis also need to develop skill in maneuvering without a prosthesis upon rising in the morning and retiring in the evening, as well as when the prosthesis is being serviced. Functional independence can make the difference between living in an institution or in one's own home. Bed mobility, transfers, and sitting balance should be achieved by the second postoperative week.

Bed mobility is the first step in regaining functional mobility, so the patient can use a bed pan, dress, bathe, and relieve pressure on sensitive tissues. Rolling onto the amputated limb may be uncomfortable immediately after surgery; rolling to the sound side may also be difficult because of the loss of the leverage of the amputated side. Rolling may be accomplished first in the easier direction for the patient, but moving in both directions should be mastered during the initial postoperative phase. Proprioceptive neuromuscular facilitation of trunk movements, using momentum generated by the three intact limbs and the use of bed rails can make rolling easier. Caution must be taken to avoid striking the amputated limb on the bed rails or other hard surfaces.

General Conditioning

Getting out of bed is expected of virtually all patients, regardless of ambulatory status. If orthostatic hypotension is evident, long sitting followed by transferring to a chair will provide the opportunity to develop tolerance for the upright position. If sitting is not tolerated initially, the health care staff should tilt the bed gradually, or use a reclining wheelchair or a tilt table to help the patient acclimate to the erect posture. Ankle pumps and seated stepping prior to standing can facilitate venous return and thus minimize orthostasis. Upright sitting assists swallowing, decreasing the chance of aspiration pneumonia.

Transfers from one surface to another can be facilitated through the use of momentum, anterior trunk weight shift, use of furniture and assistive equipment, and assistance provided by a caregiver. The stand-pivot is a common technique. Performed with or without assistance, the patient comes to standing on the sound foot, pivots on that foot to face away from the new surface, then slowly sits. Caution must be exercised, because pivoting on the sound foot creates shear force under the metatarsal heads, which is potentially damaging. Thus the patient should wear a shoe. The patient can reduce weight on the sound foot by pushing with the hands on the arms of the chair or on an assistive device, and taking several small hops to turn the body. The person with bilateral lower-limb amputation can use a sliding board or position the front of the wheelchair flush against the bed, then turn 180 degrees when transferring to and from the wheelchair.

Transfers to and from the wheelchair, bedside chair, commode or toilet, and to and from standing should all be mastered during the initial stage of rehabilitation. Transfer skill is a critical element of functional ability, which may indicate the person's suitability for prosthetic use.[52]

Nearly all people with amputations use a wheelchair during rehabilitation, and many rely on a wheelchair for primary or auxiliary transportation permanently. Wheelchair use allows the patient to travel beyond the confines of the hospital room for social interaction and treatment in the physical therapy department. Early mobilization helps the person avoid the physical complications of prolonged bed rest and the psychosocial consequences of lack of acceptance of the amputation, depression, and withdrawal from interpersonal exchanges all of which are negatively associated with prosthetic use.[52,53] Once the patient is independent in safe wheelchair use, greater distances and faster speeds can be encouraged to develop upper-limb strength and cardiopulmonary endurance. Wheelchair use should include travel on ramps and irregular terrain.

Several features of wheelchair design pertain to people with amputations. Reclining backrests suit those who have difficulty tolerating prolonged upright posture. Antitip bars should be used to prevent backward tipping if the hospital or home environment includes ramps. The patient's center of gravity is higher than normal, particularly with bilateral transfemoral amputations. The rear uprights should be set posteriorly to accommodate the altered position of the center of gravity when the individual is seated. An elevating leg rest, residual limb board, or a specialized leg rest can support the transtibial amputated limb in knee extension to prevent flexion contracture. These devices must be high enough to prevent the knee from flexing when the patient is seated in a resting position. The person with unilateral amputation should have swing-out leg rests to support the sound limb thereby preventing dependent edema and undue gravitational pull on the amputated limb. The swinging feature facilitates transfers. Leg and foot rests are unnecessary for people with bilateral amputations who are not wearing prostheses. The wheelchair seat should have a 3- to 4-inch thick foam plastic or rubber cushion to prevent decubitus ulceration of the buttocks. The individual who is insensate or will spend most of the day in the wheelchair should have a pressure-relieving cushion. Patients with marked upper-limb weakness, severe arthritis, or high amputation benefit from a powered wheelchair.

One-legged ambulation with a walker or a pair of crutches is practical, even for those who will receive a prosthesis. Such walking is more convenient for trips to the bathroom at night as well as maneuvering around the bedroom as the person gets dressed. Such ambulation should be limited, as excessive stress on the sound limb in the presence of peripheral vascular disease is risky. The patient should always wear a shoe on the sound foot whenever walking.

EMOTIONAL ADJUSTMENT

Psychological adaptation is a key priority during the postoperative period because it powerfully affects patient compliance and can determine adaptation to the amputation and the prosthesis. Adaptation and pre-prosthetic training may be the most powerful determinants of outdoor active use of the prosthesis and together with pulmonary condition and amputation level accounted for a third of the variance that explained the amount of weekly prosthetic use.[53] The patient who has just had an amputation will need to grieve and find an inner motivating drive to rehabilitate. Motivation may be even more important than amputation level as the determinant of successful outcome. Once the therapist has developed the patient's trust and has started to help the person adjust to the new state, physical rehabilitation goals follow more easily.

The person who has had recent amputation may resist seeing or touching the amputated limb, avoid visits with family and friends, and not want to discuss prosthetic fitting. The rehabilitation team should empathize with the person's distress and provide opportunities to speak about the amputation. The behavior of the staff is a powerful factor in the patient's response, with calm acceptance of the altered appearance of the limb and the initial difficulties the patient experiences. Introducing the new patient to someone who has completed rehabilitation and providing educational materials can help the patient and family realize that amputation does not preclude a satisfying life. The Amputee Coalition of America (www.amputee-coalition.org) is a good source for support and educational materials. Chapter 6 provides substantial insight into understanding the individual's emotional reactions.

READINESS FOR PROSTHETIC FITTING

The physical status of the amputated limb, the patient's overall health, as well as the person's emotional behavior, determine suitability for prosthetic fitting. The ability to extend the hip or knee of the amputated limb to within 15 degrees of full extension is desirable for fitting and optimal prosthetic function. Although contractures can be accommodated, the socket is bulkier and is likely to impose gait compensations. Hip extension and abduction strength in both limbs, and bilateral knee extension strength in transtibial amputation, are major determinants of prosthetic gait and function.[6,54] Ability to perform recumbent amputated limb exercises for these muscle groups may indicate whether the person has sufficient strength for prosthetic use.

The patient with severe cardiopulmonary disease, although not a candidate for a prosthetic ambulation, may benefit from prosthetic fitting to facilitate transfers. In any event, the individual should be taught bed mobility, transfers, wheelchair maneuvering, and as much self-care as tolerated. A prosthesis for cosmetic purposes may be appropriate. Other physical disorders, such as cerebrovascular accident, arthritis, and blindness, do not preclude prosthetic fitting, but do influence prosthetic components and rehabilitation.

In addition to physical status, psychosocial factors such as motivation, cognition, and adaptation to the amputation have a major impact on later prosthetic function. Assuming reasonable physical health, the person who wants to walk with a prosthesis and understands the degree of personal effort involved in the rehabilitation process is ready to be referred to a prosthetist. A highly motivated individual is likely to progress further than an unmotivated person regardless of physical factors. Cognition is essential for prosthetic use, because much education is needed for the use and care of the prosthesis and amputated limb.

Age, one-legged balance, and short-term memory (as measured with a 15-word recall test) explained 64% of the variance on an activities of daily living disability scale.[51] Duration of preprosthetic care is a strong determinant of community ambulation.[52]

Case Study

A 65-year-old accountant with impending right transtibial amputation secondary to diabetic complications of arteriosclerosis, was evaluated preoperatively for immediate postoperative prosthesis use. His sound ankle was deformed secondary to Charcot neuropathic ankle, and both feet were insensate. He weighed 275 pounds. He had full passive excursion of both lower limbs and good manual dexterity. Muscle power was within normal limits, although he complained of early fatigue. The skin on the right lower leg was scarred from two attempts at vascular reconstruction. He and his wife live in a single-family house with four steps between the sidewalk and the front door. Both of them rejected placement in a skilled nursing facility. The patient was cognitively intact. Prior to the onset of arteriosclerosis he engaged in leisure walking in the park near his home several times a week.

The surgeon initially decided not to prescribe an immediate postoperative prosthesis, doubting that this patient could limit weight bearing to 25 pounds until suture removal endangering wound healing.

Surgery involved midtibial amputation with myodesis. Recovery was uneventful, except that when his Foley catheter was removed he was unable to urinate sitting but could do so standing in a walker assisted by two people. The rehabilitation team decided to fit him with an Aircast Air-Limb immediate postoperative prosthesis (Aircast, Summit, NJ). The risk of damage to the surgical site was balanced with the risk of falling while standing to urinate and ascending the steps into his home. He had 4 days of inpatient physical therapy to learn to use the Air-Limb.

Two weeks later he was fully independent with the Air-Limb and a walker. He attempted to limit his weight bearing on the prosthesis; however, it was evident that he was placing more than the recommended amount of weight on the amputated side, because he had a 1-cm abrasion on his amputated limb over the anterodistal tibia. Treated with gel padding, the abrasion healed within 10 days. At 6 weeks postoperatively, he was fitted with a definitive prosthesis using a gel liner with pin suspension and a dynamic response foot. He made a fast and easy transition to the new prosthesis and ambulated in the community at various cadences with a cane.

Discussion: Although not initially considered a candidate for any type of early ambulation, the patient's personal circumstances and environmental factors warranted taking a risk with the hope that he would obtain improved function. The risks of early ambulation were explained to the patient before obtaining his consent to fit the immediate postoperative prosthesis. Pivotal to the decision was his willingness and ability to follow instructions.

Criteria for readiness for prosthetic fitting include: 1) stable medical status, 2) healing incision with no open areas larger than 1 cm, 3) ability to stand on the intact leg, 4) adequate extensor strength, and 5) adequate short-term memory.

TEAM APPROACH

There is general agreement in the rehabilitation community that prosthetic patients are best served by a multidisciplinary team approach. This allows for the development of a unified treatment plan with each professional adding their expertise. This approach works best when the entire team can be brought together in a clinic setting. However, outside of an in-patient rehabilitation hospital, care can be fragmented especially if the patient moves from a hospital to nursing facility and then to their home during the postoperative period. If no one team member takes responsibility for following the patient, care can be delayed and problems can go untreated. A new system for following patients from amputation and throughout rehabilitation is available to insure quality and continuity of care.

The Empower SMART program (Standardised Multi-disciplinary Amputee Rehabilitation and Training [Empower-Health Care Solutions AB, Växjö, Sweden]) is a quality assurance program for the rehabilitation of new amputees. It follows ISO standards and national regulations for health and welfare in Denmark, Germany, Japan, Norway Sweden, the United Kingdom, and the United States. The program includes process management, standardized procedures for the whole rehabilitation process from preoperative considerations, patient information, amputation, acute therapy, wound care, compression therapy, physiotherapy, prosthetic fitting, and follow up. All members of the team use the same program, with synchronized checklists for documentation, online registration for communication and measurable outcomes to record indicators for improvement of clinical pathways.[54]

The Web-based SMART Online also includes a PDA applications for mobile documentation. This application makes it possible for the team to share vital information and improve efficiency during amputee rehabilitation. The PDA application enables a multidisciplinary team of practitioners to access and update patient information at any location and any time.

Empower SMART Advantages

The Empower SMART program improves the quality of care and clinical outcomes through a validated system of protocols, communication, and documentation.[55] By tracking measurable goals and a joint nonconformity reporting system, users can continuously improve the rehabilitation process. Proven benefits of the program are: increased numbers of amputees becoming walkers, increase in more distal amputations (transtibial vs transfemoral), decreased number of days from amputation to delivery of first definitive prosthesis, decrease in length of stay in both acute and rehab hospitals, as well as reduction of total rehabilitation cost.[56]

Financial Disclosure: John Rheinstein, CP is co-inventor of the Aircast Air-Limb™.

REFERENCES

1. Smith DG, McFarland LV, Sangeorzan BJ, Reiber GE, Czerniecki JM. Postoperative dressing and management strategies for transtibial amputations: a critical review. *J Rehabil Res Dev*. 2003;40:213-224.

2. Pollack CV, Kerstein MD. Prevention of post-operative complications in the lower-limb amputee. *J Cardiovasc Surg (Torino)*. 1985;26:287-290.

3. Knetsche RP, Leopold SS, Brage ME. Inpatient management of lower extremity amputations. *Foot Ankle Clin*. 2001;6:229-241.

4. Eneroth M. Factors affecting wound healing after major amputation for vascular disease: a review. *Prosthet Orthot Int*. 1999;23:195-208.

5. Choudhury SR, Reiber GE, Pecoraro JA, Czerniecki JM, Smith DG, Sangeorzan BJ. Postoperative management of transtibial amputations in VA hospitals. *J Rehabil Res Dev*. 2001;38:293-298.

6. Malone, JM et al. Immediate, early, and late postsurgical management of upper-limb amputation. *J Rehabil Res*. 1984;21:33-41.

7. May BJ. Postsurgical management. In: May BJ, ed. *Amputations and Prosthetics: A Case Study Approach*. 2nd ed. Philadelphia, Pa: FA Davis; 2002:74-108.

8. Menzies H, Newham J. Semirigid dressings: the best for lower extremity amputees. *Physiother Canada*. 1978;30:225-228.

9. Mueller MJ. Comparison of removable rigid dressings and elastic bandages in preprosthetic management of patients with below-knee amputations. *Phys Ther*. 1982;62:1438-1441.

10. Isherwood PA, Robertson JC, Rossi A. Pressure measurements beneath below-knee amputation stump bandages: elastic bandaging, the Puddifoot dressing and a pneumatic bandaging technique compared. *Br J Surg*. 1975;62:982-986.

11. Mooney V, Harvey JP Jr, McBride E, Snelson R. Comparison of postoperative stump management: plaster vs. soft dressings. *J Bone Joint Surg Am*. 1971;53:241-249.

12. Kane TJ III, Pollack EW. The rigid versus soft postoperative dressing controversy: a controlled study in vascular below-knee amputees. *Am J Surg*. 1980;189:244-247.

13. Little CE, Kirby RL, Conner M. Spandex shorts to assist stump shrinkage in lower-limb amputees: a pilot study. *Physiother Canada*. 1997;49:126-128.

14. Manella KJ. Comparing the effectiveness of elastic bandages and shrinker socks for lower extremity amputees. *Phys Ther*. 1981;61:334-337.

15. Ghiulamila R. Semirigid dressing for postoperative fitting of below-knee prosthesis. *Arch Phys Med Rehabil*. 1972;53:186-190.

16. MacLean N, Fick GH. The effect of semirigid dressings on below-knee amputations. *Phys Ther*. 1994;74:668-673.

17. Sterescu LE. Semirigid (Unna) dressing for amputation. *Arch Phys Med Rehabil*. 1974;55:433-434.

18. Fish S. Semirigid dressing for stump shrinking. *Phys Ther*. 1976;56:1376.

19. Wong CK, Edelstein JE. Unna and elastic postoperative dressings: comparison of their effects on function of adults with amputation and vascular disease. *Arch Phys Med Rehabil*. 2000;81:1191-1198.

20. Bonner FJ Jr, Green RF. Pneumatic Airleg prosthesis: report of 200 cases. *Arch Phys Med Rehabil*. 1982;63:383-385.

21. Kerstein MD. Utilization of an air splint after below-knee amputation. *Am J Phys Med*. 1974;53:119-126.

22. Sher MH. The air splint: an alternative to the immediate postoperative prosthesis. *Arch Surg*. 1974;108:746-747.

23. Ham R, Richardson P, Sweet A. A new look at the Vessa PPAM aid. *Physiotherapy*. 1989;75:494-495.

24. Lein S. How are physiotherapists using the Vessa pneumatic post-amputation mobility aid? *Physiotherapy*. 1992;78:318-322.

25. Redhead RG, Davis BC, Robinson KP, Vitali M. Post-amputation pneumatic walking aid. *Br J Surg*. 1978;65:611-612.

26. Rausch RW, Khalili AA. Air splint in preprosthetic rehabilitation lower extremity amputated limbs: a clinical report. *Phys Ther*. 1985;65:912-914.

27. Burgess EM, Romano RL. The management of lower extremity amputees using immediate postsurgical prostheses. *Clin Orthop*. 1968;57:137-146.

28. Sarmiento A, May BJ, Sinclair WF. Immediate postoperative fitting of below-knee amputations. *Phys Ther*. 1970;50:10-18.

29. Baker WH, Barnes RW, Shurr DG. The healing of below-knee amputations: a comparison of soft and plaster dressings. *Am J Surg*. 1977;133:716-718.

30. Schon LC, Short KW, Soupiou O, Noll K, Rheinstein J. Benefits of early prosthetic management of transtibial amputees: a prospective clinical study of a prefabricated prosthesis. *Foot Ankle Int*. 2002;23:509-514.

31. Cummings V. Immediate rigid dressing for amputees: advantages and misconceptions. *NY State J Med*. 1974;74:980-983.

32. Woodburn KR, Sockalingham S, Gilmore H, et al. A randomised trial of rigid stump dressing following transtibial amputation for peripheral arterial insufficiency. *Prosthet Orthot Int*. 2004;28:22-27.

33. Cohen SI, Goldman LD, Salzman EW, Glotzer DJ. The deleterious effect of immediate postoperative prosthesis in below-knee amputation for ischemic disease. *Surgery*. 1974;76:992-1001.

34. Wu Y, Keagy RD, Krick HJ, Stratgios JS, Betts HB. An innovative removable rigid dressing technique to below-the-knee amputation. *J Prosthet Orthot*. 1979;61:724-729.

35. Cutson TM, Bongiorni D, Michael JW, et al. Early management of elderly dysvascular below-knee amputees. *J Prosthet Orthot*. 1994;6:62-66.

36. McArdle WD, Katch FI, Katch VL. *Exercise Physiology*. Philadelphia, Pa: Lea & Febiger; 1991.

37. Isakov E, Burger H, Gregoric M, Marincek C. Isokinetic and isometric strength of the thigh muscles in below-knee amputees. *Clin Biomech*. 1996;11:233-235.

38. McNair PJ, Marshall RN, Maguire K. Swelling of the knee joint: effects of exercise on quadriceps muscle strength. *Arch Phys Med Rehabil*. 1996;77:896-899.

39. Wong CK, Wade CK. Reducing iliotibial band contractures in patients with muscular dystrophy using custom dry flotation cushions. *Arch Phys Med Rehabil*. 1995;76:695-700.

40. Hall C, Brody LT. *Therapeutic Exercise: Moving Toward Function*. Philadelphia, Pa: Lippincott; 1999.

41. Sale DG. Neural adaptation to resistance training. *Med Sci Sports Exerc*. 1988;20:S135-S145.

42. Colby LA, Kisner C. *Therapeutic Exercise: Foundations and Techniques*. 4th ed. Philadelphia, Pa: FA Davis; 2002.

43. Carpinelli RN, Otto RM. Strength training: single versus multiple sets. *Sports Med*. 1998;26:73-84.

44. Berger RA. Effect of varied weight-training programs on strength. *Res Q*. 1962;33:168-181.

45. Gailey RS, Clark CR. Physical therapy. In: Smith DG, Michael JW, Bowker JH, eds. *Atlas of Prosthetics: Surgical, Prosthetic, and Rehabilitation Principles*. 3rd ed. Rosemont, Ill: American Academy of Orthopaedic Surgeons; 2004: 589-620.

46. Nadollek H, Brauer S, Isles R. Outcomes after trans-tibial amputation: the relationship between quiet stance ability, strength of the hip abductor muscles and gait. *Physiother Res Int*. 2002;7:203-214.

47. Perry J. *Gait Analysis: Normal and Pathological Function*. Thorofare, NJ: SLACK Incorporated; 1992.

48. Isakov E, Keren O, Benjuya N. Transtibial amputee gait: time-distance parameters and EMG activity. *Prosthet Orthot Int*. 2000;24:216-220.

49. Powers CM, Boyd LA, Fontaine CA Perry J. The influence of lower-extremity muscle force on gait characteristics in individuals with below-knee amputations secondary to vascular disease. *Phys Ther*. 1996;76:369-377.

50. Hamalainen H, Ronnemaa T, Halonen JP, Toikka T. Factors predicting lower extremity amputations in patients with type 1 or type 2 diabetes mellitus: a population-based 7-year follow-up study. *J Intern Med*. 1999;246:97-103.

51. Schoppen T, Boonstra A, Groothoff JW, de Vries J, Goeken LN, Eisma WH. Physical, mental, and social predictors of functional outcome in unilateral lower-limb amputees. *Arch Phys Med Rehabil*. 2003;84:803-811.

52. Gauthier-Gagnon C, Grise MC, Potvin D. Enabling factors related to prosthetic use by people with transtibial and transfemoral amputation. *Arch Phys Med Rehabil*. 1999;80:706-713.

53. Gauthier-Gagnon C. Predisposing factors related to prosthetic use by people with a transtibial and transfemoral amputation. *J Prosthet Orthot*. 2000;10:99-109

54. Löwenadler CM. Evidenced based practice with a multidisciplinary approach. *AAOP Journal of Proceedings*. 2005.

55. Larsson G-U, Johannesson A. Lower Extremity: A Controlled Active Protocol. 25th Academy Annual Meeting And Scientific Symposium, Hyatt Regency, New Orleans, LA, March 3-6, 1999.

56. Johannesson A, Larsson G-U, Öberg T. From major amputation to prosthetic outcome: a prospective study of 190 patients in a defined population. *Prosthet Orthot Inter*. 2004;28:9-21.

Chapter 4

Pain Management

Marisol A. Hanley, PhD; Dawn M. Ehde, PhD; Douglas G. Smith, MD

OBJECTIVES

1. Compare models of pain
2. List the components of pain
3. Distinguish among phantom limb sensation, phantom limb pain, residual limb pain, and back pain, indicating their relative prevalence
4. Explore the etiology of amputation-related pain, as well as other sources of pain
5. Specify the impact of pain on overall function and quality of life
6. Discuss the risk factors for chronic pain
7. Describe the clinical assessment of pain
8. Survey treatments of amputation-related pain

INTRODUCTION

Individuals with acquired amputations must adjust to a major life change, as well as cope with pain. Although almost all people experience some pain immediately after amputation, pain becomes an unwanted, chronic companion for many. Living with chronic pain can impact all facets of life, including one's mood, relationships, activity level, and general well-being. However, individuals can empower themselves to overcome, rather than be overcome, by pain following limb loss.

Research on pain following limb loss, especially phantom limb pain, has increased sharply in the past two decades. The purpose of this chapter is to provide a summary of current knowledge regarding the nature, scope, and treatment of pain in those with limb loss. First, a brief discussion of several relevant conceptual issues is presented, followed by a summary of the research literature concerning specific types of pain after acquired amputation. In this review, the etiology of pain, risk factors for development of chronic pain, and aspects of pain assessment will be discussed. The last section of the chapter focuses on treatment for pain

associated with amputation, both pharmacologic and rehabilitative approaches, highlighting the most important points for clinicians to know and communicate to their patients.

MODELS OF PAIN

Chronic vs Acute Pain

Distinguishing between acute and chronic pain is essential for determining appropriate intervention strategies. Acute pain may be defined as pain elicited by the activation of nociceptive transducers at the site of local tissue damage due to injury, surgical procedures, or disease.[1] By definition, acute pain is experienced for a limited time immediately following damage, and remits as the underlying pathology resolves.[2] In contrast, chronic pain can be defined as recurrent or persistent pain that is present for 6 months or longer.[1] Chronic pain may begin as acute pain with an obvious cause, or it may have a more insidious and unknown onset. Chronic pain may persist beyond expected healing time, and there may be no remaining detectable

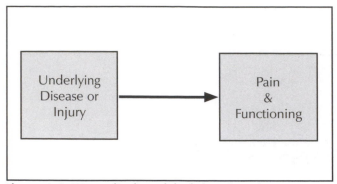

Figure 4-1. Biomedical model of chronic pain.

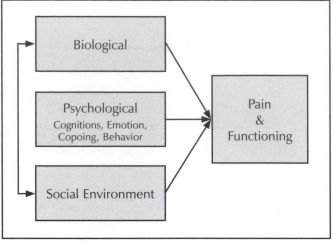

Figure 4-2. Biopsychosocial model of chronic pain.

damage, therefore, chronic pain differs from acute pain both in time duration and pathology. There are at least three subtypes of chronic pain. An ongoing disease process, such as chronic pancreatitis or cancer, may directly cause chronic pain. Alternatively, changes in or injury to the central or peripheral nervous system may be responsible for persistent chronic pain even after superficial healing has taken place, as in phantom limb pain. Lastly, there are some chronic pain conditions for which the underlying pathophysiology is undetectable or cannot fully explain the symptoms of pain or level of disability, such as chronic back pain or fibromyalgia. Some types of pain in individuals with limb loss may fall into this last category.

Biomedical Model of Pain

The traditional *biomedical model* (Figure 4-1) is rooted in the perspective of mind-body dualism, in which symptoms are viewed as either organic or psychogenic in origin despite no empirical evidence for this dichotomy. Pain is viewed as a sensory experience dependent on the degree of noxious stimuli impinging on a person; in other words, if one hurts, there must be a corresponding degree of harm or damage. In this model, diagnosis is accomplished through objective tests, and treatment focuses on correcting the organic dysfunction. The biomedical model has long been criticized for failing to recognize the influence of psychosocial variables and their interactions with the pathophysiology of chronic pain.[2-4] This model also lacks explanatory power for chronic pain states in which no organic cause can be identified. For example, early researchers on phantom pain assumed that physiological explanations were impossible because the amputated limb was gone. Phantom pain was once viewed as a manifestation of either mental-emotional or personality problems, which we now know to be untrue.[5] In the past, such assumptions may have led patients to underreport pain to their physicians due to fears of being thought to have psychological problems.[6]

Gate Control and Biopsychosocial Models

The *gate control theory* of pain was an influential development that radically changed the way researchers and clinicians thought about pain.[7,8] This theory proposed the existence of neurophysiologic gating mechanisms in the brain and spinal cord that could be excited or inhibited ("opened" or "closed") by a variety of influences, including motivational-affective, cognitive-evaluative, and sensory-physiologic components, thus suggesting a physiologic basis for the influence of psychological factors on pain perception. Subsequent physiological research based on this model has demonstrated that psychological variables can indeed modulate pain perception.[9,10] The gate control theory emphasized that there is not necessarily a one-to-one relationship between organic pathology and pain symptoms, and that pain is not an exclusively physiologic experience.

The *biopsychosocial model* (Figure 4-2) is often considered an extension of the gate control theory, and emphasizes the complex, dynamic interactions among biological, psychological, and social variables that can influence pain and a person's response to that pain.[4,11,12] Biopsychosocial models of pain acknowledge the essential role of biological factors, but also emphasize a role for psychosocial variables in determining pain expression and functioning, regardless of the source of pain or the presence or absence of psychopathology. Biopsychosocial models are appropriate for understanding the diversity often seen in expressions of and responses to chronic pain because of the inherent dynamic feedback among physical and psychological variables that is likely to occur over time.[12] Moreover, such models have shown a superior ability over more simple biologic models in predicting pain and behavioral responses to chronic pain.[4] Biopsychosocial mod-

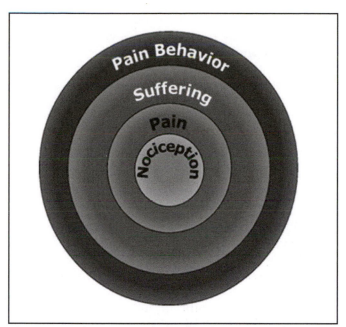

Figure 4-3. The separate but related concepts of nociception, pain, suffering, and pain behavior.

els of chronic pain propose that social environmental factors (eg, responses of significant others to pain behaviors),[13] cognitions (eg, pain-related beliefs),[14] and coping behaviors[15] may all influence aspects of the pain experience, including pain-related disability, distress, and health care utilization.[14,16]

COMPONENTS OF PAIN

The pain experience can be conceptualized as consisting of four separate components, illustrated in Figure 4-3. *Nociception* refers to the afferent pain signal from the site of damage to the central nervous system, specifically the activation of A delta and C fiber axons from the area of noxious stimuli. Nociception typically leads to *pain*, which refers to the sensation experienced by the individual once the nociceptive signal is processed. As suggested by gate control and biopsychosocial models, the perception of pain involves a perpetual integration and modulation of a number of efferent and afferent processes, influenced by one's level of conscious awareness and by processes of selective abstraction, appraisal, ascribing meaning, and learning. Pain often leads to *suffering*, which refers to the affective or emotional responses produced in the brain in response to pain, such as fear, anxiety, irritation, and occupational or interpersonal distress or disruption. The degree of suffering is influenced by one's interpretation of the pain and appraisal of its negative impact on functioning. Lastly, *pain behavior* refers to any visible behaviors that communicate to an observer (whether intentionally or not) that an individual is experiencing pain. Examples

of these include such diverse behaviors as grimacing, holding or rubbing the painful body part, guarding the painful part, resting, talking about pain, and asking for medication.[13,17,18]

These four components form separate but related parts of the pain experience, which may not necessarily be experienced at the same time. There is a great deal of individual and situational variation in the way pain is manifested. For example, an athlete with an injury during a crucial point in the game may have nociception from the site of damage, but may not experience pain, suffering, or pain behavior until he realizes he is injured after the game is over. In contrast, an individual with phantom limb pain may experience considerable pain and suffering without any active nociception. Because pain and suffering are separate components of the pain experience, individuals with chronic pain may take steps to reduce their suffering via the use of adaptive coping techniques, such as relaxation exercises and distraction techniques.

Pain is often conceptualized and assessed as a unidimensional construct. Individuals may be asked to rate their pain on a numerical scale (eg, 0 to 10, 0 to 100) ranging, for example, from no pain to the worst pain imaginable. Although important, these rating scales assess only pain intensity, or one's subjective rating of how much it hurts, which can be thought of as the "volume" of pain. Pain specialists now recognize the importance of other dimensions of pain as well, including pain duration, frequency of pain episodes, and pain-related disability. Frequency and duration of pain episodes are especially relevant for phantom limb pain due to its commonly episodic nature. These dimensions will be described in the review that follows.

TYPES AND PREVALENCE OF PAIN AND SENSATIONS

Several types of pain and sensations may be present in individuals with amputations. To illustrate the multidimensional nature of pain in this population, the case studies on the following page present two cases of individuals with multiple pain problems.

Nonpainful Phantom Limb Sensations

In addition to the various types of pain experienced by individuals with limb loss, *nonpainful phantom limb sensations* (NPLS), defined as sensations in the missing (phantom) limb that are not painful, may also be present. Prevalence estimates suggest that the large majority of persons with limb loss experience NPLS.[19-23] Common feelings include the sensation that a missing foot is wrapped in cotton or that a missing limb is actually present. These sensations may include such feelings as touch, pressure, temperature, itch, posture,

Case Studies

Grant is a 36-year-old man with a transhumeral amputation due to a motor vehicle collision 4 years previously. He is married with two young children, and his elderly parents live next door. He works full-time and uses a functional prosthesis mainly for household chores. He has intense phantom limb pain episodes a few times per week, more often at night, typically reaching levels of 7 to 8 on a 0 to 10 scale; this pain interferes with his sleep. Grant has noticed that these episodes are worse following arguments with his wife or parents. He also feels pain and tightness in his back and neck, also worse at the end of the day. He often becomes moody and irritable when in pain and worries about snapping at his children. Grant has tried many over-the-counter painkillers, which do not work well for him.

Anne is a 67-year-old woman who underwent a transtibial amputation 3 months previously due to peripheral vascular disease. Her husband is deceased, and she lives alone, although she has frequent visits from her children and grandchildren. She is experiencing moderate, intermittent residual limb and phantom limb pain, which have interfered with her prosthesis training. She has been reluctant to ambulate on her own with her prosthesis due to fear of bringing on pain episodes, as well as fear of falling. She is also worried by the sensation that her phantom limb is growing shorter. Although her activity level was not high before the amputation, she has almost ceased going out to visit friends or to do errands.

or location in space.[24,25] Sensations may also involve feelings of movement in the phantom limb, such as the sensation that the distal part of the phantom limb is moving progressively closer to the residual limb, referred to as "telescoping."[26] Although by definition, these sensations are not perceived as painful, there has been no research, to our knowledge, regarding what impact, if any, NPLS may have on the lives and functioning of individuals who experience them.

Phantom Limb Pain

Phantom limb pain (PLP), one of the most frequently discussed consequences of amputation, is defined as painful sensations perceived in the missing portion of the amputated limb.[25] Although early research suggested the incidence of PLP was low, we now know that the majority of persons with amputations experience PLP. At least 60%,[27] but possibly as many as 85%,[19,28,29] of individuals with amputation report PLP, which may persist for many years after amputation.[23,30] No differences in phantom pain have been found in relation to age, site or level of amputation, or presence of a previ-

ous amputation.[31,32] In addition, phantom pain has been found to be equally present in persons with traumatic and vascular amputations.[28,30] The majority of studies have found that PLP is most often intermittent and episodic in nature, with only a few individuals reporting constant pain.[21,29,32] Based on a synthesis of their research, Sherman et al[5] suggest that continuous pain may be an intensified version of nonpainful sensations, whereas intermittent pain may have other origins.

Conclusions regarding prevalence and characteristics of PLP are influenced by the way PLP is defined and measured. For instance, studies that ask participants to report "any PLP" may include data from persons for whom PLP is occasionally present, but not particularly problematic. Therefore, it is important to determine the extent to which reported pain is bothersome and disabling. Recent research suggests that PLP is present but not highly disabling for the majority, but may be troublesome for a significant subset of persons with amputation. For example, 23% of a community-dwelling sample of persons with lower-limb amputation (N=255) reported that PLP was significantly disabling and moderately to severely limited their functioning.[19] Pezzin and colleagues[33] found that 22% of persons with limb loss secondary to trauma reported severe PLP in the past month, with severe defined as being "extremely" or "very" bothered by this pain.

The onset of PLP typically occurs during the first week after amputation[20,34], and patients who do not develop early PLP are less likely to develop PLP in the future.[35] There are some conflicting findings regarding the usual course of PLP, possibly due to population and methodological differences.[36] Some studies have found that PLP diminishes or disappears during the first 2 years postamputation,[20,34] whereas others have found that PLP persists over periods of years or decades.[30,37] It cannot be assumed that PLP will diminish over time; therefore, it should be assessed periodically even if the amputation occurred many years before.

Episodes of PLP may last from a few seconds to weeks, but most commonly are reported in terms of minutes or hours. Using a prospective daily diary method, a British study of 89 adults with amputations found that 84% of the sample reported pain on each of the 7 study days, and 16% reported PLP on 3 to 5 days of the study period. Regarding frequency of episodes, 71% reported more than one episode of PLP per day, and of these, 75% reported experiencing 4 to 5 episodes per day. Regarding duration of episodes, 80% experienced PLP for 6 to 10 hours each day, with only 11% reporting an average of 12 or more hours of PLP each day.[38]

Average pain intensity in this same diary study was found to vary across the 7-day study period from 3 to 8 on a 0 to 10 numerical rating scale (NRS) (mean=4.5, standard deviation [SD]=4.6).[38] Average pain intensity in a large, cross-sectional survey study was reported to be somewhat higher (mean=5.6 on a 0 to 10 NRS, SD=3.9).[6,30] A more recent survey study (N=255) found a similar level of average pain intensity (5.1, SD=2.6).[19] Although there is variability across studies, average pain intensity at this level (5 to 6 on a 0 to 10 NRS) is generally classified as moderate.[39]

Descriptors of PLP vary, but painful phantom sensations are commonly reported as shooting, burning, stabbing, boring, squeezing, and throbbing.[27] In other studies, they have been described as squeezing, burning, knifelike, and throbbing,[20] as well as sharp, tingling, shooting, and stabbing.[19] Phantom limb pain occurs most frequently in the hand or foot and is often most intense in these areas.[5] Both the sensory and motor cortices of the brain are organized with areas corresponding to each part of the body. The amount of cortex dedicated to each body part is not proportional to the size of the body part, but rather, is determined by the sensitivity and complexity of movement required by that body part. Therefore, the thigh has a small representation compared to the large representation of the hand. This may, in part, explain why more intense and vivid sensations and pain are perceived in a phantom hand or foot, compared to a knee or elbow.

Most of the research has been conducted on samples comprised mostly or completely of individuals with lower-limb amputations. Upper-limb amputation is less common, and prevalence data for upper PLP are harder to find. Two recent community survey studies have found rates of PLP of 41% (N=99)[40] and 51% (N=72)[21] in samples of persons with upper-limb loss. The latter study also found that 48% of those with pain experienced it on a daily basis, and the presence of phantom sensations was associated with a greater relative risk of PLP. In a clinic sample (N=76) of adults with upper-limb amputation, 69% reported PLP.[41]

Residual Limb Pain

Residual limb pain (RLP) refers to pain in the portion of the amputated limb that is physically present. Acute RLP is a natural consequence of amputation; optimally, acute RLP will remit with healing of the wound. Unfortunately, RLP becomes chronic for some people. Prevalence rates vary from 13% to 71% of persons with limb loss[22]; this wide variation is most likely due to differences in study populations (clinic vs community) and methodology (study design, definition of RLP). Because such discrepancies hamper conclusions about RLP, longitudinal epidemiologic studies that clearly define RLP are needed to clarify the issue.

Similar to PLP, several studies have found RLP to be intermittent and episodic in nature.[5,19,23,42] For example, Gallagher and colleagues[42] found that of the 48% of their sample (N=104) who reported RLP, 13% experienced an episode of RLP once or twice in the week preceding the survey, 63% experienced an episode more

than twice, and 13% experienced constant RLP. Similar to PLP, several studies suggest that RLP is typically in the range of mild to moderate intensity, although a significant subset of individuals (15% to 35% across different studies) report RLP in the severe range (7 to 10 on a 0 to 10 scale).[19,23,33] Several studies suggest that RLP can interfere significantly with functioning.[42,43] Of the persons reporting RLP in the survey study by Gallagher et al, almost 40% reported that RLP interfered "moderately" to "a lot" with activities, compared to 17% who reported the same level of interference from PLP.

In one of the few studies to examine pain in those with upper-limb amputation, Kooijiman and colleagues[21] found that 48.6% of their sample of Dutch adults reported chronic RLP. Another study found that 55% of a sample of persons with upper-limb amputation (N=76) reported current RLP, with 75% of those with RLP describing their pain as intermittent and 25% as continuous.[41]

Back Pain

Recent research suggests that back pain may be fairly common in persons with lower-limb amputations, and may contribute to pain-related impairment and function.[43] Ehde and colleagues[19] found that 52% of a community sample of persons with lower-limb amputations (N=255) reported back pain, a rate much higher than the prevalence of chronic back pain in the general population (estimated point prevalence of 15% to 25%).[44] Smith and colleagues[23] found a 71% rate of back pain in a sample of persons with lower-limb loss (N=92). In addition, back pain was rated as more bothersome than other types of pain. Persons with transfemoral amputations rated back pain as more frequent and intense than those with transtibial amputations. A study of individuals with unilateral transfemoral amputations due to nonvascular causes found that 47% of the sample (N=97) reported back pain.[45] In these studies, however, it is not known if back pain was a premorbid condition or developed as a consequence of limb loss. Although the cause may often be unclear, back pain appears to be a fairly common, yet often overlooked, issue for individuals with limb loss. It may be reduced with gait training or other rehabilitative interventions, although these possibilities have not yet been empirically examined. Individuals with upper-limb amputations may also experience back and neck pain, due in some cases to biomechanical factors such as shoulder hiking and positional scoliosis.

Youth With Amputation

There is relatively little research regarding the prevalence of pain and NPLS in youth with amputations. Although a review article in 1993 suggested that children and adolescents with limb loss or limb deficiency may not experience chronic PLP,[46] this conclusion may have been premature given the lack of empirical tests of this assumption at that time. More recent research suggests that chronic PLP may be as prevalent in youth with acquired amputations as in adults.[47,48] Wilkins and colleagues[49] found that the majority (70%) of youth with surgical amputations reported phantom limb sensations and roughly half (49%) reported PLP, whereas relatively few youth with congenital limb deficiency experienced phantom limb sensations (7%) or PLP (4%). Similarly, the majority (70%) of youth in the surgical group reported residual limb pain, compared to 33% of youth in the congenital group.[49]

ETIOLOGY OF AMPUTATION-RELATED PAIN

Central and Peripheral Mechanisms of Phantom Limb Pain

The presence of a perceived phantom limb (whether painful or not) for the majority of individuals with limb loss suggests the existence of innate neural networks in the brain able to generate all of the qualities of experience believed to originate in the body. Melzack[26] has proposed the concept of the neuromatrix, a neural network widely extending throughout selective areas of the entire brain, including the somatic, visual, and limbic systems. The output pattern from the hypothesized neuromatrix may account for the sensory, affective, and cognitive dimensions of pain experience and behavior.[50] According to this theory, input from the body is not necessary for the perception of sensation to occur, as demonstrated by PLP.[26]

Both central and peripheral neural mechanisms are thought to contribute to the development of PLP.[51] Although central abnormalities may be more important for the maintenance of chronic PLP, the initiating event in the development of PLP is probably peripheral. One hypothesis is that the massive barrage of noxious afferent stimuli during injury or amputation may initiate central processes that later generate pain. Alternately, the sudden loss of peripheral input may trigger central changes that result in deafferentiation pain. Possible central processes include spinal sensitization and cortical reorganization. Spinal cord sensitization refers to the sensitization of dorsal horn neurons in the spinal cord after amputation, possibly as a result of the loss of high threshold input to the dorsal horn neurons.[22,52] This sensitization may result in spontaneous neuronal activity and increased sensitivity to afferent input.[51] Cortical reorganization occurs when the topographic representation of the lost limb after amputation is taken over by sensory input from other areas of the body, a process that illustrates the plasticity of the nervous system.[53] For example, the representation of the mouth or face in the motor and sensory areas of the cortex could shift into the zone formerly represented by the now amputated hand or arm.[54] The functional role of cortical reorganization is unknown, but one study found that greater cortical reorganization was associated with higher intensity PLP ($r=0.93$), suggesting that cortical reorganization may play a causal role.[55]

Peripheral mechanisms implicated in amputation-related pain include neural activity originating from afferent fibers in a neuroma and spontaneous activity in injured dorsal root ganglion neurons.[56] Persons with RLP are more likely to have PLP than persons who do not experience RLP,[6,31] suggesting that peripheral neuronal activity may help generate both types of pain.[57]

Other Sources of Pain

In addition to the mechanisms described above, there are other possible etiologies of pain and discomfort for persons with limb loss. Causes of RLP and other types of amputation-related pain are discussed briefly below; for a more detailed discussion, the reader is referred to a recent review.[58]

Neuromata

Amputation necessitates the transsection of a number of major nerves and countless smaller sensory and fine motor nerve branches. When a nerve is transsected, the axons within the nerve will attempt to regenerate and grow to eventually reinnervate the distal limb. In amputation, however, the axon will attempt to grow, but will instead form an intertwined mass of scar and nerve tissue, which is called an amputation *neuroma*. The free end of every divided nerve heals by forming a neuroma, but not every neuroma will cause pain. Some neuromata become painful in response to pressure, stretching, or other types of physical manipulation. Even when undisturbed, electrical potentials may arise within the neuroma, causing both local and distant sensory and motor phenomena. These sensations are sometimes experienced as bothersome and painful. Afferent activity originating from the neuroma may be one of the peripheral factors contributing to PLP. Clinical[59] and experimental[57] evidence indicates that percussion of a symptomatic neuroma can induce both RLP and PLP. However, central factors involved in PLP may become more important over time than activity in the periphery.[60]

Techniques to prevent or minimize neuroma formation have not proved highly successful and have not been associated with lower rates of symptomatic neuromata or PLP. As neuroma formation is inevitable, the generally accepted surgical technique during amputation remains to draw the large nerves distally, section them, and allow them to retract away from areas of pulsating vessels, pressure, and scarring. The surgeon's goal is to position the nerve ending in a well-cushioned soft tissue site where irritation from outside sources of contact and pressure will be minimized. In this way, neuromata might be prevented from causing pain. Knowledge of prosthetic designs and areas of contact and pressure will aid the surgeon in nerve placement.

Bone Spurs and Heterotopic Bone

The surgical technique of beveling can help avoid irregular or prominent areas of bone, but it does not prevent the formation of bone spurs and heterotopic bone. When bone is transsected, small slips of periosteum can ossify into spurs (also called spikes) of bone, causing areas of high pressure and pain when the weight bearing into the prosthetic socket pushes soft tissue into bone. In individuals with trauma and burns, the damaged muscle can also form areas of heterotopic bone. The irregular surface and edges of this bone can cause pressure and pain. Bone spurs and heterotopic bone can be diagnosed with plain radiographs. The first step of treatment is to make prosthetic modifications to minimize pressure on the area. If pain persists, surgical resection of the bone spur or heterotopic bone may be indicated.

Overuse Musculoskeletal Pain

This is a general term for pain resulting from the natural increases in stress and wear on anatomic structures due to limb loss. Even the most carefully constructed residual limb subjects the body to tremendous forces for which it was not designed, leading to overuse of certain joints and muscles that may become painful over time. Pain in the contralateral limb may be caused by overuse due to changes in gait pattern. One study found that severe joint pain in the contralateral limb was reported by 16.9% of a sample of persons with lower-limb loss due to trauma.[33] Similarly, pain in the back and neck may result from an unnatural gait or changes in posture, although these assumptions need to be empirically examined.

Prosthetic-Related Pain

In some cases, RLP can be minimized with a prosthetic socket designed to apply pressure in the areas that can tolerate it, while relieving and protecting more sensitive areas. An exact mold of the residual limb does not make a good socket. Instead, the skilled prosthetist modifies the limb model to increase tolerant regions' share of the load, thus relieving more sensitive areas. A poor fit can result in local pain, bruising, redness, blisters, or skin ulceration in the residual limb. The prosthetic socket should be checked periodically for changes in the location and distribution of forces caused by the changing shape of the residual limb due to factors such as normal maturation, muscle atrophy, and weight loss or gain.

IMPACT ON FUNCTIONING AND QUALITY OF LIFE

Chronic pain syndromes are frequently accompanied by changes in physical, emotional, social, and vocational functioning. Few studies have empirically examined the impact of pain on quality of life in individuals with amputation. As with other chronic pain conditions, research suggests that pain in this population may have serious consequences for health, functioning, and quality of life, even when pain is episodic. In a study of individuals with lower-limb amputation (N=437), van der Schans and colleagues[61] found that those who experienced PLP had a poorer quality of life compared to those who did not experience PLP. Other research has found that higher levels of pain in persons with limb loss are associated with higher overall disability (both physical and psychosocial).[62] However, a study of individuals with lower-limb loss and PLP found that 75% of the sample could be classified as having a low level of pain-related disability, demonstrating that many individuals with limb loss and pain function well despite their pain.[19]

The functional consequences of pain in individuals with limb loss can include interference in prosthetic training and walking ability[63] and reduced likelihood of employment and social activities.[34,64] Disability associated with severe PLP, as well as lesions in the residual limb, are associated with employment difficulties after amputation.[33]

Chronic pain can be associated with depression and psychological distress.[65] Compared to persons with limb loss who do not experience pain, those with pain are more likely to report depressive symptoms[66,67] and anxiety.[30] In addition, a longer duration of amputation-related pain has been associated with increased levels of psychological distress.[37] Consistent with a biopsychosocial model, increases in depression, stress, and anxiety are correlated with intensified PLP episodes.[68]

To summarize, pain can potentially contribute to problems in rehabilitation, employment, daily activities, and psychosocial functioning for individuals with limb loss, although we cannot assume that pain always leads to such problems, given that many individuals with limb loss and pain have low levels of suffering and disability. The research has tended to focus on lower-limb loss and PLP, although RLP and back pain have also been shown to significantly impact functioning. More research is needed to explore factors that distinguish individuals who function well despite pain and those who encounter difficulties.

RISK FACTORS FOR CHRONIC PAIN

Acute Pain

Acute pain has been suggested as a risk factor for chronic pain in several pain populations, including persons with PLP.[69] Given what we know about the etiology of PLP, it appears likely that acute surgical and post-amputation pain (PLP and RLP) could play a role in the development of chronic pain.[70] Effective post-amputation pain control could potentially reduce the risk of chronic PLP. However, these assumptions, to our knowledge, have not yet been tested empirically.

Preamputation Pain

According to current pain theories, long-term and/or intense preamputation pain may create a somatosensory pain memory in the brain that leaves an individual at risk for similar pain after amputation. Several studies have explored the relationship between preamputation pain and the development of PLP, producing complex and sometimes contradictory findings. As with other aspects of research on amputation-related pain, methodological variability may contribute to the differing findings, which preclude definite conclusions at this time. A prospective study by Nikolajsen and colleagues[35] of 56 patients undergoing lower-limb amputation found that intensity, rather than duration, of preamputation pain was predictive of PLP at 1 week and 3 months after amputation. In addition, preamputation pain increased the risk of RLP in the first week. Preamputation pain was not predictive, however, of either RLP or PLP at 6 months.[35] Similarly, in a prospective study of 58 patients (mainly participants with lower-limb loss), Jensen and colleagues[31] found that preamputation pain was related to PLP during the first 6 months after amputation, but was not predictive of persistent PLP at 2-year follow-up. PLP was more likely when the duration of preamputation pain was longer than 1 month.

In contrast, a cross-sectional survey study of British veterans (N=590) found no relationship between preamputation pain and PLP.[32] In general, a prospective study design, in which participants are assessed at multiple time points (eg, pre- and postamputation, follow-up), is a stronger research design than a cross-sectional retrospective study, which asks participants to recall events in the past. The two prospective studies described above[31,35] suggest that preamputation pain may be more strongly related to PLP in the short-term than in the long-term.

Psychosocial Factors

We now know a great deal about psychosocial risk factors for the development of chronic pain. Although PLP is clearly not the result of psychopathology, the recent emphasis on physiological mechanisms runs the risk of overlooking psychosocial factors that may play a role in exacerbating pain or decreasing adaptive functioning. The chronic pain literature has shown, for example, that people who believe they can control their pain, who believe they are not severely disabled, and who avoid negative thoughts about their condition function better than those who do not.[15] Social support[23,71] and personality factors can also play a role in adjustment to chronic pain.

Few studies have examined the role of psychosocial factors specifically in relation to chronic pain following limb loss. Similar to the more general chronic pain literature, this research has shown that pain catastrophizing (excessive negative and unrealistic thoughts about pain, such as "this pain is awful" or "I can't stand this") stands out as a significant risk factor. For example, Hill and colleagues[37,72] found strong associations between pain catastrophizing and measures of both pain severity and psychological distress in samples that included people with upper- and lower-limb amputation. A prospective, longitudinal study of 70 persons after lower-limb amputation found that pain catastrophizing was predictive of pain interference and depressive symptoms at 1 and 2 years after amputation. Social support was also associated with adjustment to amputation and PLP.[73]

Pain-Related Anxiety

Living with chronic pain syndromes can be associated with higher levels of stress and anxiety. Because both PLP and RLP may be experienced intermittently, individuals with limb loss and pain may experience anxiety related to their anticipation of the next pain episode. In our clinical experience, severe pain episodes, even if they occur infrequently, may increase overall levels of stress. In addition, some individuals, especially older people with lower-limb loss, experience a fear of falling that may serve to increase their general muscle tension.[74] Both the effects of stress over time and increased muscle tension may exacerbate the perception of pain.

CLINICAL ASSESSMENT OF PAIN

The first step in managing pain is to conduct a thorough and accurate assessment of pain, including biologic and psychosocial factors that are contributing to the experience of nociception, pain, suffering, and pain behavior. In recent years, there has been an increased recognition of the impact of pain on a person's life, and a call for pain and suffering not to be overlooked or ignored. The American Pain Society has created the phrase "Pain: the fifth vital sign" to increase awareness of the importance of routine pain assessment,[75] and the American Pain Foundation publishes the *Pain Care Bill of Rights* (Table 4-1).[76] The use of reliable and valid stan-

Table 4-1

PAIN CARE BILL OF RIGHTS

As a person with pain, you have:

- The right to have your pain taken seriously and to be treated with dignity and respect by doctors, nurses, pharmacists, and other health care professions.
- The right to have your pain thoroughly assessed and promptly treated.
- The right to be informed by your doctor about what may be causing your pain, possible treatments, and the benefits, risks, and costs of each.
- The right to participate actively in decisions about how to manage your pain.
- The right to have your pain reassessed regularly and your treatment adjusted if your pain has not been eased.
- The right to be referred to a pain specialist if your pain persists.
- The right to get clear and prompt answers to your questions, take time to make decisions, and refuse a particular type of treatment if you choose.

Adapted from American Pain Foundation. *Pain Action Guide*. Baltimore, Md: American Pain Foundation; 2001

dardized instruments is recommended. For more information on pain assessment, the reader is referred to the *Handbook of Pain Assessment* by Turk and Melzack.[18]

Pain Intensity

Standardized pain intensity rating scales provide patients and clinicians with a simple method to quantify pain intensity and track changes over time. One of the most widely used rating scales is the 0 to 10 NRS, where 0 refers to "no pain" and 10 refers to "pain as bad as it can be." Research has shown that the numbers on this scale are interpreted similarly across individuals and medical conditions. When pain intensity is classified based on its interference with daily functioning, pain in the 0 to 4 range is typically classified as "mild" pain, 5 to 6 as "moderate," and 7 to 10 as "severe."[39]

Because the impact of pain on an individual's life will depend on many factors, pain assessment extends beyond a simple rating of pain intensity. We recommend asking patients to distinguish between PLP, RLP, and any other types of pain they may have. Clinicians will want to assess the frequency and duration of pain episodes, as well as the type of sensations experienced, which may help to pinpoint the cause of pain. For example, pain from ambulating on a bone with minimal soft tissue covering may be described as throbbing or pulsating. Sherman[5] suggests that burning, tingling, or throbbing PLP may be associated with reduced blood flow to the residual limb, and cramping or squeezing PLP may be associated with increased muscle tension in the residual limb, whereas shocking or shooting PLP may have no identified physiological correlates. Individuals with limb loss are strongly encouraged to keep a home log of pain to identify factors (eg, prosthesis use, physical or mental stress, excretion, diet, or

changes in weather) associated with their pain.[5]

Standardized measures can be built into assessment procedures in most clinical settings and typically can be self-administered quickly and easily. Benefits include the ability to track patient progress over time and to make comparisons between different settings, populations, and interventions. We encourage clinicians to assess pain interference to provide a clearer picture of the impact of pain on daily activities and general functioning. An excellent standardized self-report measure of pain interference is the Pain Interference Scale of the Brief Pain Inventory,[77] which assesses the impact of pain on a variety of daily activities, including sleep, work, self-care, and recreational activities, as well as mood and relationships. This scale may serve as a valuable tool for examining the impact of pain on daily life.

Dimensions of functioning in persons with lower-limb amputations can be assessed with either of two well-known validated self-report measures: the Trinity Amputation and Prosthesis Experience Scales (TAPES)[78] and the Prosthesis Evaluation Questionnaire (PEQ).[79] The TAPES was designed to measure multiple dimensions of adjustment to amputation and lower-limb prostheses; items pertaining to pain assess the presence, frequency, duration, and intensity of PLP and RLP, as well as the extent to which pain interferes with daily life. The PEQ was developed to measure the prosthesis function and quality of life of persons with lower-limb amputations; the 12-item pain scale assesses the frequency, intensity, and bothersomeness of NPLS, PLP, RLP, and back pain.

A number of standardized, self-reported measures of pain, although not designed specifically for pain associated with limb loss, have been used successfully in many medical settings and may enable comparisons with other pain populations. For example, the Graded Chronic Pain Scale (GCPS)[80] is a simple, reliable, and valid measure that can provide information about several dimensions of pain, including a classification, or "grade," of an individual's level of pain-related disability. The GCPS has been used with diverse pain populations, including at least one sample with limb loss.[19]

Medical Assessment

Thorough medical examination is especially important for identification of musculoskeletal issues, problems with the residual limb, and vascular issues that may contribute to pain. Many of these problems, once identified, may be resolved or improved. The proximal neurologic system is the easiest to overlook when examining a person with limb loss. Medical examination should explore for neurologic signs and symptoms that indicate radicular pain from the neck or low back, as well as nerve compression etiologies. A change in the severity of PLP in a person with upper-limb loss may suggest cervical stenosis, disc herniation, or thoracic outlet syndrome. Likewise, PLP or other bothersome sensations in an amputated foot may suggest lumbar disc herniation or spinal stenosis. The physical examination is complicated by the fact that certain usual clues, such as focal changes in motor units or changes in sensation in the hand or foot, may not be relevant for an individual with limb loss. In addition, traditional nerve traction tests, such as the straight leg test to examine for sciatic nerve irritation, are more difficult to perform and interpret in individuals with limb loss.

Mechanical or local pain can be explored with physical examination of the amputation site itself. Neuromata, bone spurs, heterotopic bone, local nerve compression, muscle compression, and muscle herniation are all possible direct local etiologies of pain. Neuromata can often be diagnosed when pain is reproduced by deep palpation of a nodule or when Tinel's phenomenon is experienced (tingling or distinct reproduction of electrical pain with tapping over the end of the nerve). Imaging studies, particularly magnetic resonance imaging (MRI), may assist with diagnosis of neuromata, although not every neuroma revealed by MRI is symptomatic. Correlation between the imaging study and the pain location is necessary to confirm that the pain is caused by an entrapped, scarred, or irritated nerve end. The prosthetic socket may contribute to nerve irritation, which may remain symptomatic for some time even after modification of the socket.

Mechanical pain from bone spurs or heterotopic bone can be suspected from crepitance of the tissue as it is moved over the end of the irregular bone surface, or compressed onto a bone spur. Radiological findings of irregular bone may support these findings, although irregular bone formation near the amputation site is common and may be asymptomatic. Again, correlation with the physical examination is needed prior to intervention. Often the first intervention is a modification of the prosthesis to remove pressure or transfer load from that area. Surgical excision should be considered only when nonoperative treatment has failed, and both the physical examination and the imaging study confirm the presence of bone spurs or heterotopic bone as the cause of pain.

Peripheral vascular disease may be considered as a cause of claudication or rest pain when the patient reports that the pain ceases immediately upon stopping walking or removal of the prosthesis. Examination of the proximal pulses, texture, and temperature of the amputated limb must be conducted. Occasionally, the prosthetic socket or suspension system can induce venous congestion or arterial occlusion in static or dynamic use of the device. If the pain began after a change to a new type of socket or suspension system, one must consider this etiology. Individuals with transtibial amputations may experience popliteal compression only when sitting, and may find that the pain is relieved with standing, removal of the device, or even simple release of a distal locking mechanism.

Prosthetic Assessment

Prosthetic assessment includes gait assessment and examination of the prosthetic socket and suspension system. Pain specific to one area may suggest regions of the socket or suspension system causing undue pressure or irritation at the anatomic site. Common areas of pain due to excessive pressure include the crest of the tibia and the fibular head.[81] The thorough clinician should consider how the device contacts the body at rest, sitting, and in dynamic situations of use. A device that appears to be causing no local pressure at rest can be observed to piston and cause repeated irritation of a particular region while in use. For example, an upper-limb prosthesis can change contact areas and loading when used to carry a weight or when involved in a specific position or activity.

Assessment for pain complaints should include an observation of limb length and the alignment of the pelvis while the patient stands. Improper prosthetic length can cause gait deviations that may be improved with adjustment of the device.[82] Gait assessment should include observation of symmetry, balance, proportion of time in stance and swing phase on each limb, and deviations of the trunk, hips, knees, and feet. In persons with transfemoral amputations, insufficient socket flexion may result in excessive lordosis during ambulation to compensate for this imbalance. Clinical experience suggests that chronic gait deviations may cause or aggravate back pain, although this assumption has not been empirically tested.

Table 4-2

PHQ-9: Measure

Over the last 2 weeks, how often have you been bothered by any of the following problems?

	Not at all	Several days	More than half the days	Nearly every day
A. Little interest or pleasure in doing things	☐	☐	☐	☐
B. Feeling down, depressed, or hopeless	☐	☐	☐	☐
C. Trouble falling or staying asleep, or sleeping too much	☐	☐	☐	☐
D. Feeling tired or having little energy	☐	☐	☐	☐
E. Poor appetite or overeating	☐	☐	☐	☐
F. Feeling bad about yourself—or that you are a failure or have let yourself or your family down	☐	☐	☐	☐
G. Trouble concentrating on things, such as reading the newspaper or watching television	☐	☐	☐	☐
H. Moving or speaking so slowly that other people could have noticed? Or the opposite—being so fidgety or restless that you have been moving around a lot more than usual	☐	☐	☐	☐
I. Thoughts that you would be better off dead or of hurting yourself in some way	☐	☐	☐	☐

Adapted from Kroenke K, Spitzer RL, Williams JB. The PHQ-9: validity of a brief depression severity measure. *J Gen Intern Med*. 2001;16:606-613.

Assessment of Psychological Distress

Depression is more common in persons with chronic pain than in the general population (point prevalence of 3% to 9%)[83] or in primary care populations (point prevalence of 10% to 15%).[84] The point prevalence for depression in persons with acquired amputation appears to be somewhere between 25% and 35%.[85] Major depressive disorder (MDD) is a psychological disorder characterized by depressed mood, lack of interest or pleasure in usual activities, changes in sleep and appetite, psychomotor retardation or agitation, loss of energy or concentration, feelings of hopelessness and worthlessness, and thoughts of suicide or death.[83] Some of these symptoms must be present nearly every day for 2 weeks to meet criteria for MDD. However, individuals may experience other mood disorders or subclinical levels of depression, anxiety, or psychosocial stress.

Because depressive symptoms are easily missed in medical settings, depressive symptoms should be routinely screened for and evaluated by clinicians working with persons with limb loss. Standardized screening measures are available and effectively used in medical settings. We particularly recommend the Patient Health Questionnaire-9 (PHQ-9),[86] a brief depression screening scale. The PHQ-9 is a reliable and valid index of depressive symptoms, and can also be used to diagnose MDD. In addition, the PHQ-9 can be quickly and easily self-administered. The PHQ-9, including scoring instructions appears in Table 4-2.

TREATMENT OF AMPUTATION-RELATED PAIN

Some individuals with amputation and pain may not receive treatment for their pain; at this time, we can only speculate about possible reasons. For some, pain may not be bothersome enough to warrant seeking treatment. We must also consider issues of access to treatment involving financial and geographic factors. In addition, some people with PLP may be reluctant to discuss their pain with their physicians or may encounter barriers to accessing treatment for PLP.[30] For instance, among 149 British veterans with amputations who discussed their PLP with their physicians, 49 (33%) reported being told there was no treatment to help their pain, and only 17 (11%) respondents were referred to a pain clinic.[32] Similarly, a study of American veterans (N=2694) found that 54% of the sample had discussed PLP with their physicians but only 19% were offered treatment.[6] Patients may not discuss PLP and sensations with their physicians due to worries about impacting the patient-doctor relationship or being thought "insane."[6,30] Some individuals with limb loss report that physicians have either stated directly or implied that their PLP was "just in their heads."[5] In addition, some health care providers may not be fully aware of the prevalence of pain in individuals with limb loss, or may be reluctant to discuss the issue if they believe they have little to offer in terms of effective treatment.

Limitations of Treatments

Various treatments for PLP have been reported, but few effective treatments have been identified.[5,87,88] One review noted the existence of more than 60 different treatment strategies, including medical, psychological, surgical, and alternative medicine options, but observed that the success rates for these treatments in general have rarely exceeded the expected placebo response rate of 25% to 30%.[5] Additionally, methodological concerns, such as small sample sizes, lack of controls, lack of blinding, heterogeneous populations, and short follow-up periods, have hampered drawing strong conclusions regarding the efficacy of many treatments currently in use. For example, one review of PLP treatment found some support for the efficacy of several types of medication (anticonvulsants, tricyclic antidepressants, and neuroleptics), as well as for spinal cord stimulation and transcutaneous electrical nerve stimulation (TENS), but as the authors noted, most of the literature they reviewed consisted of case reports or small, uncontrolled studies.[29] One exception was a randomized, controlled trial of TENS as a treatment for PLP, which found TENS to be ineffective in reducing chronic PLP.[89]

The bulk of the literature has tended to focus exclusively on PLP, or has failed to distinguish between PLP and RLP, making firm conclusions regarding the management of RLP difficult. Phantom limb pain and RPL should be carefully differentiated; RLP may be more responsive to treatment if a specific cause can be identified.[90]

When patients display many pain behaviors and high levels of distress and suffering, clinicians may feel pressure to fix the pain problem quickly. However, treatment may not result in long-term pain eradication or even consistent reduction. The key term in this case is *management* of pain. A highly important goal of patient education is to help individuals switch their model of pain from a biomedical perspective to a biopsychosocial one. Individuals may benefit from learning that, although there may be no cure for chronic pain, they may be able to reduce their pain intensity and/or suffering by learning techniques to manage chronic pain. Pain management requires that individuals learn to be active self-managers, which requires skills such as effective communication and collaboration with health care providers.[91]

Preventive Approaches

As discussed above, central sensitization of dorsal horn neurons of the spinal cord around the time of amputation is thought to contribute to the development of PLP.[24,27,55,92,93] This theory has prompted research into novel approaches aimed at preventing the development of chronic PLP. Several studies have examined the use of perioperative epidural anesthesia for the purpose of reducing the massive afferent discharge entering the central nervous system from the periphery as a result of preamputation pathology, the amputation itself, and the immediate postoperative process.[94-98] The results of efforts to prevent central sensitization have been mixed. One study supported this approach for preventing PLP,[95] whereas others studies have not been able to demonstrate any long-term prophylactic effects.[94,96-98] Because these investigations vary greatly in terms of methodology, sample size, anesthesia techniques, and amputation etiologies, more research is needed before making any definite conclusions regarding the efficacy of preventive approaches.[70]

Although we do not yet fully understand the mechanisms involved in the development of chronic PLP, severe acute pain may result in central representations of pain that persist independently after healing.[69] Katz[70] suggests that traditional postoperative pain control is sometimes inadequate because pain is treated only after it is well entrenched. The use of preemptive analgesics or local anesthetics before the start of surgery is recommended both to increase patient comfort and reduce noxious afferent input that may contribute to central sensitization. During the postoperative period, patients may benefit from patient controlled analgesia (PCA), in which patients are able to self-administer, as needed, doses of a narcotic analgesic within the limits of a set dosing schedule. Use of PCA may also help individuals to have a greater sense of control and to reduce their anxiety about pain relief, setting the stage for smoother rehabilitation and adjustment to limb loss. It is important to develop a plan for tapering off the narcotic analgesic, thus achieving a balance between providing effective short-term pain relief and preventing negative consequences of long-term narcotic use.

Reversal of Cortical Reorganization

Some researchers have focused on establishing a functional link between cortical reorganization and PLP. Several studies have tested interventions for reversing the cortical reorganization that may have occurred around the time of amputation. In one study, six patients with PLP underwent anesthesia of the amputation limb by brachial plexus blockade. The three patients who experienced PLP relief during this procedure showed substantial reduction in cortical reorganization, whereas the three patients who did not experience PLP relief did not have concurrent reductions in cortical reorganization.[99] Similarly, Flor and colleagues[54,100] have attempted to reduce chronic PLP by providing feedback (sensory discrimination training) to brain areas altered by somatosensory pain memories. Individuals with upper-limb amputations and PLP participated in 10 sessions of feedback-guided sensory training in which their task was to discriminate the frequency or location of high intensity nonpainful electric stimuli applied to the amputation limb. Pre- to post-treatment changes in cortical reorganization, measured by neuroelectric source imaging, and in pain intensity ratings were compared to a control group who received usual medical treatment. The group treated with sensory discrimination training had significant reductions in PLP and cortical reorganization compared to the control group. This promising line of research merits confirmation with additional trials.

Ramachandran and colleagues have reported preliminary success with a treatment for severely painful involuntary clenching spasms in phantom arms and hands based on visual illusion. The treatment involves placement of a midvertical sagittal mirror in front of the individual, so that the person sees the reflection of the intact limb optically superimposed on the felt location of the phantom limb, resulting in the optical illusion that the phantom limb is now present. In one study, six of 10 patients claimed they could feel movements emerging from the phantom limb based on the visual feedback from the intact limb viewed in the mirror. Four of these patients reported being able to "unclench" the phantom hand and relieve the spasms, and one patient reported a permanent and complete disappearance of the painful phantom arm after repeated use of the mirror for 2 weeks.[93,101] If these preliminary results could be consistently replicated, this technique could be a noninvasive option for individuals with similar sensations. More research concerning the central and peripheral processes of the nervous system will hopefully lead to new interventions for PLP that are more consistently effective than any treatment attempts thus far.

Pharmacological Treatment

Tricyclic Antidepressants

Although tricyclic antidepressants (TCAs) have long been used to treat PLP, trials evaluating the efficacy of TCAs for PLP have been nonexistent until recently. One meta-analysis of 39 placebo controlled trials of antidepressants for chronic pain concluded that antidepressants were beneficial for a variety of types of chronic pain, however, pain after limb loss was not included in this meta-analysis.[102] The efficacy of TCAs in the treatment of painful peripheral neuropathies has been supported.[103] Given that amputation requires the severing of multiple peripheral nerves, it is plausible that TCAs may be helpful in treating amputation-related pain as well. To our knowledge, only one randomized controlled clinical trial examined the efficacy of TCAs for relieving chronic amputation-related pain. This study of adults (N=39) with either PLP or RLP compared the effects of amitriptyline to an active placebo (benztropine mesylate) and found no significant benefit for either type of pain.[104]

Anti-Seizure

Anti-seizure drugs are commonly used to combat neuropathic pain due to their effectiveness in calming excited nerves. They have been prescribed for PLP based, in part, on clinical impressions that they may minimize the number of episodes of PLP. Two recent double-blind, placebo-controlled, crossover studies of gabapentin for PLP have been completed. One of these studies (N=14 completers) found that gabapentin resulted in significantly greater pain intensity reduction compared with placebo after a 6-week trial.[105] In contrast, another study (N=24) did not find a significantly greater reduction in pain intensity during the gabapentin phase compared to the placebo phase. However, a greater proportion of patients reported a meaningful pain reduction during the gabapentin phase.[106] This research suggests that gabapentin might be effective for certain subgroups of patients, but more clinical trials are needed to explore the use of gabapentin.

Non-Narcotic Analgesics

The most commonly used medications for any type of chronic pain are non-narcotic analgesics. To our knowledge, there is no specific research on their efficacy for amputation-related pain, but they may serve as a starting point because they are unlikely to be hazardous to the patient.[22]

Narcotic Analgesics

Use of narcotic analgesics for the treatment of neuropathic pain remains controversial and has generated intensive debate regarding the role of opioids in the management of chronic neuropathic pain and the consequences of long-term use.[56] One study found that the majority of patients with chronic nonmalignant pain had concerns regarding physiological dependence on narcotics and the potential for abusing these medications.[107] Narcotics are very effective in the short-term, and are recommended during the immediate postoperative period. Effective control of acute pain may even reduce the risk of developing chronic pain. However, long-term use of narcotics can result in dependence and increasing tolerance to higher dosages, leading to poorer pain control and greater disability and depression over time.[22] In addition, narcotics are not likely to erase the pain, but only to calm reactions and make the pain seem less bothersome. Traditional narcotics have a fast onset and a high initial peak effect, but they wear off quickly and pain recurs. Common unpleasant side effects include constipation, sedation, and nausea.[108] In addition, narcotic use is associated with an array of safety risks, such as drowsiness, decreased reaction time, clouded judgment, and, in large doses, inhibited respiration that may make breathing difficult or impossible.

New, longer-acting narcotics (eg, OxyContin [Purdue Pharma LP, Stamford, Conn]) are designed to take effect more slowly and linger in a person's system for an extended time, avoiding a rapid peak and drop-off, and hopefully minimizing tolerance effects as well. However, misuse of these drugs is a risk, because their longer-acting structure can be easily altered by crushing the pills, potentially turning them into street drugs used for a powerful high.

In support of narcotics, however, a recent study found preliminary evidence that opioids may influence cortical reorganization in individuals whose cortical reorganization is not yet irreversibly chronic. This double-blind crossover trial (N=12) of oral retarded morphine sulphate (MST) for PLP found a significant pain reduction (50% decrease) in 42% of patients over the 4-week trial. In addition, this study found evidence of reduced cortical reorganization with MST in three patients, concurrent with reductions in pain intensity.[109] Although a promising line of research, larger clinical trials are needed that can also examine long-term consequences of narcotic use. For now, clinicians must balance the needs of the patient with the potential for harm over time. If drug intake increases or activity levels decrease, patients may need to be titrated off of narcotic medication.

Surgical Interventions

Surgical section of peripheral nerves or total spinal anesthesia have not been shown to relieve PLP, strengthening the conclusion that peripheral input is not the main cause of chronic PLP.[29] Surgical revision may be indicated for selected patients with RLP only when pain is clearly due to a pathological process in the residual limb, such as a bone spur, heterotopic bone, or symptomatic neuroma.[22] For example, neuroma resection may be warranted when symptoms can be attributed to mechanical pressure on the neuroma based on thorough physical examination consistent with imaging studies. Neuroma resection may result in symptomatic relief of RLP but is unlikely to affect PLP, a fact that should be clearly communicated to patients prior to surgery. Failure to obtain pain relief with neuroma resection indicates that this procedure should not be reattempted. Other procedures, such as rhizotomy, cordotomy, and dorsal column stimulation have not been supported,[22,110] and only limited early support has been found for dorsal root entry zone lesions.[110] In conclusion, none of the current surgical procedures has a high likelihood of success, and may be most appropriate for clearly defined problems in the residual limb.

Rehabilitation Interventions

Rehabilitation approaches are recommended for individuals with limb loss and pain, particularly for those with higher levels of pain interference. Early rehabilitation may even help reduce the likelihood of chronic severe pain. For instance, Pezzin and colleagues[33] found that higher intensity inpatient rehabilitation of persons with amputations was associated with lower levels of bodily pain at long-term follow-up, as well as increased physical functioning and vitality. The most accepted rehabilitation approach is multidisciplinary and is based on a biopsychosocial model of pain. Interventions address not only the pathophysiologic processes, but also the psychological, social, and behavioral factors associated with pain, distress, and pain-related disability. Modalities for rehabilitation therapies include physical therapy, occupational therapy, prosthetic intervention, vocational rehabilitation, and psychological approaches. For individuals with especially high levels of suffering and disability, referral to a multidisciplinary pain rehabilitation program is an option if such a program is available in the area. Such programs have strong empirical support for their effectiveness when chronic pain is the primary disability,[111] but have not been empirically tested for pain in individuals with limb loss.

Early rehabilitation goals include maintaining muscular strength and preventing contractures, both of which may decrease the likelihood of severe long-term pain. Contractures can develop as a result of inactivity (eg, prolonged sitting), muscle imbalance, fascial tightness, protective withdrawal reflex into hip and knee flexion, and loss of plantar stimulation in extension. After lower-limb amputation, it is important to maintain full mobility in the hips and knees. Overall, an exercise program that is begun early and maintained by the individual is ideal for maintaining strength and preventing pain. Patients can be encouraged to begin ambulating as early as possible with crutches or temporary prostheses.[74] Patient education should emphasize the importance of an ongoing exercise routine.

As described above, back pain can be a significant source of pain in persons with lower-limb loss that tends to be overlooked in the literature. Physical therapists, prosthetists, and other care providers should pay careful attention to gait patterns that may contribute to back pain. Although not yet examined in the literature, neck pain may be another possible consequence of deviations in posture or gait.

INTERVENTIONS FOR RESIDUAL LIMB PAIN

Early postoperative residual limb care is crucial for managing acute pain and possibly for preventing severe long-term pain.[90] Use of rigid postoperative dressings and aggressive edema control help manage acute RLP. In addition, these dressings may facilitate early prosthesis fitting and ambulation, which have also been associated with decreased risk of PLP.[29] Given that most hospital stays after amputation are brief, patients will require education about performing proper residual limb care independently.

Possible interventions for RLP include heat, icing, massaging the residual limb, and early use of a prosthesis.[90] Percussion or vibration of the residual limb has been sporadically reported as helpful for some patients.[22] Some individuals report that ultrasound of the residual limb is helpful, but, to our knowledge, there are no data in the literature regarding the use of ultrasound for RLP. Alleviating factors will vary among individuals and types of RLP, but patients can experiment with these simple physical methods, given that they are noninvasive and unlikely to have harmful effects. The most important targets for reducing prosthetic-related pain are alleviating poor socket fit, inappropriate suspension, excessive distal residual-limb weight bearing, and painful adductor roll in transfemoral amputations.[25]

Psychological and Behavioral Interventions

Individuals with pain may be at increased risk for depressive symptoms or anxiety, although one cannot assume that someone with pain will experience psychological distress. If a person meets criteria for a depressive disorder, the disorder may also be a target of treatment. Appropriate goals for psychological intervention can include reducing pain and suffering, targeting negative thoughts about pain, increasing use of proactive coping strategies (eg, problem solving, engaging in enjoyable activities, attending support groups), and decreasing fear or anxiety. Cognitive-behavioral interventions, for instance, typically consist of multiple components,[112] such as relaxation training, changing negative thoughts about pain and function, and increasing use of positive affirmations. People who more frequently catastrophize may be at greater risk for increases in pain and suffering over time.[37,72,73,113] Individual or group psychotherapy may help decrease negative thoughts and increase the frequency of reassuring, positive thoughts. Psychologists can also play a helpful role in providing consultation to other members of the rehabilitation team and assisting in developing behavior plans.

Complementary and Alternative Modalities

A growing number of individuals with pain or chronic health problems are exploring complementary and alternative modalities. One study found that 29% of rehabilitation patients in an outpatient clinic had used some form of alternative treatment in the past 12 months.[114] Most of these treatments have not yet been empirically tested in controlled studies and are discussed in the literature mostly in the context of case reports. For example, some recently published case reports for treatment of PLP include therapeutic touch,[115] hypnotic imagery,[116] and acupuncture.[117] To our knowledge, there are no published reports of magnet therapy for pain associated with amputation; however, a recent double-blind trial of magnet therapy for chronic low back pain found no significant effect.[118]

Although alternative treatments, for the most part, have not yet been proven more effective than placebo, some researchers have argued for more explicitly using the benefits of the placebo effect itself.[119] Alternative treatments may serve as an adjunct to more traditional medicine and may help increase an individual's sense of being an active self-manager. Patients should be discouraged from expecting miracle cures, and potential benefits should be weighed against the lack of empirical evidence and any potential harm that may result. The thorough clinician will want to assess for use of complementary and alternative treatments to be sure that none are contraindicated for a particular individual.

SUMMARY AND CONCLUSIONS

We revisit the two cases presented earlier to illustrate patient-centered, multidisciplinary approaches to pain management.

Case Studies

At his latest visit to the amputation clinic, Grant informs his physician of the extent and intensity of his pain, and mentions the link between pain and emotional stress. His physician refers him to the physical therapist and the rehabilitation psychologist on the team. Grant works with his physical therapist on stretching and strengthening exercises to help his back and neck pain. With his psychologist, he learns several techniques to prevent and cope with stress, including neutralizing negative thoughts that make his pain more difficult to deal with. He also becomes skilled at using a relaxation imagery technique based on memories of a camping trip. Grant's physician prescribes a narcotic analgesic as needed, which Grant uses infrequently when his pain episodes are most severe.

continued

Table 4-3

CHAPTER SUMMARY

Phantom Limb Pain (PLP)

- Common consequence after amputation with potential to become chronic
- Effective pain control before, during, and immediately after amputation may reduce the risk of chronic PLP
- Prevalence estimates: 60% to 85%
- Multiple causes are likely: central and peripheral neural mechanisms
- Not caused by psychiatric or personality disturbance, but may be exacerbated by stress
- Few effective, empirically validated treatments have been identified

Residual Limb Pain (RLP)

- Natural consequence after amputation
- Prophylactic postoperative pain control is recommended
- Ideally, will remit with wound healing, but may become chronic
- Prevalence estimates for chronic RLP vary greatly (13% to 71%)
- May be more responsive to treatment than PLP if a specific cause (eg, neuroma, heterotopic bone, prosthetic-related) can be identified

Pain Assessment

- Pain should be routinely assessed: "the fifth vital sign"[75]
- Distinguish among nonpainful sensations, RLP, PLP, and other pain
- Assess multiple components of pain: intensity, interference, frequency, duration, suffering, pain behaviors
- Other types of pain may be present (eg, back or neck pain)
- Assess posture, gait, pressures on the residual limb, and back and neck health

Chronic Pain Management

- Early prosthesis training: emphasize ambulation and return to functioning
- Chronic pain requires ongoing management; neither clinicians nor patients should expect a "cure"
- Balance maintenance of hope with realistic expectations
- Flexible, interdisciplinary, patient-centered approach is best
- Patient education is crucial
- Help patients switch to biopsychosocial model of pain
- Help patients become active self-managers

---

continued

Anne's physical therapist and prosthetist notice her difficulty ambulating with her new prosthesis and talk to Anne about her pain. During a subsequent meeting with Anne, the rehabilitation team members aim to help Anne find ways to increase her sense of control over her rehabilitation. Based on Anne's feedback, her prosthetist makes several adjustments to her prosthesis that increase her comfort. In addition, her physical therapist consults with the team psychologist, and together they create a behavior plan to decrease her fears of falling and of pain by gradually increasing her length of time ambulating independently. They also teach Anne to alternate moderate activity with scheduled rest periods without her prosthesis to help prevent more severe episodes of pain. Anne realizes that she feels better overall with a moderate level of activity.

Table 4-3 summarizes of important points for clinicians to know and communicate to their patients about pain in limb loss. Some pain immediately after amputation is inevitable while healing takes place, but can be well-controlled by attending to pain before it becomes intense. Great strides have been made over the past several decades in our ability to define and measure pain, although there is still much work to be done. At this time, we cannot eliminate or even reduce all types of pain. When pain becomes chronic, there may be no "cure," and therefore a pain management approach may be necessary. Given the amount of research on amputation and pain, researchers may soon develop more consistently effective interventions. The scientific and medical communities will continue to work cooperatively with individuals with limb loss and pain to improve their quality of life.

Acknowledgement: This work was partially supported by the grant "Management of Chronic Pain in Rehabilitation" (PO1 HD/NS33988) from the National Institute of Child Health and Human Development and the National Institute of Neurological Disorders and Stroke.

REFERENCES

1. IASP. International Association for the Study of Pain Task Force on Taxonomy. In: Merskey H, Bogduk N, eds. *Classification of Chronic Pain*. Seattle, Wash: IASP Press; 1994:209-214.

2. Bonica JJ. *The Management of Pain.* 2nd ed. Vol 2. Philadelphia, Pa: Lea & Febiger; 1990.

3. Engel GL. The need for a new medical model: a challenge for biomedicine. *Science.* 1977;196:129-136.

4. Novy DM, Nelson CV, Francis DJ, Turk DC. Perspectives of chronic pain: an evaluative comparison of restrictive and comprehensive models. *Psychol Bull.* 1995;118:238-247.

5. Sherman RA. *Phantom Pain.* New York, NY: Plenum Press; 1997.

6. Sherman RA, Sherman C. Prevalence and characteristics of chronic phantom limb pain among American veterans. Results of a trial survey. *Am J Phys Med.* 1983;62:227-238.

7. Melzack R, Wall PD. Pain mechanisms: a new theory. *Science.* 1965;150:971-979.

8. Melzack R, Wall PD. *The Challenge of Pain.* New York, NY: Basic Books; 1982.

9. Baum A, Gatchel RJ, Krantz D. *An Introduction to Health Psychology.* 3rd ed. New York, NY: McGraw-Hill; 1997.

10. Fordyce WE, Steger JC. Chronic pain. In: Pomerleau OF, Brady JP, eds. *Behavioral Medicine: Theory and Practice.* Baltimore, Md: Williams & Wilkins; 1979:125-153.

11. Loeser JD, Fordyce WE. Chronic pain. In: Carr JE, Dengerink HA, eds. *Behavioral Science in the Practice of Medicine.* New York, NY: Elsevier; 1983:331-345.

12. Turk DC, Flor H. Chronic pain: a biobehavioral perspective. In: Gatchel RJ, Turk DC, eds. *Psychosocial Factors in Pain: Critical Perspectives.* New York, NY: The Guilford Press; 1999:18-34.

13. Fordyce WE. *Behavioral Methods for Chronic Pain and Illness.* St Louis, Mo: Mosby Year Book Inc; 1976.

14. Jensen MP, Romano JM, Turner JA, Good AB, Wald LH. Patient beliefs predict patient functioning: further support for a cognitive-behavioral model of chronic pain. *Pain.* 1999;81:95-104.

15. Jensen MP, Turner JA, Romano JM, Karoly P. Coping with chronic pain: a critical review of the literature. *Pain.* 1991;47:249-283.

16. Jensen MP, Turner JA, Romano JM, Lawler BK. Relationship of pain-specific beliefs to chronic pain adjustment. *Pain.* 1994;57:301-309.

17. Loeser JD. What is chronic pain? *Theor Med.* 1991;12:213-225.

18. Turk DC, Melzack R, eds. *Handbook of Pain Assessment.* 2nd ed. New York, NY: Guilford Press; 2001.

19. Ehde DM, Czerniecki JM, Smith DG, et al. Chronic phantom sensations, phantom pain, residual limb pain, and other regional pain after lower limb amputation. *Arch Phys Med Rehabil.* 2000;81:1039-1044.

20. Jensen TS, Krebs B, Nielsen J, Rasmussen P. Phantom limb, phantom pain, and stump pain in amputees during the first 6 months following limb amputation. *Pain.* 1983;17:243-256.

21. Kooijman CM, Dijkstra PU, Geertzen JHB, Elzinga A, van der Schans CP. Phantom pain and phantom sensations in upper limb amputees: an epidemiological study. *Pain.* 2000;87:33-41.

22. Loeser JD. Pain after amputation: phantom limb and stump pain. In: Bonica JJ, ed. *The Management of Pain.* 2nd ed. Philadelphia, Pa: Lea & Febiger; 1990:244-256.

23. Smith DG, Ehde DM, Legro MW, Reiber GE, del Aguila M, Boone DA. Phantom limb, residual limb, and back pain after lower extremity amputations. *Clin Orthop.* 1999;361:29-38.

24. Melzack R. Phantom limbs. *Sci Am.* 1992;266:120-126.

25. Davis RW. Phantom sensation, phantom pain, and stump pain. *Arch Phys Med Rehabil.* 1993;74:79-91.

26. Melzack R. Phantom limbs and the concept of a neuromatrix. *Trends in Neurosciences.* 1990;13:88-92.

27. Nikolajsen L, Jensen TS. Phantom limb pain. *Br J Anaesth.* 2001;87:107-116.

28. Houghton AD, Nicholls G, Houghton AL, Saadah E, McColl L,. Phantom pain: natural history and association with rehabilitation. *Ann R Coll Surg Engl.* 1994;76:22-25.

29. Iacono RP, Linford J, Sandyk R. Pain management after lower extremity amputation. *Neurosurgery.* 1987;20:496-500.

30. Sherman RA, Sherman CJ, Parker L. Chronic phantom and stump pain among American veterans: results of a study. *Pain.* 1984;18:83-95.

31. Jensen TS, Krebs B, Nielsen J, Rasmussen P. Immediate and long-term phantom limb pain in amputees: incidence, clinical characteristics and relationship to pre-amputation pain. *Pain.* 1985;21:267-278.

32. Wartan SW, Hamann W, Wedley JR, McColl I. Phantom pain and sensation among British veteran amputees. *Br J Anaesth.* 1997;78:652-659.

33. Pezzin LE, Dillingham TR, MacKenzie EJ. Rehabilitation and the long-term outcomes of persons with trauma-related amputations. *Arch Phys Med Rehabil.* 2000;81:292-300.

34. Parkes CM. Factors determining the persistence of phantom pain in the amputee. *J Psychosom Res.* 1973;17:97-108.

35. Nikolajsen L, Ilkjaer S, Christensen JH, Kroner K, Jensen TS. Randomised trial of epidural bupivacaine and morphine in prevention of stump and phantom pain in lower-limb amputation. *Lancet.* 1997;350:1353-1357.

36. Hill A. Phantom limb pain: a review of the literature on attributes and potential mechanisms. *J Pain Symptom Manage.* 1999;17:125-142.

37. Hill A. The use of pain coping strategies by patients with phantom limb pain. *Pain.* 1993;55:347-353.

38. Whyte AS, Niven CA. Variation in phantom limb pain: results of a diary study. *J Pain Symptom Manage.* 2001;22:947-953.

39. Jensen MP, Smith DG, Ehde DM, Robinson LR. Pain site and the effects of amputation pain: further clarification of the meaning of mild, moderate, and severe pain. *Pain.* 2001;91:317-322.

40. Dijkstra PU, Geertzen JH, Stewart R, van der Schans CP. Phantom pain and risk factors: a multivariate analysis. *J Pain Symptom Manage.* 2002;24:578-585.

41. Fraser CM, Halligan PW, Robertson IH, Kirker SG. Characterising phantom limb phenomena in upper limb amputees. *Prosthet Orthot Int.* 2001;25:235-242.

42. Gallagher P, Allen D, Maclachlan M. Phantom limb pain and residual limb pain following lower limb amputation: a descriptive analysis. *Disabil Rehabil.* 2001;23:522-530.

43. Marshall HM, Jensen MP, Ehde DM, Campbell KM. Pain site and impairment in individuals with amputation pain. *Arch Phys Med Rehabil.* 2002;83:1116-1119.

44. Andersson GBJ, Pope MH, Frymoyer JW, Snook S. Epidemiology and cost. In: Pope MH et al, eds. *Occupational Low Back Pain: Assessment, Treatment, and Prevention.* St Louis, Mo: Mosby Year Book; 1990:95-113.

45. Hagberg K, Branemark R. Consequences of non-vascular trans-femoral amputation: a survey of quality of life, prosthetic use and problems. *Prosthet Orthot Int.* 2001;25:186-194.

46. Wesolowski JA, Lema MA. Phantom limb pain. *Reg Anesth.* 1993;18:121-127.

47. Katz J. Children do experience phantom limb pain. *Reg Anesth.* 1997;22:291-293.

48. Krane EJ, Heller LB. The prevalence of phantom sensations and pain in pediatric amputees. *J Pain Symptom Manage.* 1995;10:21-29.

49. Wilkins KL, McGrath PJ, Finley GA, Katz J. Phantom limb sensations and phantom limb pain in child and adolescent amputees. *Pain.*1998;78:7-12.

50. Melzack R. From the gate to the neuromatrix. *Pain.* 1999;(Suppl 6):S121-S126.

51. Nikolajsen L, Jensen TS. Phantom limb pain. *Current Reviews in Pain.* 2000;4:166-170.

52. Howe JF. Phantom limb pain—a re-afferentation syndrome. *Pain.* 1983;15:101-107.

53. Elbert T, Flor H, Birbaumer N, et al. Extensive reorganization of the somatosensory cortex in adult humans after nervous system injury. *Neuroreport.* 1994;5:2593-2597.

54. Flor H. The modification of cortical reorganization and chronic pain by sensory feedback. *Appl Psychophysiol Biofeedback.* 2002;27:215-227.

55. Flor H, Elbert T, Knecht S, et al. Phantom-limb pain as a perceptual correlate of cortical reorganization following arm amputation. *Nature.* 1995;357:482-484.

56. Wu CL, Tella P, Staats PS, et al. Analgesic effects of intravenous lidocaine and morphine on postamputation pain: a randomized double-blind, active placebo-controlled, crossover trial. *Anesthesiology.* 2002;96:841-848.

57. Nikolajsen L, Hansen CL, Nielsen J, et al. The effect of ketamine on phantom pain: a central neuropathic disorder maintained by peripheral input. *Pain.* 1996;67:69-77.

58. Czerniecki JM, Ehde DM. Chronic pain after lower extremity amputation. *Critical Reviews in Physical Medicine and Rehabilitation.* 2003;15:309-332.

59. Jensen TS, Nikolajsen L. Pre-emptive analgesia in postamputation pain: an update. *Prog Brain Res.* 2000;129:493-503.

60. Nikolajsen L, Ilkjaer S, Jensen TS. Relationship between mechanical sensitivity and postamputation pain: a prospective study. *Eur J Pain.* 2000;4:327-334.

61. van der Schans CP, Geertzen JH, Schoppen T, Dijkstra PU. Phantom pain and health-related quality of life in lower limb amputees. *J Pain Symptom Manage.* 2002;24:429-436.

62. Marshall M, Helmes E, Deathe AB. A comparison of psychosocial functioning and personality in amputee and chronic pain populations. *Clin J Pain.* 1992;8:351-357.

63. Carabelli RA, Kellerman WC. Phantom limb pain: relief by application of TENS to contralateral extremity. *Arch Phys Med Rehabil.* 1985;66:466-467.

64. Millstein S, Bain D, Hunter GA. A review of employment patterns of industrial amputees—factors influencing rehabilitation. *Prosthet Orthot Int.* 1985;9:69-78.

65. Rudy TE, Kerns RD, Turk DC. Chronic pain and depression: toward a cognitive-behavioral mediation model. *Pain.* 1988;35:129-140.

66. Lindesay JE. Multiple pain complaints in amputees. *J R Soc Med.* 1985;78:452-455.

67. Sherman RA, Sherman CJ, Bruno GM. Psychological factors influencing chronic phantom limb pain: an analysis of the literature. *Pain.* 1987;28:285-295.

68. Arena JG, Sherman RA, Bruno GM, Smith JD. The relationship between situational stress and phantom limb pain: cross-lagged correlational data from six month pain logs. *J Psychosom Res.* 1990;34:71-77.

69. Dworkin RH. Which individuals with acute pain are most likely to develop a chronic pain syndrome? *Pain Forum.* 1997;6:127-136.

70. Katz J. Phantom limb pain. *Lancet.* 1997;350:1338-1339.

71. Goldberg GM, Kerns RD, Rosenberg R. Pain-relevant support as a buffer from depression among chronic pain patients low in instrumental activity. *Clin J Pain.* 1993;9:34-40.

72. Hill A, Niven CA, Knussen C. The role of coping in adjustment to phantom limb pain. *Pain.* 1995;62:79-86.

73. Hanley MA, Jensen MP, Ehde DM, et al. Psychosocial predictors of long-term adjustment to lower-limb amputation and phantom limb pain. *Disabil Rehabil.* 2004;26:882-893.

74. May BJ. Assessment and treatment of individuals following lower extremity amputation. In: O'Sullivan SB, Schmitz TJ, eds. *Physical Rehabilitation: Assessment and Treatment.* 4th ed. Philadelphia, Pa: F.A. Davis Company; 2001:619-644.

75. American Pain Society. *Pain: the fifth vital sign.* Available at: http://www.ampainsoc.org/advocacy/fifth.htm. Accessed December 12, 2004.

76. American Pain Foundation. *Pain Action Guide.* Baltimore, Md: American Pain Foundation; 2001.

77. Cleeland CS, Ryan KM. Pain assessment: global use of the Brief Pain Inventory. *Ann Acad Med.* 1994;23:129-138.

78. Gallagher P, Maclachlan M. Development and psychometric evaluation of the Trinity Amputation and Prosthesis Experience Scales (TAPES). *Rehabilitation Psychology.* 2000;45:130-155.

79. Legro MW, Reiber GD, Smith DG, del Aguila M, Larsen J, Boone D. Prosthesis evaluation questionnaire for persons with lower limb amputations: assessing prosthesis-related quality of life. *Arch Phys Med Rehabil.* 1998;79:931-938.

80. Von Korff M, Ormel J, Keefe FJ, Dworkin SF. Grading the severity of chronic pain. *Pain*. 1992;50:133-149.

81. Seymour R. Examination of the patient with an amputation and the patient requiring an orthosis. In: Seymour R, ed. *Prosthetics and Orthotics: Lower Limb and Spinal*. Philadelphia, Pa: Lippincott Williams & Wilkins; 2002:36-50.

82. Lee RY, Turner-Smith A. The influence of the length of lower-limb prosthesis on spinal kinematics. *Arch Phys Med Rehabil*. 2003;84:1357-1362.

83. American Psychiatric Association. *Diagnostic and Statistical Manual of Mental of Mental Disorders*. 4th ed. Washington, DC: American Psychiatric Association; 1994.

84. Coyne JC, Fechner-Bates S, Schwenk TL. Prevalence, nature, and comorbidity of depressive disorders in primary care. *Gen Hosp Psychiatry*. 1994;16:267-276.

85. Rybarczyk B, Szymanski L, Nicholas JJ. Limb amputation. In: Frank RG, Elliott TR eds. *Handbook of Rehabilitation Psychology*. Washington, DC: American Psychological Association; 2000:29-47.

86. Kroenke K, Spitzer RL, Williams JB. The PHQ-9: validity of a brief depression severity measure. *J Gen Intern Med*. 2001;16:606-613.

87. Sherman RA, Sherman CJ, Gall NG. A survey of current phantom limb pain treatment in the United States. *Pain*. 1980;8:85-99.

88. Williams AM, Deaton SB. Phantom limb pain: elusive, yet real. *Rehabil Nurs*. 1997;22:73-77.

89. Finsen V, Persen L, Lovlien M, et al. Transcutaneous electrical nerve stimulation after major amputation. *J Bone Joint Surg Br*. 1988;70:109-112.

90. Finnoff J. Differentiation and treatment of phantom sensation, phantom pain, and residual-limb pain. *J Am Podiatr Med Assoc*. 2001;91:23-33.

91. Gatchel RJ, Turk DC. Interdisciplinary treatment of chronic pain patients. In: Gatchel RJ, Turk DC, eds. *Psychosocial Factors in Pain: Critical Perspectives*. New York, NY: Guildford Press; 1999:435-444.

92. Postone N. Phantom limb pain. A review. *Int J Psychiatry Med*. 1987;17:57-70.

93. Ramachandran VS, Rogers-Ramachandran D. Phantom limbs and neural plasticity. *Arch Neurol*. 2000;57:317-320.

94. Nikolajsen L, Ilkjaer S, Kroner K, Christensen JH, Jensen TS. The influence of preamputation pain on postamputation stump and phantom pain. *Pain*. 1997;72:393-405.

95. Bach S, Noreng MF, Tjellden NU. Phantom limb pain in amputees during the first 12 months following limb amputation, after preoperative lumbar epidural blockade. *Pain*. 1988;33:297-301.

96. Jahangiri M, Jayatunga AP, Bradley JW, Dark CH. Prevention of phantom pain after major lower limb amputation by epidural infusion of diamorphine, clonidine and bupivacaine. *Ann R Coll Surg Engl*. 1994;76:324-326.

97. Lambert AW, Dashfield AK, Cosgrove C, Wilkins DC, Walker AJ, Ashley S. Randomized prospective study comparing preoperative epidural and intraoperative perineural analgesia for the prevention of postoperative stump and phantom limb pain following major amputation. *Reg Anesth Pain Med*. 2001;26:316-321.

98. Nikolajsen L, Ilkjaer S, Jensen TS. Effect of preoperative extradural bupivacaine and morphine on stump sensation in lower limb amputees. *Br J Anaesth*. 1998;81:348-354.

99. Birbaumer N, Lutzenberger W, Montoya P, et al. Effects of regional anesthesia on phantom limb pain are mirrored in changes in cortical reorganization. *J Neurosci*. 1997;17:5503-5508.

100. Flor H, Denke C, Schaefer M, Grusser S. Effect of sensory discrimination training on cortical reorganization and phantom limb pain. *Lancet*. 2001;357:1763-1764.

101. Ramachandran VS, Rogers-Ramachandran D. Synaesthesia in phantom limbs induced with mirrors. *Proc Biol Sci*. 1996;263:377-386.

102. Onghena P, Van Houdenhove B. Antidepressant-induced analgesia in chronic non-malignant pain: a meta-analysis of 39 placebo-controlled studies. *Pain*. 1992;49:205-219.

103. Max MB. Antidepressant drugs as treatment for chronic pain: efficacy and mechanisms. In: Bromm B, Desmedt JE, eds. *Advances in Pain Research and Therapy—Issue of Pain and the Brain: From Nociception to Cognition*. Vol 22. New York, NY: Raven Press Ltd; 1995:501-515.

104. Robinson LR, Czerniecki JM, Ehde DM, et al. Trial of amitriptyline for relief of pain in amputees: results of a randomized controlled study. *Arch Phys Med Rehabil*. 2004;85:1-6.

105. Bone M, Critchley P, Buggy DJ. Gabapentin in postamputation phantom limb pain: a randomized, double-blind, placebo-controlled, cross-over study. *Reg Anesth Pain Med*. 2002;27:481-486.

106. Smith DG, Ehde DM, Hanley MA, Campbell KM, Jensen MP, Robinson LR. Efficacy of gabapentin in treating chronic phantom and residual limb pain. *J Rehabil Res Develop*. In press.

107. Jamison RN, Anderson KO, Peeters-Asdourian C, Ferrante FM. Survey of opioid use in chronic nonmalignant pain patients. *Reg Anesth*. 1994;19:225-230.

108. Dworkin RH, Backonja M, Rowbotham MC, et al. Advances in neuropathic pain: diagnosis, mechanisms, and treatment recommendations. *Arch Neurol*. 2003;60:1524-1534.

109. Huse E, Larbig W, Flor H, Birbaumer N. The effect of opioids on phantom limb pain and cortical reorganization. *Pain*. 2001;90:47-55.

110. Saris SC, Iacono RP, Nashold BS. Dorsal root entry zone lesions for post-amputation pain. *J Neurosurg*. 1985;62:72-76.

111. Turk DC, Okifuji A. Treatment of chronic pain patients: clinical outcomes, cost-effectiveness, and cost-benefits of multidisciplinary pain centers. *Critical Reviews in Physical and Rehabilitation Medicine*. 1998;10:181-208.

112. Haythornthwaite JA, Benrud-Larson LM. Psychological aspects of neuropathic pain. *Clin J Pain*. 2000;16(Suppl):S101-S105.

113. Jensen MP, Ehde DM, Hoffman AJ, Patterson DR, Czerniecki JM, Robinson LR. Cognitions, coping and social environment predict adjustment to phantom limb pain. *Pain*. 2002;95:133-142.

114. Wainapel S, Thoms A, Kahan B. The use of alternative therapies by rehabilitation outpatients. *Arch Phys Med Rehabil*. 1998;79:1003-1005.

115. Leskowitz ED. Phantom limb pain treated with therapeutic touch: a case report. *Arch Phys Med Rehabil*. 2000; 81:522-524.

116. Oakley DA, Whitman LG, Halligan PW. Hypnotic imagery as a treatment for phantom limb pain: two case reports and a review. *Clin Rehabil*. 2002;16:368-377.

117. Xing G. Acupuncture treatment of phantom limb pain: a report of 9 cases. *J Tradit Chin Med*. 1998;18:199-201.

118. Collacott EA, Zimmerman JT, White DW, Rindone JP. Bipolar permanent magnets for the treatment of chronic low back pain: a pilot study. *JAMA*. 2000;283:1322-1325.

119. Benson H. Harnessing the power of the placebo effect and renaming it "remembered wellness." *Annu Rev Med*. 1996;47:193-199.

Chapter 5

Skin Disorders and Their Management

Clay M. Kelly, MD

OBJECTIVES

1. Describe the anatomy and physiology of normal skin
2. Trace the healing process
3. Relate prosthetic wear to various skin disorders
4. Differentiate among the grades of ulceration, including their management
5. Indicate the most common types of skin infection and dermatitis and their management

INTRODUCTION

The skin is the largest organ of the human body, accounting for 16% of total body weight. Without adequate skin no one could survive. Skin is dynamic and adaptable; its form and function vary by location and usage requirements. Perhaps the most remarkable characteristic of skin is its ability to heal itself. Not only has the person with amputation lost skin, but the person will soon submit some skin to unaccustomed stresses. Weight bearing and confining the amputated limb in an enclosed environment in contact with unfamiliar materials are major stressors. It is no wonder that some patients develop skin ailments. This chapter reviews problems experienced by some people with amputation, particularly adults with lower-limb amputation.

NORMAL SKIN

Anatomy

Normal skin consists of three layers, each of which serves specific purposes (Figure 5-1). The first, or outermost, layer is the epidermis. This is the visible skin that directly interacts with the environment. The epidermis is divided into four strata: the corneum, lucidem, granulosum, and germinativum. Epidermal cells are continually moving outward from the basal, germinativum layer. The epidermis is nonvascular and has no nerve endings. Skin on the palm of the hand and the sole of the foot is specialized and has thicker epidermis than most of the other skin in the body.

The dermis lies beneath the basal layer and is comprised of collagen and elastic fibers, microvascular elements, glands, and nerve endings. This is the biologically active part of the skin. Hair follicles with their erector pilae muscles traverse this area. Connective tissue supports the other constituents of the skin and accounts for it elasticity. Two types of glands, sebaceous and sweat, function in this part of the skin. Sebaceous glands are generally near hair follicles and secrete oils, keeping the hair and skin well lubricated. Sebaceous production peaks at puberty and remains constant until old age, when it begins to decrease. Sweat glands are subdivided into apocrine and eccrine varieties. Apocrine glands are larger and are found in the axilla and anogenital areas. They secrete a milky material, which may dry. Bacteria will subsequently degrade apocrine secretions and account for odors in these areas. Eccrine glands are smaller and are generally known as sweat glands. The ducts open to the skin and are not near hair follicles. They secrete a thin hypotonic solution, which aids in thermoregulation. They respond to temperature and emotional stimuli.

Below the dermis is the subdermis, which includes connective tissue, fat, nerves, and blood vessels. This level provides physiological and mechanical support for the more superficial skin elements.

Function

Skin functions several ways to help insure homeostasis. The most obvious function is its direct exposure to the environment. In this capacity, it is exposed to, and protects one from light (especially ultraviolet irradiation) and mechanical trauma, temperature extremes, bacteria, and other microorganisms. In addition to shielding underlying tissue from electrolytic liquids, it also protects the body from loss of vital fluids. The skin also interacts with the endocrine and immunologic systems.

Environment

Bacteria and other microorganisms are ubiquitous. Several are normal inhabitants of the skin. Staphylococcal and streptococcal species are common normal flora, yet if given free access to bodily structures beneath the skin can become lethal quickly. On an ongoing basis, healthy, unbroken skin tolerates these microorganisms while shielding deeper organs from them. A system of buffering, mediated through the sweat glands, renders the skin inhospitable to some bacteria, and allows the skin to respond to environmental changes in acidity. Normal Ph is between 4.2 and 5.6. Exposure to dilute acids or alkali changes local skin acidity, which soon returns the normal mildly acidic state.

Skin also carries an electrical charge, typically negative. A change to more alkalinity on the skin increases the negativity, whereas a shift to more acidity shifts the polarization to a more positive state. Normally, bacteria that are negatively charged are repelled from the skin surface.

Skin is permeable to fat-soluble substances and some gases, whereas electrolytic solutions and other gases will not pass through the skin.

When in sunlight, the skin is bombarded with light rays, which include ultraviolet rays. Skin intercepts these rays, increasing its quantity of melanin pigment in the melanocytes in response to continual exposure. Melanin has the unique ability to absorb light over a broad range of light waves. Overexposure to these rays may cause permanent changes and damage to the skin.

Temperature Regulation

Human beings survive in a narrow temperature range. A change of core temperature of 4° in either direction requires medical attention. The skin, with its vascular and eccrine elements, plays a major role in

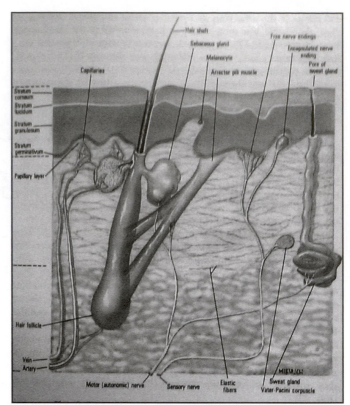

Figure 5-1. Skin cross-section. Reprinted with permission from Levy WS. *Skin Problems of the Amputee.* St. Louis, Mo: Warren H. Green; 1982.

temperature regulation. When core temperature rises, the small vessels in the skin dilate, allowing more blood to flow near the surface, dissipating heat into the surrounding environment. At warm temperature, sweating occurs to help dissipate heat. Eccrine glands secrete their hypotonic solution onto the skin's surface. As sweat on the skin surface evaporates, heat is consumed, effectively lowering the surrounding temperature. Each gram of water that evaporates from the skin uses 580 calories of heat. Inside a prosthetic socket, the skin of the amputated limb loses this mechanism. Conversely, when core temperature lowers, blood flow to the skin is decreased, thereby conserving heat.

Sensation

The sense of touch is conveyed through the microscopic neural elements of the dermis. These include free, as well as specialized, sensory nerve endings that detect deep pressure, vibration, warmth, and cold. Skin sensation protects the individual from hostile elements in the environment, such as bee stings and fire. Sensory loss may lead to skin ulceration, particularly when the skin is exposed to high compressive and shear stress.

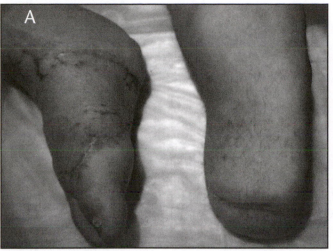
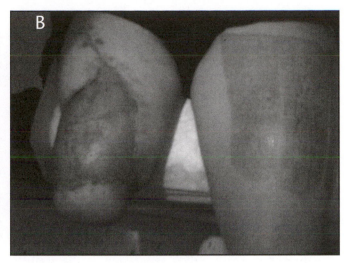

Figures 5-2A & B. Full and split thickness grafts.

HEALING

Scar Formation

The skin has the unique ability to repair itself. Partial thickness injuries do not extend through the basal layer. They cause the skin to form superficial eschar (scab) and epithelial advancement. Shallow wounds heal faster than full-thickness wounds. If the basal layer is broached (full-thickness injury), healing occurs through four stages—hemostasis, inflammation, scar formation (fibroproliferation), and scar remodeling. Scar tissue lacks the neural, glandular, and vascular elements of normal skin, and never has more than 80% of normal skin's tensile strength

All people with acquired amputation have some scarring. Problems with scars include its propensity to adhere to other tissues, primarily bone. Hypertrophic scars and keloids may occur. Hypertrophic scars tend to occur relatively early, usually about 4 weeks after surgery, and may regress with time. Keloids have a mean time of appearance of 30 weeks, and appear to be a more exuberant hypertrophic scar. Some keloids are pigmented; pain, burning, and itchiness are often associated with them, although malignant transformation is rare.

Dermatologic treatment includes moisturizers and deep tissue massage for adherent scars. Among the numerous interventions for hypertrophic scars and keloids are corticosteroid injection, laser therapy, cryogenic therapy, radiation, medications, and surgical excision by a plastic surgeon or a dermatologist. Keloids, rather than hypertrophic scars, are more likely to recur after excision. Prosthetic adjustments to relieve pressure in areas of scarring may be necessary. Newer materials, such as gel liners and socks, may be beneficial.

Grafts

When the deficit in skin coverage is extensive, as in the trauma patient with deep abrasions or degloving injuries, the plastic surgeon may need to provide skin coverage via split-thickness or full-thickness grafts (Figures 5-2A & B). Split-thickness grafts have epidermis and part of the dermis. They are usually taken from another part of the patient's intact skin, typically the contralateral thigh or abdomen. These have good survival potential but poor appearance, often resembling chicken skin. Full-thickness skin grafts, such as the filet of sole pedicle flap used to preserve transtibial level amputations in trauma, include epidermis, dermis, and some subcutaneous tissues. Although they have more tenuous survival, the cosmetic outcome and pressure tolerance is better, especially inside the prosthetic socket.

Healing of skin grafts usually takes 6 to 12 weeks. Prosthetic fitting should be delayed until the graft heals because unhealed grafts are pressure intolerant.

MECHANICAL CONDITIONS OF THE SKIN RELATED TO PROSTHETIC WEAR

Maceration

Areas of persistent friction or pressure, when combined with increased moisture inside the prosthetic socket, can cause the outer keratin layer of skin to begin to peel. Local burning pain is typical. Treatment usually consists of prosthetic adjustments to relieve pressure concentration, plus protection from further irritation with a Duoderm wafer (ConvaTec, Princeton, NJ), or similar material. Patients who have excessive sweating (hyperhydrosis) may need to use a socket fitted over several cotton socks to absorb the moisture. Local

BOTOX (Allergan, Irvine, Calif) injections have been anecdotally noted to help control sweating in individuals with amputation.

Intertriginous Dermatitis

Skin folding can lead to superficial dermatitis within the folds. Intertrigo results from moisture and friction. A common example is seen in transfemoral amputations where a proximomedial flesh roll develops. Maceration may be followed by local yeast or bacterial infection. Treatment with topical antibiotics or antifungals is indicated. Good hygiene and socket modifications to eliminate the flesh roll should remedy the problem.

Blister

A blister is a fluid-filled separation of the stratum corneum from the underlying layers. Blisters are often seen on the amputated limb, especially early in prosthetic rehabilitation (Figure 5-3). Common sites include the margins of the socket brim, where skin excursion, and therefore, shear, may be greater, and around the surgical incision. The patient fitted with a suction socket may develop blisters where suction pockets develop. Treatment is geared toward eliminating socket pressure, gapping, and friction. Temporary cessation of prosthetic wear may be necessary. Blisters should not be lanced. The deflated skin of a resolving blister acts like a moist dressing on a clean wound. It will take 10 to 20 days for the skin to repair itself once the offending agent is removed.

Abrasion and Erosion

Abrasion refers to the scraping away of the skin, such as after persistent scratching of an itchy area. Erosion refers to wearing away of the skin often at points of high pressure within the prosthesis. In the transtibial amputated limb, the infrapatellar ligament, anterodistal limb end, and hamstring tendons are likely sites. The transfemoral amputated limb may have abrasions or erosions at the ischial seat, groin, and on the distal end of the thigh. Prosthetic alignment and fit need to be adjusted to alleviate undue pressure and shear force.

Atrophy

Atrophy describes the decrease in size or "wasting away" of cell tissue. Although atrophy is uncommon in the epidermis, it occurs in subcutaneous tissues, fat, and muscle from long-term prosthetic wear. Muscle atrophy results from disuse. Atrophy can lead to change in amputation limb shape with increased prominence of underlying bones. Ongoing socket modifications and strengthening exercise are indicated to avoid skin problems associated with atrophy.

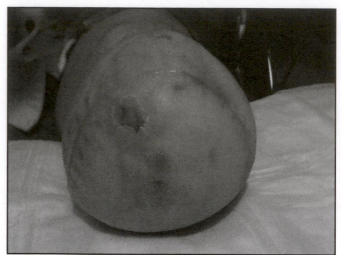
Figure 5-3. Blisters.

Ulceration

Skin ulceration refers to a defect in the epidermis. It may be caused by pressure, shear, laceration, or failing circulation (ischemia). Numerous diseases, particularly diabetes, also may lead to ulceration. Ulceration on the amputated limb, not present on other parts of the body, may be considered due to local friction or pressure. The pressure ulcer grading system is useful in the nonischemic ulcer caused by pressure.

Grade 1

Grade 1 ulceration is an area of unblanchable erythema in an area of pressure or shear caused by the prosthesis. Although the skin is not broken, deeper tissue injury may be present. Treatment is primarily reduction of pressure and shear inflicted by the socket. Prosthesis wearing time should be limited until the redness decreases. Hydrocolloidal dressings (eg, Duoderm), which are thin and adhere to the skin and help protect it from pressure and shear, may be effective, especially if there is discomfort. Silicon or gel impregnated socks are also helpful.

Grade 2

Grade 2 ulcerations extend through the epidermis and dermis into the subdermal layer (Figure 5-4). They do not penetrate the fascial plane beneath the subdermis, and thus represent a partial thickness loss. They respond well to coverage with hydrocolloidal dressings. The thin variety of hydrocolloid dressing is more desirable for areas within the socket. Typically, dry dressings are too bulky and do not maintain the correct position within the prosthesis. Thin transparent films can be used in the patient who is not wearing a prosthesis, but, when the prosthesis is worn, films tend to lose position and retain excessive fluids against the wound. Fluid retention may lead to skin maceration. Prosthetic

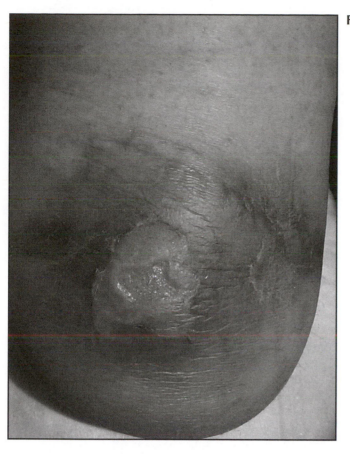

Figure 5-4. Grade 2 ulceration.

modifications, including silicon or gel impregnated socks, may be beneficial.

Grades 3 and 4

Grade 3 ulcerations penetrate the subdermal layer to the fascia. Grade 4 extends into the muscle, bone, ligament, tendon, or joint capsule. Management requires cessation of prosthetic wear until the ulcer heals. The risk of infection is greater in severe ulcerations. Deep infections, such fasciitis and osteomyelitis, are hard to eradicate. These wounds should be examined for possible extensions into other parts of the soft tissues. The condition of the ulcer dictates the treatment. A simple, but effective, management tool remains the "red, yellow, black" wound management algorithm.

The red wound is clean, with a granulation base. A moist occluded environment is indicated to optimize the healing process. This can be achieved with saline dressings, hydrocolloids, thin transparent film, and hydrogels. Topical healing agents, such as silver sulfadiazine, may speed healing by providing a moist occluded environment and inhibiting bacterial proliferation.

The yellow wound is covered with exudative and fibrinous material. This wound needs to progress to the red state. Saline wet-to-dry dressings allow for progressive debridement of exudates, which dries and adheres somewhat to the exudates. When the dressing is removed, some of the exudate will be removed with it. Topical fibrinolytic agents may speed this process. Alginates, with their absorptive capabilities, are also useful.

The black wound is covered with eschar, devitalized tissue, which needs to be removed either by mechanical debridement or prolonged application of fibrinolytic agents. The goal is to progress to the red wound state, and then provide a moist occlusive environment.

WOUND APPLICATIONS

Evidence of thoughtful care of wounds dates back at least to 2200 BCE. The "three healing gestures" of cleansing the wound, preparing topical dressings, and bandaging are still practiced, albeit it a more modern way. In general, wound healing is optimized by providing a warm, moist, occluded environment. As wounds vary in area, depth, bacterial content, and amount and type of exudates, no one dressing is sufficient for every wound. Several types of dressings are shown in Table 5-1.

Non-adhering dressings include Xeroform (Kendall, Mansfield, Mass), Vaseline gauze (Kendall), Telfa (Kendall), and Adaptic (Johnson & Johnson, New

Table 5-1

Wound Dressings

Type of Dressing	Examples
Nonadherent fabrics	Telfa
• Absorbtive	
- Gauze	Kerlix
- Foams	
Occlusive	
• Nonbiologic	
- Films	Tegaderm, Op-Site
- Hydrocolloids	Duoderm, Tegasorb
- Alginates	Calcicare, Sorbsan, Kaltostat
- Hydrogels	Hydrogel, Intrasite Gel
• Biologic	
- Homograft	
- Xenograft	Pig skin
- Amnion	
- Skin Substitute	Graftskin
Creams, ointments, solutions	
• Antibacterial	Silvadene, Bacitracin
• Enzymatic	Collagenase, Accuzyme
• Other	Normal Saline (0.9%), Betadine

Adapted from Lionelli GT. Wound dressings. *Surg Clin North Am*. 2003; 83(3):617-638.

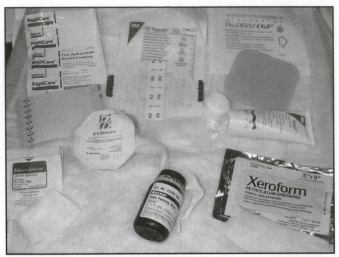

Figure 5-5. Sample wound dressings.

Hydrocolloids may be the ideal wound dressing for the prosthesis wearer. These dressings are made of pectin, gelatin, carboxymethylcellulose and similar materials.. They come in powders, pastes and adhesive wafers. The wafer is low profile, occlusive, and yet will absorb some moisture which allows for wearing the prosthesis and healing concomitantly. Duoderm and Tegasorb (3M) are examples.

Hydrogels also provide a moist occlusive environment and are used for clean, dry wounds. Ulcers that cannot be treated "in prosthesis" may respond well to hydrogels.

Biologic occlusive dressings include autograft (skin from the patient), homograft (skin from another person), xenograft (skin from an animal, usually pig), and amnion (from human placentas). Such dressings are used in burns or larger full-thickness wounds, with homografts and xenografts considered temporary. Synthetic biologic skin substitutes may have components that incorporate into healing skin. This class of dressing has been used in some individuals with amputation with anecdotal success.

ULCERATION DUE TO DISEASE

Ulceration due to medical causes is most often circulatory failure, either arterial or venous disease. Numerous disease states can produce ulceration. Typically, the ischemic limb is cold to touch, with pulses not palpable. The ulceration is distal on the amputated limb and may be confined to the anterior or posterior flap of the limb. Management includes laboratory studies and referral to the vascular surgeon for definitive diagnosis and management. The patient cannot use a prosthesis until the ulcer heals.

Brunswick, NJ). These may be coated to improve occlusion, nonadherence, or bacteriostatic properties. (Figure 5-5)

Absorptive dressings are used in exudative wounds to help avoid wound maceration from an overly moist environment. Numerous brands may be used. The wet-to-dry dressing for wounds requiring debridement uses this type of dressing with a moistened inner layer and dry absorptive outer layer. Alginates are derived from the calcium salt of alginic acid, a product of seaweed. These dressings have excellent absorptive ability, suitable for exudative wounds. They are not appropriate for use within the prosthesis as the moist environment quickly exhausts the absorptive capability of the dressing.

Occlusive dressings provide a warm, moist environment in which clean wounds will heal most efficiently. Occlusive films include Tegaderm (3M, St Paul, Minn) and Op-site (Smith & Nephew, Memphis, Tenn). Typically, they are a poor choice for the prosthesis-wearing patient as sweat and other fluids tend to accumulate beneath the dressing and may cause wound maceration.

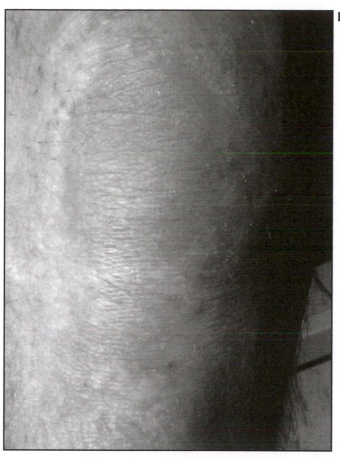

Figure 5-6. Lichenification.

Table 5-2

BACTERIAL SKIN INFECTIONS OF THE AMPUTEE

Infection	Description	Treatment
Folliculitis	Papular or pustular inflammation of hair follicles	Benoyl Peroxide, Topical antibiotics
Furuncle	Painful, firm or fluctuant abscess originating from a hair follicle	Drain and pack
Carbuncle	A network of furuncles connected by sinus tracts	Drain and pack. May be loculated
Cellulitis	Painful, erythematous infection of deep skin with poorly demarcated borders	Oral or IV antibiotics
Osteomyelitis	Erythematous skin locally, and a draining sinus	IV antibiotics and/or surgical resection

Adapted from Stulberg DL. Caring for common skin conditions: common bacterial skin infections. *American Family Physician*. 2002;66(1):119-124.

SKIN THICKENING

Skin will eventually adapt to chronic friction and pressure, thickening to form a callus well-circumscribed from the area of pressure. This is beneficial where tolerance to pressure is desired, such as the infrapatellar ligament. Corns are circumscribed thickening of skin that may occur on the amputated limb. They are caused by localized pressure and can be treated by soaking, application of salicylic acid, or paring. Sometimes after soaking, a corn can be removed with blunt dissection or with a forceps.

Lichenification is the leathery thickening of skin from persistent mechanical injury to the skin (Figure 5-6). There can be increased pigmentation. Often the thickened skin develops "crisscrossed" marking. Itchiness and burning are usually present. Socket adjustments are the key to reducing lichenification, together with topical corticosteroids.

INFECTION

Infection is the state produced by the establishment of an infective agent in or on a host. Skin may have several manifestations of bacterial infections (Table 5-2).

Folliculitis

Folliculitis is the most benign skin infection and is caused by pyoderma centered on the hair follicle, resulting from *Staphylococcus aureus*, *Pseudomonas aeruginosa*, or *Candida*. It presents as a series of raised, red, painful lesions on the amputated limb. Local discomfort is usually the only complaint. Folliculitis may be initiated by physical or chemical irritation or bacterial proliferation. The patient is liable to develop folliculitis because all three conditions may be present within the prosthesis. Treatment includes cleanliness of the skin, prosthesis, and socks or liners. Prosthetic adjustments to decrease physical irritation are indicated. Topical agents include benzoyl peroxide and antibiotics such as clindamycin and erythromycin.

Furuncles and Carbuncles

A furuncle is a follicular infection that has progressed deeper and extends beyond the follicle. This is an abscess, commonly known as a boil. They are tender, erythematous, compressible to firm masses filled with purulent material (pus) and are distinct. They have a predilection for areas exposed to friction; consequently, the prosthesis-enclosed limb is a likely target. The pathogen is usually *S aureus*. Boils will typically open spontaneously to the skin surface and drain, which is usually curative.

Carbuncles are coalesced furuncles connected through multiple tracts. They are often loculated, and thus more difficult to drain completely. Treatment consists of incising the tip of the boil and allowing it to drain. Patients are ill-advised to lance themselves. Packing with a sterile or Iodoform-impregnated gauze applied with gentle pressure, and changed daily aid healing. Antibiotics need to be considered in cases where systemic symptoms, such as fever and malaise, are encountered. Severe cases may require intravenous antibiotics.

Cellulitis

Cellulitis is a skin infection characterized by redness, warmth, and swelling (Figure 5-7). It may occur at skin openings such as ulcers, surgical wounds, and sites of maceration, laceration, and yeast infections. The most common pathogens are Group A *Streptococcus* and *Staphylococcus*. The legs are the most common-

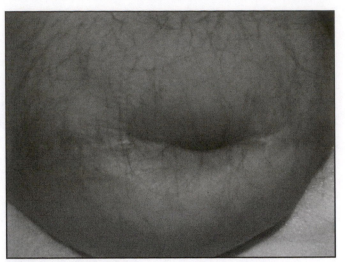

Figure 5-7. Cellulitus.

ly affected. The lower amputated limb has ongoing stressors from the prosthesis, which may lead to skin openings. Treatment emphasizes scrupulous hygiene and antibiotics, such as Augmentin (GlaxoSmithKline, Philadelphia, Pa), erythromycin, tetracycline, Keflex, and ciprofloxacin Table 5-3. Although uncomplicated cellulitis frequently improves quickly, often within 1 day, the patient needs to take the full course of antibiotics. Cases in which the dermis is thickened may take longer to respond. Intravenous antibiotics need be considered in patients who have diabetes, are immunocompromised, or have infections unresponsive to oral therapy.

Osteomyelitis

Osteomyelitis is infection of the bone, most often from *S aureus*. People with amputation are prone to subacute or chronic osteomyelitis at the level of bony amputation. The skin manifestation is usually a small draining sinus that does not heal. Prolonged intravenous antibiotics are required, and surgical skin resection and amputated limb remodeling may be necessary. In the absence of associated skin and soft tissue infection, or edema, the patient may wear the prosthesis, but should apply a thin absorbent dressing over the affected area. If there is moderate or marked drainage, the dressing should be changed several times per day.

Fungus

Tinea infections are common on the amputated limb and areas under suspension sleeves. As with many other skin conditions, moisture, closely fitting garments, and shear and compression force are predisposing factors. Although "tinea stumpis" has not been defined, it is similar to tinea pedis and tinea cruris. The area infected is initially very red and sharply demarcated. Pruritis (itchiness) may be very intense. Scaliness may develop

Table 5-3

ORAL ANTIBIOTICS FOR CELLULITIS

Antibiotic	Generic	Class	Dosage	Duration
Amoxicillin	amoxicillin	penicillins	500 mg q 12 hours	7 to 14 days
Augmentin	amoxicillin/clavulanate	penicillins	500 mg q 12 hours	7 to 14 days
Keflex	cephalexin	cephalosporins	500 mg q 12 hours	7 to 14 days
Erythromycin	erythromycin	macrolides	500 mg q 12 hours	7 to 14 days
Cipro	ciprofloxacin	floroquinolones	500 mg q 12 hours	7 to 14 days

Table 5-4

COMMON TOPICAL DRUGS FOR FUNGAL SKIN INFECTIONS

Drug	Strength	Brand	Per day	Dermatitis?
Clotrimazole	1%	Lotrimin	2	Yes (Y)
		Desenex	2	Y
		Mycelex	2	Y
Econazole	1%	Spectazole	1	Y
Ketoconazole	2%	Nizoral	2	Y
Nystatin	100K u per ml/cc	Nystatin	2	Rare (R)
		Mycolog	2	R
		Mycostatin	2	R
Terbinafine	1%	Lamisil	2	Y
Tolnaftate	1%	Tinactin	2	R

There are several other topical antifungal. Please refer to PDR or similar source

Adapted from AAP. *2000 Red Book. Report of the Committee on Infectious Diseases.* 25th ed. Elk Grove Village, Ill: American Academy of Pediatrics; 2000.

and later lichenification. The lesion may become less red with time and smaller satellite lesions may appear in the region. Treatment involves improving hygiene and application of topical antifungal medications (Table 5-4).

DERMATITIS OF THE AMPUTATED LIMB

According to Lyon, 34% of people with amputations experience a skin problem. He found that dermatitis was the most common skin condition in a review of 63 cases. Although there is no way to distinguish contact irritant dermatitis from allergic dermatitis, allergic contact is presumed responsible for approximately one third of patients. Lyon performed skin testing and found that the materials used in the prosthesis may cause contact dermatitis.

Contact Dermatitis

Contact dermatitis refers to skin irritation from substances that cause an irritative reaction on the first exposure. A mild reaction may consist only of local reddening with itching, burning, or both. A more severe reaction may include local inflammation, blister formation, and serous draining (eczematous reaction). Table 5 lists potential allergens in the prosthesis-wearing patient.

Allergic dermatitis requires a preliminary sensitizing exposure to establish the skin's ability to react to the allergen. Thus, the first exposure does not result in a dermatitic reaction. Sensitization also has a variable period, and may take years to develop. Therefore, a patient may comment that a substance was incorporated in the socket before and had not previously caused a problem.

Table 5-5

POTENTIAL ALLERGENS IN PROSTHETIC WEARING PATIENTS

Allergen	Where
Benzoyl Peroxide	Resin hardener
PTBP	Neoprene adhesive
Neoprene	Suspension sleeve
Potassium Dischromate	Leather liners
para-Phenylenediamine	Rubber in valve
Fragrance	Detergents
	Creams
	Lotions
Silicon	Socks and sleeves
Sulfa	Silvadene
Hydrocortisone	Topical OTC cortisone

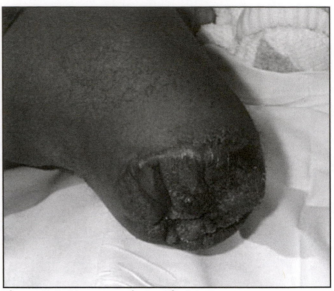

Figure 5-8. Verrucous hyperplasia.

Case Study

A 69-year-old man with a new transtibial amputation from vascular disease presented to the clinic with an itchy, reddened area of skin on his thigh. He had been fitted with a prosthesis 8 weeks prior and was making progress in gait training. Examination revealed circumferential raised skin about the thigh in the area of direct contact with the neoprene suspension sleeve. He changed to a gel-lined sleeve, and applied Lidex topically for 7 days. He was able to continue gait training with no further skin disorder.

Case Study

A 19-year-old college student presented to the clinic shortly after moving into town, complaining of a "skin problem." She noted that the problem began shortly after her most recent prosthesis was delivered. She could not address the problem because of her impending move. Examination revealed skin thickening, with hyperpigmentation, and wart-like changes. The amputated limb was malodorous, which was out of character for her general grooming and dress. Verrucous hyperplasia was easily diagnosed (Figure 5-9).

A 7-day course of antibiotics was prescribed to cover skin pathogens, and a pad inserted in the bottom of her socket. The prosthetist modified the socket to decrease proximal tightness and improve total contact throughout. When the antibiotics were finished, a topical steroid cream was started. At 3-week follow-up, she felt, looked, and smelled considerably better (Figure 5-10).

Identification and removal of the offending agent is the key to resolving the skin inflammation (Table 5-5). Where dermatitis is located adjacent to specific material, simply replacing the material with a functionally equivalent substance may suffice. Topical corticosteroids may speed resolution and aid in symptomatic relief. In refractory cases, skin testing by the dermatologist and definitive treatment may be necessary.

Verrucous Hyperplasia

Verrucous hyperplasia is a skin condition almost confined to people who wear prostheses (Figure 5-8). The name refers to "wart-like skin thickening." There is no true wart formation or other viral activity, but rather partitioned thickening of the skin. The conditions that lead to this are constriction, moisture, suction, and poor hygiene. Levy determined that distal pressure is required to help resolve this problem.

Epidermal Cyst

The epidermal, or sebaceous, cyst is typically found on the face, around the eyes, behind the ears, or on the back. It also can be found on the amputated limb. In the transfemoral amputated limb, this is usually in the inguinal fold, and in the transtibial amputated limb, the popliteal fossa. The cyst wall forms keratin, producing a round protruding mass, referred to as a "skin pearl." Treatment involves incision, drainage, and removal of the epithelial wall. For small lesions, this can be done with a small gauge hypodermic needle; larger cysts may need a scalpel. Prevention is via hygiene and maintenance of optimal prosthetic fit and alignment

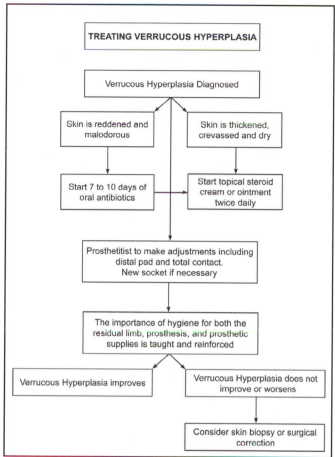

Figure 5-9. Treatment of verrucous hyperplasia.

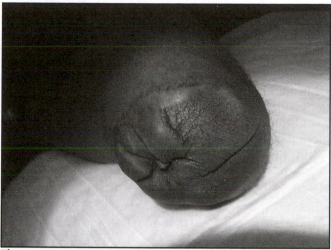

Figure 5-10. Verrucous hyperplasia at follow-up.

Psoriasis

Psoriasis occurs in up to 3% of the population. It is transmitted genetically and is characterized by recurrent exacerbations. Although having an amputation does not predispose one to having the disease, limb loss may precipitate a local outbreak in the amputated limb. Lesions begin as red, scaly papules that come together to form oval plaques. The scale is adherent, silvery white, and friable; bleeding may occur when it is removed. It occurs on extensor surfaces more than on flexor surfaces. Plaques are apt to develop at sites of physical trauma. Topical steroids are the first line of treatment. Topical tar solutions are also useful.

Eczema

"Eczema" derives from the Greek word for "boil out." It is not a diagnostic but rather a descriptive term. A skin condition having blisters, serous drainage and oozing, crust formation, and erythema would be aptly termed eczematous. Treatment consists of searching for the cause of this dermatitis so that appropriate remedial measures may be taken.

Edema

Edema is excess fluid in tissue due to increased fluid pressure, decreased oncotic pressure, or increased capillary permeability. It is common in the amputated limb postoperatively. In cases of severe trauma with multiple local injuries and limb salvage, edema may be massive. Common causes of regional edema in the amputated limb include deep vein thrombosis, reactive hyperemia from initial prosthetic wearing, cellulitis, trauma, and allergic or hypersensitivity reaction. Generalized edema has numerous medical causes including vascular disease, malnutrition, heart failure, anemia, and renal failure with fluid overload. Reactive hyperemia is common in patients who are in the early stage of wearing a prosthesis. The skin and subcutaneous structures in the amputated limb are not designed for weight bearing. Placed in a rigid socket and repeatedly loaded and unloaded may increase local circulation. Treatment includes using elastic shrinker socks and progressive prosthesis wearing.

Follicular Hyperkeratosis

Hair follicles in intertriginous areas may be subject to rubbing when the prosthesis is applied. If the follicles become plugged with keratinous material, follicular hyperkeratosis results. Dilatation of the follicle causes discomfort and inflammation. Secondary folliculitis may occur also. Treatment is aimed at decreasing friction and pressure and establishing good hygiene to keep the pores from further plugging. Benzoyl peroxide, salicylic acid, and warm bathing may be helpful.

Itchiness

Itchiness and burning are saved for last as they are not truly conditions of the skin, but rather side effects from skin or nerve disorders. Damage to peripheral nerves may lead to burning, itching, or other painful sensations. Swelling, hypersensitivity, allergic dermatitis, local infection, abrasion, maceration, lichen planus, and dry skin (xerosis) are all potential causes of discomfort. Medications such as narcotic analgesics may cause itchiness, as may numerous medical conditions such as thyroid disorder, uremia in the patient with kidney failure, liver disease, and several types of malignancy. Emotional stress can cause psychogenic itching. Treatment is aimed at determining the cause of itchiness and rectifying it. Antihistaminic agents, both oral and topical, may be useful.

SUMMARY

The person with amputation, particularly lower-limb amputation, of necessity exposes the skin of the amputated limb to many factors that can cause or exacerbate skin disorders. Pressure and shear, as well as the occlusive intrasocket environment, cause many skin problems. Appropriate selection of socket and liner materials, ongoing maintenance of prosthetic fit and alignment, and meticulous hygiene are the first line in avoiding these problems. Appropriate diagnosis and treatment are necessary when problems persist.

BIBLIOGRAPHY

AAP 2000 Red Book: Report of the Committee on Infectious Diseases, 25th ed. American Academy of Pediatrics; 2000.

Canale ST. *Campbell's Operatve Orthopaedics*. 10th ed. St. Louis, Mo: Mosby; 2003.

Carek PJ. Diagnosis and management of Osteomyelitis. *American Family Physician*. 2001;63(12):2413-20.

Choucair MM, Fivenson DP. Leg ulcer diagnosis and management. *Dermatology Clinics*. 2001;19(4);659-78.

Dubay DA. Acute wound healing: the biology of acute wound failure. *Surgery Clinics of North America*. 2003;83(3):463-81.

Goldman L, Ausiello D. *Cecil's Textbook of Medicine*. 22nd ed. Philadelphia, PA: WB Saunders; 2004.

Habif TP. *Clinical Dermatology*. 4th ed. St. Louis: Mosby-Year Book; 2004.

Horn WA. Graftskin heals an ulcer on an amputation stump. *Dermatologic Surgery*. 2001;26(10):946-8.

Karakozis S. Carcinoma arising in an amputation stump. *American Surgeon*. 2001;67(5):495-7.

Levy SW. *Skin Problems of the Amputee*. Warren Green Inc, St. Louis, Mo: 1983.

Levy SW. Skin care determines prosthetic comfort. *Biomechanics*. 1999;45-54.

Lionelli GT. Wound dressings. *Surgical Clinics of North America*. 2003;83(3):617-38.

Lyon CC, Kularni J, Zimerson E, et al. Skin disorders in amputees. *Journal of the American Academy of Dermatology*. 2000;42(3):501-7.

Luba MC. Caring for common skin conditions: common benign skin tumors. *American Family Physician*. 2003; 67(4):729-38.

Mandell EL, Bennett JE, Dolin R. *Principles and Practice of Infectious Diseases*. 6th ed. New York, NY: Churchill Livingstone; 2005.

Mostow EN. Wound healing: a multidisciplinary approach for dermatologists. *Dermatology Clinics*. 2003;21(2):371-87.

Noble J. *Textbook of Primary Care Medicine*. 3rd ed. St. Louis, Mo: Mosby; 2001.

Robson MC. Proliferative scarring. *Surgical Clinics of North America*. 2003;83(3):557-69.

Shafer JJ, Taylor SC, Cook-Bolden F. Keloidal scars: a review and a critical look at therapeutic options. *Journal of the American Academy of Dermatology*. 2002;46(2 Suppl Understanding):S63-97.

Strauss RM, Harrington CI. Stump acne: a new variant of acne mechanica and a cause of immobility. *British Journal of Dermatology*.2001;144(3);647-8.

Stulberg DL. Caring for common skin conditions: common bacterial skin infections. *American Family Physician*. 2002; 66(1):119-24.

Valencia IC. Inpatient dermatology: skin grafting. *Dermatology Clinics*. 2000;18(3):521-32.

Wooten M. Management of chronic wounds in the elderly. *Clinics in Family Practice*. 2001;3(3);599-626.

Chapter 6

Psychological Consequences of Amputation

Pamela G. Forducey, PhD, ABPP; William D. Ruwe, PhD, PsyD;
Kawaljeet Kaur, MD

OBJECTIVES

1. Highlight common psychological consequences after amputation
2. Relate the age of the patient to emotional adjustment to limb loss
3. Recommend interventions to reduce negative responses to amputation

INTRODUCTION

Amputation, whether catastrophic or secondary to a chronic disease process, results in a personal loss, both real and symbolic. Disability after amputation is not limited to the physical realm but also affects the psychological health of the individual. Health care providers who work with individuals with disability should explore what has drawn them to this particular field of endeavor. An understanding of their own thoughts and feelings surrounding disability will heighten their awareness and sensitivity about the psychological challenges patients and their families encounter as they attempt to reorganize their lives following an amputation.

The reality is that individuals, irrespective of age, often experience psychological distress after undergoing an amputation. Among the most frequently reported emotional problems are generalized sadness, anxiety, crying spells, and insomnia.[1] Subsequent to amputation, people are faced with the issues of adjustment to, and acceptance of, the loss of their limb and related functional limitations.[2] The health care provider can facilitate the psychological adjustment of the person with an amputation by possessing a basic knowledge of the following aspects: condition that led to the amputation; premorbid physical, cognitive, psychological, social, and spiritual functioning of the person; current social support systems; economic situation; awareness of and access to both medical and community-based resources; and what abilities and limitations the person currently possesses.

This chapter focuses on common psychological consequences of amputation (ie, grief and adjustment reactions, depression, anxiety, and post-traumatic stress disorder [PTSD]). Special populations (ie, children/adolescents, adults, older adults), body image, sexual functioning, and self-efficacy also are discussed. Interventions that have demonstrated effectiveness are explored, including brief psychotherapy, cognitive behavioral therapy (CBT), pain management (eg, biofeedback and relaxation training), advocacy/peer support groups, and family response. Mind/Body/Spirit connections also are considered. Optimal treatment for the comprehensive rehabilitation and biopsychosocial management of the patient with amputation involves the multidisciplinary team in which the patient and his or her primary care givers are the nucleus. Psychological treatment is most beneficial when it is provided in this milieu.

COMMON PSYCHOLOGICAL CONSEQUENCES AFTER AMPUTATION

The psychological effects of amputation are highly variable and depend on the person's age, level of maturity, personality traits, coping skills, flexibility, available social support, coexisting medical conditions, and whether the amputation was planned or sudden. Gallagher and MacLachlan[3] surveyed 200 patients who were fitted with a prosthesis to investigate coping strategies with respect to age and length of time with a prosthesis. The Coping Strategy Indicator, a self-reported measure, was used. It has three scales: problem-solving, seeking social support, and avoidance. Avoidance scores were considerably higher in individuals whose amputation resulted from trauma as opposed to disease or congenital causes. This is consistent with the theory that individuals who do not have adequate time to prepare mentally for the surgery react with denial.

Cheung et al[4] concluded that in comparison to the lower limb, upper-limb traumatic amputations are associated with a significantly increased incidence of PTSD and depression. These authors noted that the upper limb plays a greater role in self-expression, self-care, and communication, resulting in a more profound functional loss than that following amputation of the lower limb. Complaints of pain were elevated more for those with lower-limb amputations than the upper limb but the difference was not statistically significant. The study was limited by small sample size, potential experimenter bias, potential cultural differences in the two groups, and primarily male participants. Bhojak et al[5] demonstrated that persons with amputation experience significantly greater alienation, neuroticism, and body distortion than their nondisabled counterparts. Dissatisfaction with current life and disillusionment about the future are more prevalent.

Grief Reactions

The emotional reaction to amputation may be characterized by a myriad of emotions.[3] Initial grief and depression are common and have been encountered frequently when patients are asked to complete self-report measures.[6-8] Loss of a limb is often equivalent to the death of a loved one, and frequently entails a period of grieving. The grief reaction, conceptualized by Kubler-Ross,[9] may include the stages of denial, anger, bargaining, depression, and acceptance. However, these stages might not occur in a fixed sequence. Somatic symptoms predominate during the early stages. Some people try to suppress their emotions; therefore grief facilitation is helpful at this stage to prevent resurfacing of these emotions later when they can interfere with rehabilitation and adjustment.

Adjustment Reaction

Postamputation adjustment is not limited to the physical aspects of amputation, but encompasses emotional, psychosocial, and vocational factors. Because most patients receive a prosthesis, adjustment to it is a major concern. In general, lower-limb prostheses are more readily accepted by the patient than upper-limb prostheses because of better function and cosmetic acceptability. Adjustments depend on the patient's age, gender, and the perceived extent of their disability.[3] Identity and social acceptance are the primary issues for young adults. Women are especially concerned with creating an illusion of an intact body, whereas function is a more important consideration for men. Comfort and balance while standing, the feel of the prosthesis against the skin, prosthetic odor, and the energy required to ambulate are greater concerns for women.[10] Such gender-specific issues must be addressed during post-amputation counseling.

Minimal research has been conducted to determine what qualities are likely to result in a positive adjustment to amputation,[2] although some investigators have reported a philosophical shift in a positive direction.[11-13] Individuals may develop new priorities, focus on more meaningful relationships, gain a new perspective on life, or recognize the value and tenuous nature of physical health. Dunn[14] found that 77% of 138 participants reported that they had experienced a positive aspect of the amputation; those making such reports also exhibited a lower rate of depression. From the cognitive perspective, such reframing also may be operating in those who view themselves as fortunate to be alive and enjoying greater health than others despite their limb loss. Rybarczyk and colleagues[2] indicated that the use of humor, identifying positive aspects of the experience, effective social comparisons and role models, as well as the belief that they are doing well despite the loss of their limb, are effective coping strategies that may contribute to enhanced adjustment subsequent to an amputation.

Factors that generally do not appear to affect adjustment include medical cause of the amputation (eg, vascular disease, traumatic injury, or cancer) and length of time since amputation.[2] It is not altogether true that greater physical impairment caused by the amputation leads to poorer psychological adjustment. Rybarczyk et al[2] conclude, "the degree of impairment, irrespective of other factors, is too simplistic to serve as an important predictor or an individual's overall adjustment." However, the extent to which an individual's activities are restricted by the amputation correlates highly with adjustment.[15] Thus, individuals who were very active prior to the amputation may find that the loss of the limb dramatically impedes their ability to perform many former activities. When those activities are essential to a person's sense of identity and self-worth, the patient may experience greater feelings of demoralization and depression.[2] Other factors that relate to poor adjustment after amputation include little or no previous history of medical problems, the presence of chronic phantom limb pain, marked restriction in activities of daily living, adolescence, enduring concerns about body image, social stigma, and feelings of vulnerability.

MacBride et al[16] reported that approximately 23% of people with amputation characterize the initial period after the amputation as the most distressing time. Many regard the time when they are fitted with a prosthesis as the most psychologically distressful, when confronted with a prosthesis that does not function as well or look as realistic as they had expected.[2]

Depression

After an amputation, many individuals suffer from clinically significant depression, with an estimated 21% to 35% of patients developing depressive symptoms.[6,8,17,18] Studies using standardized self-report measures also indicate that post-amputation clinical depression rates range from 21% to 35%.[1,7] Following amputation, patients should be regularly screened for depression. Rates of postamputation depression are highly variable and depend on the premorbid function, as well as the patient's perceived sense of helplessness. Differentiation between depression, grief reaction, and adjustment disorders is often difficult in the initial phase. Depression necessitates prompt medical and psychological help, whereas grieving is a normal reaction. Pharmacotherapy often is advisable for the adjunctive treatment of depression, and selective serotonin reuptake inhibitors (SSRI) are the first line of antidepressants. Selective serotonin reuptake inhibitors are preferred over the tricyclic antidepressants (TCA), especially in the elderly, as they lack the anticholinergic side effects of TCAs. A therapeutic trial period of 4 to 6 weeks with the antidepressant is necessary to determine its efficacy. Cognitive disorders such as delirium and dementia, which can masquerade as depression in the elderly, should be ruled out.

Rybarczyk et al[2] suggested that individuals with amputations generally have developed a coping style at or about the time they are being fitted with a prosthesis. Assessment for depressive symptomatology and level of adjustment would be most appropriate at that critical time. Cognitive-behavioral interventions implemented at that time and directed towards changing the patient's faulty self-evaluations and perceptions of others may lead to enhanced adjustment to the loss of the limb.

Adequate pain management in the postoperative period facilitates earlier ambulation and an improved mood. Available social support also influences the patient's mood. A study of individuals with complex regional pain syndromes indicated that depressed mood lessened with higher ratings of perceived social support.[19] Therapy also should focus on developing healthier coping strategies.

Rates of depression vary among different populations. A study conducted in Turkey demonstrated the prevalence of depression to be 34.7% in a traumatic group versus 51.4% in a surgical group.[20] These authors attributed the differential levels of depression to the fact that surgical patients were older and had concurrent chronic medical illnesses. Some of them had multiple amputations. Rates of depression also correlated with advanced age, unmarried status, lower education level, and poor economic status. Further, greater functional ability was associated with lower rates of depression.

Anxiety

Mild to moderate anxiety is a normal response to the hospitalization and the amputation procedure itself.[1,21,22] The hospital environment is an anxiety-provoking environment for many individuals. Anxiety is aggravated by a feeling of lack of control. Inflexible coping strategies are often the root of severe anxiety reactions. Symptomatic relief of anxiety may be achieved by intermediate acting benzodiazepines such as lorazepam. At the psychological level, adequate counseling and desensitization to the procedure is often beneficial. Patients should be encouraged to verbalize their feelings, and adequate social support should be provided by family members, caregivers, and/or peers.[23]

Anxiety may develop at any time during the period surrounding the amputation. If the amputation is the result of trauma, patients may experience considerable anxiety as they are hospitalized on an emergent basis and find themselves in an unfamiliar environment. Feelings of anxiety may arise, or be heightened, as the patient develops greater awareness of the loss of the limb and begins to evaluate the immediate and long-term implications of the loss.[23] Frequent interactions with the medical staff, exposure to numerous, sometimes painful, medical procedures, perceived loss of control, and the overwhelming uncertainties regarding their future may elicit profound feelings of anxiety. Anxiety reactions also may be triggered by thoughts about future "mutilation" or by concerns of being separated from loved ones and familiar, comfortable surroundings.[24] Livneh and colleagues[24] found pronounced postamputation anxiety most common among younger individuals who had only recently experienced the amputation and who exhibited higher levels of cognitive disengagement.

Anxiety also may develop during the post-acute period as the individual makes a transition into more normal life routines. For example, as the patients begin to prepare for returning to work and resuming their role in the family, significant feelings of anxiety may arise secondary to concerns and fears generated by the inevitable questions about the impact the amputation might have on their functional abilities. How will the amputation affect the individual's ability to perform essential job functions? How will coworkers and family members respond to the amputation? How will the loss affect one's capacity for sexual expression and intimacy?

If the patient develops or continues to experience depression, concomitant feelings of anxiety are expected.[25] Rybarczyk and colleagues,[16] however, reported that both depression and anxiety tend to decrease with time after the amputation. They also noted that the patient's perceived quality of life similarly improves over time. In contrast, Fisher and Hanspal[26] asserted that time from amputation was not highly associated with anxiety and depression, noting that only a "few patients" reported emotional distress. However, they indicated that anxiety was reported more often that depression. The presence of depression and/or anxiety may influence the amount of amputation limb pain reported by an individual.[27]

Post-Traumatic Stress Disorder

One form of anxiety disorder that also occurs, especially following traumatic amputation, is PTSD. Obviously, in such circumstances, the traumatic event has caused serious injury, and often is accompanied by intense feelings of fear, helplessness, or horror. An acute distress disorder or, more chronically, PTSD may occur, in which the patient persistently re-experiences the traumatic event in the form of intrusive thoughts, flashbacks, or nightmares. In addition, patients with PTSD exhibit intense distress and symptoms of increased autonomic arousal or a sympathomimetic response when reminded of the trauma, and actively avoid those stimuli that evoke thoughts of the event.[23] Post-traumatic stress disorder can develop days to months after the initial event.

Group psychotherapy is often helpful in the treatment of PTSD, where the patient is encouraged to verbally relive the experience. Gradually, the patient is desensitized and can think about the situation without experiencing the distress reaction. Adequate pain control is essential to avoid the precipitation of distress by the noxious stimuli.

Body Image

Emotional problems related to distorted body image and altered perception of the self are frequent in the initial post-amputation period. Patients are often faced with their own mortality as they may view a part of themselves as already "dead." Acceptance of altered body image might be difficult for some due to our society's enormous emphasis on personal appearance.

People commonly define themselves by their physical appearance and disturbance of body image and an inability to cope with the changed body may profoundly affect the individual's psychological status. Those with amputation must contend with three different body images: before the amputation, without a prosthesis and with a prosthesis. Patients often feel incomplete and distressed by their appearance and assume that others have similar perceptions, leading the patient to use avoidance as a defense mechanism.[23] Self and/or social stigmatization are frequent following amputation and play a significant causal role in maladjustment to amputation by enhancing negative body image.[18]

The development of self-stigmatization is characterized by feelings of embarrassment, shame, or revulsion.[18] Rybarczyk and colleagues[8,18] suggested that the self-stigmatization was predictive of depression, lower levels of adjustment (by external raters), and decreased quality of life. These investigators further differentiated self-stigmatization from the "grief over loss of a part of the self" that occurs immediately following the amputation. They noted that self-stigmatization is not uncommon even years after the amputation procedure.[18]

In addition, individuals with amputation may perceive that other people view them as inferior in ways other than the physical loss of a limb.[2] People who feel more stigmatized generally are more likely to be depressed,[18] and the perceived social stigma also culminates in lower levels of adjustment. Although in some studies,[8,18] no relationship between gender and concerns about body image were found, one group of investigators[17] indicated that women are more susceptible to depression than men following amputation.

Difficulty accepting the new body image and perceived social stigma further depends on the patient's sense of vulnerability and defenselessness, thereby leading to increased adjustment problems and decreased quality of life.[28] Many individuals who have undergone an amputation feel more vulnerable and have significantly greater fears of being victimized.[29] The sense that they may be at greater risk for violence or criminal acts can lead to social avoidance, decreased quality of life, and poorer health status.[30,31] Deconditioning, which often occurs after amputation, may lead to a heightened sense of vulnerability.

Despite widespread educational measures, some individuals without disabilities experience inhibition and awkwardness when interacting with a person with a disability, leading to additional challenges for the patient. The sense of vulnerability is similar to other post-traumatic experiences, and should be addressed by assisting patients to develop coping skills, encouraging them to participate in previously avoided activities to enhance the feelings of self-efficacy, and by discussing the issues of damaged body image.

Sexual Functioning

One area that is typically not addressed with patients with amputation is sexual functioning. Primary health care professionals, especially physicians, rarely initiate an open and forthright discussion about the sexual concerns, which may further complicate and confound the problem. Although some professionals are uncomfortable with the topic, others may believe that they lack adequate knowledge to address the patient's sexual issues.

Williamson and Walters[32] found that less than 10% of the patients they evaluated were provided information or opportunities to ask questions about sexual functioning subsequent to amputation, which is characteristic of the neglect of sexuality in health care settings.

Sexual functioning after amputation may be affected by vascular, neurological, physical, and mechanical causes. Vascular and neuropathic problems resulting from chronic disease conditions, such as diabetes and peripheral vascular disease, hinder normal erectile response. The patient might also have positioning problems during the act due to loss of range of motion and balance.[23] Psychological factors may play a significant role in sexual dysfunction following amputation. Psychological sources of erectile dysfunction include depression, altered body image, fear of rejection by the partner, low self-esteem, and performance anxiety.

A study conducted at Houston Veterans Affairs Medical Center explored the effect of amputation on various aspects of sexual behavior.[33] Of 30 men with various levels of lower-limb amputation, 67% reported erectile dysfunction and 19% stated orgasmic problems. Fifty-three percent engaged in sexual intercourse or oral sex at least once a month. Despite problems with the sexual act itself, over 90% of the patients reported interest in sex as "high." Preamputation sexual functioning or spousal input was not obtained in the study.

Health care professionals, especially physicians, should always discuss these issues with the patient; if addressing the patient's concerns is beyond the physician's area of expertise, a referral to a sex therapist or psychologist should be made.

Self-Efficacy

Self-efficacy has a major impact on the individual's coping skills and post-amputation quality of life.[34] By exercising control over one's habits, the patient can modify the lifestyle and reduce or eliminate destructive habits that exacerbate poor health. The individual's coping ability and self-efficacy directly influence the ability to exert control over modifiable health behaviors and environmental variables that affect health status. Self-efficacy underscores the importance of multifaceted strategies that address issues in addition to the physi-

cal or medical components of medicine and focuses on the psychological empowerment of the individual. Three phases of personal change are the adoption of new behavior patterns, their generalized use under different circumstances, and finally, their maintenance over a prolonged period of time. Initiation or adoption is highly dependent on the person's motivation and willingness to change. Similarly, lack of motivation can culminate as detrimental habits. Although the patient's sense of self-efficacy is an inherent attribute, health care professionals can aid by imparting education about the methods of regulating and changing behavior. This process is similar to promotion of disease management for chronic medical conditions.

AGE-RELATED ISSUES

Children and Adolescents

Young children adjust relatively well to the loss of a limb.[35] Some factors that may contribute to the child's positive adjustment to amputation include family cohesion, social support, and low levels of family conflict.[36] Adolescents, in contrast, may experience greater adjustment difficulties, and specifically may be affected adversely by concerns with body image, peer relationships, and their sense of autonomy, independence, and immortality.[37] Walters[38] noted that many adolescents progress through several stages in the process of adjusting to the loss of a limb. Not surprisingly, the initial reactions include anger, depression, and discouragement. As they begin to grieve the loss of the limb, they may withdraw and become more despondent. Ultimately, adolescents usually accept the changes in body appearance and become more inclined to reintegrate within their social system.

Younger Adults

The most common cause of amputation among young adults is trauma secondary to motor vehicle accidents, assault, and industrial accidents. Often, alcohol or drugs are an accompanying factor, resulting in patient guilt that needs to be addressed. Feelings of guilt delay emotional recovery and may be detrimental to the therapeutic alliance. A sense of impotence frequently accompanies the initial emotional response. Post-traumatic stress disorder can follow days to months after any acute traumatic event. Suspicion of PTSD requires thorough evaluation, as the patient may not initiate the topic to avoid painful memories. Traumatic amputations are further complicated psychologically because the patients frequently do not have sufficient time to prepare emotionally for the sudden changes caused by the loss of the limb.

Older Adults

Older adults who undergo amputations are less likely to suffer from adjustment problems.[6,39,40] Factors that may contribute to this response include anticipated greater physical infirmities associated with the aging process, less active lifestyle, and diminished expectations regarding their mastery of their environment.[2]

Amputations among the elderly are most commonly due to effects of chronic conditions such as diabetes and vascular diseases. Cardiac, neurological, renal, and ophthalmic complications of the underlying disease process frequently complicate the clinical picture. Patients usually have concomitant disease processes making medical management challenging. They are often physically deconditioned, thus initiating physical therapy prior to the amputation can have a positive effect on their psychological health, in addition to building stamina. Candid discussion of the rehabilitation process, along with the reassurance that amputation will be a last resort, facilitates the patient's acceptance of the procedure. When possible, adequate time should be provided for the patient to prepare psychologically, as amputation is rarely an acute decision in this population. After the patient has consented, the procedure should be scheduled as early as possible, as waiting aggravates the patient's stress. For similar reasons, rescheduling the procedure is not advisable.[23]

INTERVENTIONS

A well-coordinated, comprehensive multidisciplinary team is the most effective rehabilitation approach to amputation and ideally should incorporate the expertise of a rehabilitation psychologist or counselor. If possible, preamputation counseling should be offered because it may serve to preclude some of the adverse psychological consequences. Open communication regarding emotional recovery, social and sexual adjustments, and the long-term treatment plan is important. Each patient's individual medical condition, along with current strengths, social support, psychiatric illnesses, and coping mechanisms must be considered in the effort to promote positive outcomes and high quality of life following amputation.

Interventions for individuals who have undergone an amputation should focus on normalizing their feelings and experiences.[2] Because amputation has far-reaching psychosocial, vocational, financial, and sexual effects that involve not only the patient, but also his or her family, all should be integrated into the therapeutic process.

This process can be accomplished in the context of a supportive psychotherapeutic relationship or in a group format in which individuals with similar physical conditions meet to share life experiences. Support groups offer the patient and family members an environment in which they can interact with others in a similar situation and, in that format, may find greater meaning in their experience. Bibliotherapy also may prove helpful for those with an amputation. Other potentially helpful interventions include online support groups, peer counselors, and self-monitoring tools (eg, for depression).

A British study[25] supports the beneficial effect of counseling for amputation patients. Counseling focused on the emotional and practical problems related to changes in the patient's ability to perform certain tasks. Those who received counseling during the early post-amputation period reported a positive effect on the practical problems as compared to control patients. Emotional functioning was unaffected in both groups, leading the investigators to conclude that emotional problems may become more apparent at a later stage (6 to 24 months) after amputation.

Brief Psychotherapy

A brief period of psychotherapy may be helpful in facilitating the grieving process and addressing other emotional concerns. In our experience, six to eight sessions are usually approved by third-party payers and in general appear to be sufficient to address reactive emotional symptoms and perceived negative attitudes subsequent to amputation. Most patients and their family members are usually willing to participate in a time-limited therapy program. Discussing psychotherapeutic options with the patient is helpful as it involves the patient in the decision-making process. This provides a sense of control for the patient and facilitates the development of an effective therapeutic alliance.[23] Among the specific techniques that may be helpful are modeling, emotive therapy, relaxation techniques, and behavioral rehearsal.[35] One of the most common, well-documented therapeutic modalities is cognitive behavioral therapy (CBT) based on the cognitive model of Beck.[41]

Cognitive Behavioral Therapy

Cognitive behavioral therapy hypothesizes that it is not events, per se, that influence the patient's emotions and behaviors, but rather the individual's perception of events.[41,42] The primary goal of CBT is to help patients understand how their thinking is related to their feelings and behavior and to teach them how to modify maladaptive cognitive patterns. In so doing, the therapist instructs the patient to identify, evaluate, and replace or modify maladaptive aspects of their cognitions with more positive and realistic thoughts.

In the early stages of CBT, emphasis is placed on eliciting automatic thoughts through imagery and role-playing. Automatic thoughts are quick, evaluative thoughts that are not the result of deliberation or reasoning. They are situation-specific thoughts that reflect core beliefs. Automatic thoughts are conceived to develop so quickly and automatically that the individual is not aware of them, but instead cognizant of the negative feelings and emotions that follow. Automatic thoughts frequently lead to cognitive distortions.[42-45] Two examples of cognitive distortions include all-or-none thinking (also known as black-and-white or dichotomous thinking) and catastrophizing (also known as negative prediction or fortune telling). In all-or-none thinking, the individual views a situation in the form of two categories rather than on a continuum (eg, "Since I lost my leg, I am an incomplete person"). In catastrophizing, the individual predicts a negative future without considering other more likely outcomes (eg, "Without my leg, my boss will not let me go back to work on the assembly line").

In summary, CBT states that when an individual is confronted with a given situation, maladaptive automatic thoughts are activated. The automatic thoughts are typically replete with cognitive distortions and lead to negative thoughts about oneself, the future, and others. Cognitive distortions lead to negative emotions and ultimately serve to reinforce underlying maladaptive schemas and core beliefs.

Pain Management

Three important factors of a patient's perception and reaction to pain are cognition, coping response, and social environment. Jensen et al[46] concluded that psychosocial variables are more important than other variables when accounting for pain and functional recovery following amputation. Catastrophizing is considered the single most important predictor for future pain symptoms. The influence of the environmental and the social responses on the patient's disability follows an operant or behavioral conditioning model. For instance, solicitous responses to pain behaviors are associated with greater perceived disability and higher ratings of pain intensity.[47]

Phantom limb pain (PLP) represents a significant risk factor for poor psychological adjustment following amputation. Unfortunately, PLP affects many people with amputation, with estimates that this subjective experience occurs in 60% to 90% of all such individuals.[1,48-50] Moreover, children also experience PLP, with estimates that more than 80% of children and adolescent patients are affected.[51] Although PLP is commonly reported during the first 6 months after the amputation, many patients have no subsequent relief from the pain and may even experience an exacerbation in PLP over time.[46] Jensen et al[46] noted that if PLP persists, six common interventions include: 1) alterations in the surgical procedures (eg, administration of epidural agents prior to the surgery), 2) psychoeducation, 3) thermal imagery, 4) biofeedback, 5) relaxation therapy, and 6) pharmacological agents (eg, muscle relaxants). Other therapies that have been used to alleviate PLP include sympathetic blocks, prosthetic adjustments, transcutaneous electrical stimulation (TENS), and ultrasound treatments.[2] Physical therapy and occupational therapy can also play an important role in helping the patient reintegrate at a functional level despite the presence of PLP. Cognitive behavioral therapy has also been used in treating chronic PLP.[52] Comprehensive discussion of pain is found in Chapter 4.

Biofeedback and Relaxation Training

Biofeedback and relaxation training are the two techniques that have been demonstrated to be the most effective psychological interventions for the management of chronic pain.[53] Biofeedback is a procedure in which a patient's physiological responses (muscle tension, skin temperature, heart rate, etc) are monitored and reflected to the patient instantaneously. Such immediate feedback allows the therapist and patient to collaborate on techniques to control the patient's bodily responses and, as a result, lower the experience of pain by reducing the level of arousal. Techniques that are commonly used to achieve the desired physiological changes include diaphragmatic breathing, passive neuromuscular relaxation, guided imagery, and cognitive restructuring. As the patient becomes more adept at incorporating these skills, the therapist becomes gradually less involved until the patient is ultimately capable of achieving the desired result independently.

A small body of research also demonstrates the positive effect of hypnotic interventions in patients with amputation. McGarry[54] described a patient with an index finger amputation where hypnosis was successfully used to eliminate pain, overcome phantom sensations, maximize white blood cell flow to the area to prevent wound infection, optimize wound healing, promote reorganization of the neurosensory cortex, and deal with the altered self-image.

Group Interventions

Group participation may be especially helpful, and multidimensional interventions within the group also may promote greater coping skills and enhanced self-management. Some elements of this type of group treatment include psychoeducation, relaxation therapy, CBT (for anxiety and depression), problem-solving, and communication, which may yield important benefits.[2] Other group topics may include nutrition, sleep, and exercise.

Peer networks for people with amputation consist of rehabilitated individuals who are linked through one or more organizations. Peer support groups serve to provide emotional and educational support to new patients and their families. The preferable mode of contact is face-to-face, although it may also be through telephone, electronic mail, fax, or regular mail. Peer support is beneficial for patients of all age groups. The following comments by Larry, 25 years post-transtibial amputation of the left leg, highlight how a peer support network works:

> It was March 8, 1977, my 33rd birthday. I had given the orthopedic surgeon permission to amputate my injured left leg below the knee on the following day.
>
> March 9, 1977, would be a day that would change my life forever. All kinds of questions were buzzing through my head: Would I be too disabled to provide a living for my family? Would I be confined to a life on crutches? Would I be able to play with my kids? Would I be enough of a man to satisfy my wife? The medical people couldn't—or wouldn't—completely answer the myriad of questions I had. In the seventies, there were no support groups to call. The only person I could think to contact was a former co-worker who had lost his arm in an accident.
>
> That was 25 years and a half-dozen artificial legs ago. It is amazing how much technological progress has been made in prosthetics since then. My first leg, which looked like a plastic doll's appendage, attached to my hips with some uncomfortable straps. By the middle eighties, I was jogging, swimming and bicycling on an energy-loaded Flex Foot. I FELT LIKE SUPERMAN! I WAS ABLE TO LEAP TALL BUSHES IN A SINGLE BOUND! Well, perhaps I'm exaggerating a bit, but I was so elated with this newfound freedom I wanted to shout it with the world. I had discovered my potential! Twenty-five years ago, I was ready to resign myself to the fact that my life, at best, might be nothing more than a mere existence.
>
> In the early 90s, I answered an ad in the paper. Someone was wanting to start an amputee support group. We named the group SAFRA (Support Alliance For Recovering Amputees). The group meets quarterly at a local hospital with sponsorship from a rehab group. SAFRA members visit new amputees in the hospitals, as well as provide strength, hope, and inspiration for other members at the meetings. I have discovered that we all have different levels of achievement. Diabetics may not become joggers, but, chances are, with a healthy lifestyle, they won't be confined to a life in a wheelchair.
>
> My advice to new amputees is that they will feel overwhelmed initially. They should not close themselves off to the world. In addition to the rehabilitation care they receive in the hospital, they should seek out support from family, friends, will receive valuable advice and understanding from people who will have true empathy and encourage them to live life to their full potential. The choice is theirs… they can be overwhelmed or be strong.

Family Responses and Support

Amputation affects not only the patient, but also the entire family. This effect is more pronounced if the patient is the major financial provider. The dynamics of the family change as the patient tries to cope with disability and the caregivers adapt to their new responsibilities. Some people with amputation may perceive themselves as failures as they deal with altered body image and the perceived or real inability to fulfill financial and social obligations. As already noted, amputation also affects the patient's sexual function, thus placing a greater strain on marital relationships. Family counseling is often helpful, and family members should be aware and sensitive of the grieving process, helplessness, and frustration experienced by the patient.

Mind/Body/Spirit Connection

Fitchett et al[55] observed a strong correlation between religiosity/spirituality and positive adjustment following amputation. Although there was little evidence that such correlations held over time, a positive relationship existed between counselors who inquired about these values and the perceived helpfulness of the therapy.

Although medicine predominantly deals with the patient at the physical level, an increasing body of evidence demonstrates the profound influence of thoughts and attitudes on physical functioning. The efficacy of placebo medications in a variety of settings underscores the significant influence of mind on physical functions. Gallagher and MacLachlan[56] indicated that patients who have a positive attitude toward the amputation in terms of its character-building effect, improved coping abilities, financial benefits, change of attitude, or meeting new people, have a significantly higher rating of their health and physical capabilities ($P<0.008$) than patients who were pessimistic about the event. These observations point to the fact that changing the patient's mental perception can result in a sustainable positive outcome.

Advocacy Groups/Web-Based Education

Amputee Coalition of America

Amputee Coalition of America (ACA) is a national, not-for-profit consumer education organization founded in 1989 for people with amputation and those born with limb defects. The coalition consists of support groups for amputees and their family members. Membership consists of individuals, organizations, health care professionals, and family members. ACA focuses on imparting education to empower members to enable them to participate actively in the decision-making process regarding their health care. The coalition also serves as an advocate for people with amputations and is involved in legislation reviews and identification of new policy issues.

Internet-Based Support and Education Resources

The Internet is rapidly becoming an effective means of education and resources for patients with chronic or acute problems. Some of the prominent Internet-based resources for patients with amputation include the ACA (http://www.amputee-coalition.org), Landmine survivors network (http://www.landminesurvivors.org), and the Amputee Resource Center (http://www.usinter.net/wasa/arc.html). These sites have educational material helpful for patients and their caregivers. The resources also include peer visitation networks and other helpful links.

CONCLUSION

The psychological effects of amputation are individualized and highly variable, ranging from uncomplicated grief responses to adjustment reactions to depression and anxiety disorders including PTSD. Emotional consequences depend on a myriad of variables such as age, gender, level of maturity, premorbid personality traits, sense of self-efficacy, internal and external coping mechanisms, flexibility, available social support, coexisting medical conditions, pain tolerance, and whether the amputation was planned or sudden. Poor psychological adjustment has been associated with significant restriction of activities, and persistent body image or social stigma. Positive emotional adjustment often correlates with the individual's perception of the extent of the disability, development of new priorities, a renewed focus on meaningful relationships, and development of a new perspective on life. Other favorable coping responses that facilitate positive adjustment after amputation include identifying positive aspects of life, maintaining a sense of humor, and interacting with positive role models.

A well-coordinated, comprehensive multidisciplinary team is the most effective rehabilitation approach to amputation and ideally should incorporate the expertise of a rehabilitation psychologist or counselor. The individual and family members should be core members of this team process. Psychological and community-based interventions that have demonstrated effectiveness with this population are brief psychotherapy, CBT, pain management, advocacy/peer groups, and family support. Therapeutic interventions should focus on the negative emotional sequelae (eg, anxiety and depression) associated with the amputation and chronic pain (if present), as well as the patient's adjustment to the altered circumstances. The treatment team also should be cognizant of the needs of the family members and address them as appropriate. The multidisciplinary team format is ideally suited to address the physical, psychological, social, and occupational issues that might arise during the process of rehabilitation and reintegration into society.

Individuals with disabilities such as amputation are assuming a much more proactive role in the maintenance of their health care, and psychologists and rehabilitation counselors may serve as a conduit to make these individuals aware of community resources and information. The advent of the Internet has led to greater consumer empowerment. Consumers are more educated and aware of their rights as compared to their counterparts a decade ago. With the active participation of consumers, insurance companies and case management techniques have brought disease management to the forefront. Consumers have become equal partners with health care professionals, and decisions about health care ideally are made mutually, rather than by the more traditional medical model in which the physician dominated these interactions. These concepts gain added importance for chronic problems including amputation. This trend will continue to advance as consumers educate themselves further and assume more active roles, acting in collaborating with their health care providers to make decisions that will be most personally empowering.

REFERENCES

1. Shukla GD, Sahu SC, Tripathi RP, Gupta DK. A psychiatric study of amputees. *Br J Psychiatry.* 1982;141:50-53.

2. Rybarczyk B, Szymanski L, Nicholas JJ. Limb amputation. In: Frank RG, Elliott TR, eds. *Handbook of Rehabilitation Psychology.* Washington, DC: American Psychological Association; 2000:29-47.

3. Gallagher P, MacLachlan M. Psychological adjustment and coping in adults with prosthetic limbs. *Behav Med.* 1999;25:117-124.

4. Cheung E, Alvaro R, Colotla VA. Psychological distress in workers with traumatic upper or lower limb amputations following industrial injuries. *Rehabilitation Psychology.* 2003;248:109-112.

5. Bhojak MM, Nathawat SS, Swami DR. Psychological consequences following lower limb amputation. *Indian Journal of Clinical Psychology.* 1989;16:102-104.

6. Williamson GM, Schulz R, Bridges MW, Behan AM. Social and psychological factors in adjustment to limb amputation. *Journal of Social Behavior and Personality.* 1994;9:249-268.

7. Frank RG, Kashani JH, Kashani SR, et al. Depression among amputees. *J Clin Psychiatry.* 1983;44:256-258.

8. Rybarczyk BD, Nyenhuis DL, Nicholas JJ, et al. Social discomfort and depression in a sample of adults with leg amputations. *Arch Phys Med Rehabil.* 1992;73:1169-1173.

9. Kubler-Ross E. *On Death and Dying.* New York, NY; Simon & Schuster Adult Publishing Group; 1997.

10. Legro MW, Reiber G, del Aguila M, et al. Issues of importance reported by persons with lower limb amputations and prostheses. *J Rehabil Res Dev.* 1999;36:155-163.

11. Keany KC, Glueckauf RL. Disability and value change: an overview and reanalysis of acceptance of loss theory. *Rehabilitation Psychology.* 1993;38:199-210.

12. Taylor SE. Adjustment to threatening events: a theory of cognitive adaptation. *Am Psychol*. 1983;38:1161-1173.

13. Taylor SE. Psychosocial factors in the course of disease. Paper presented at: Annual Meeting of the Society for Behavioral Medicine; 1997; San Francisco, Calif.

14. Dunn DS. Well-being following amputation: salutary effects of positive meaning, optimism, and control. *Rehabilitation Psychology*. 1997;41:285-302.

15. Radloff LS. The CES-D scale: a self-report depression scale for research in the general population. *Applied Psychological Measurement*. 1977;1:385-401.

16. MacBride A, Rogers J, Whylie B, Freeman SJ. Psychosocial factors in the rehabilitation of elderly amputees. *Psychosomatics*. 1980;21:258-265.

17. Kashani JH, Frank RG, Kashani SR, et al. Depression among amputees. *J Clin Psychiatry*. 1983;44:256-258.

18. Rybarczyk B, Nyenhuis DL, Nicholas JJ, et al. Body image, perceived social stigma, and the prediction of psychosocial adjustment to leg amputation. *Rehabilitation Psychology*. 1995;40:95-110.

19. Feldman SI, Downey G, Schaffer-Neitz R. Pain, negative mood, and perceived support in chronic pain patients: a daily diary study of people with reflex sympathetic dystrophy syndrome. *J Consult Clin Psychol*. 1999;67:776-785.

20. Cansever A, Uzun O, Yildiz C, et al. Depression in men with traumatic lower part amputation: a comparison to men with surgical lower part amputation. *Mil Med*. 2003;168:106-109.

21. Schubert DS, Burns R, Paras W, Sioson E. Decrease of depression during stroke and amputee rehabilitation. *Gen Hosp Psychiatry*. 1992;14:133-141.

22. Marshall M, Helmes E, Deathe AB. A comparison of psychosocial functioning and personality in amputee and chronic pain populations. *Clin J Pain*. 1992;8:351-357.

23. Fitzpatrick MC. The psychological assessment and psychosocial recovery of the patient with an amputation. *Clin Orthop*. 1999;361:98-107.

24. Livneh H, Antonak RF, Gerhardt J. Psychosocial adaptation to amputation: the role of sociodemographic variables, disability-related factors and coping strategies. *Int J Rehabil Res*. 1999;22:21-31.

25. Price EM, Fisher K. How does counseling help people with amputation? *Journal of Prosthetics and Orthotics*. 2002;14:102-106.

26. Fisher K, Hanspal RS. Phantom pain, anxiety, depression, and their relation in consecutive patients with amputated limbs: case reports. *BMJ*. 1992;316:903-904.

27. Sriwatanakul K, Kelvie W, Lasagna L. The quantification of pain: an analysis of words used to describe pain and analgesia in clinical trials. *Clin Pharmacol Ther*. 1982;32:143-148.

28. Behel JM, Rybarczyk B, Elliott TR, et al. The role of perceived vulnerability in adjustment to lower extremity amputation: a preliminary investigation. *Rehabilitation Psychology*. 2002;47:92-105.

29. Goodwin LR, Holmes GE. Counseling the crime victim: a guide for rehabilitation counselors. *Journal of Applied Rehabilitation Counseling*. 1988;19:42-47.

30. Ross CE. Fear of victimization and health. *Journal of Quantitative Criminology and Health*. 1993;9:159-175.

31. Williamson GM, Schulz R. Activity restriction mediates the association between pain and depressed affect: a study of younger and older adult cancer patients. *Psychol Aging*. 1995;10:369-378.

32. Williamson GM, Walters AS. Perceived impact of limb amputation on sexual activity: a study of adult amputees. *J Sex Res*. 1996;33:221-230.

33. Bodenheimer C, Kerrigan AJ, Garber SL, Monga TN. Sexuality in persons with lower extremity amputations. *Disabil Rehabil*. 2000;22:409-415.

34. Bandura A. *Self-Efficacy: The Exercise of Control*. New York, NY: W.H. Freeman and Company; 1997.

35. Atala KD, Carter BD. Pediatric limb amputation: aspects of coping and psychotherapeutic intervention. *Child Psychiatry Hum Dev*. 1992;23:117-130.

36. Tyc VL. Psychosocial adaptation of children and adolescents with limb deficiencies: a review. *Clin Psychol Rev*. 1992;12:275-291.

37. Tebbi CK, Mallon JC. Long-term psychosocial outcome among cancer amputees in adolescence and early adulthood. *Journal of Psychosocial Oncology*. 1987;5:69-82.

38. Walters J. Coping with a leg amputation. *Am J Nurs*. 1981; 81:1349-1352.

39. Dunn DS. Positive meaning and illusion following disability: reality negotiation, normative interpretation, and value change. *Journal of Social Behavior and Personality*. 1994;9:123-138.

40. Frank RG, Kashani JH, Kashani SR, et al. Psychological response to amputation as a function of age and time since amputation. *Br J Psychiatry*. 1984;144:493-497.

41. Beck AT. Thinking and depression, II: theory and therapy. *Arch Gen Psychiatry*. 1964;10:561-571.

42. Beck JS. *Cognitive Therapy: Basics and Beyond*. New York, NY: Guilford Press; 1995.

43. Beck AT. *Depression: Cause and Treatment*. Philadelphia, Pa: University of Pennsylvania Press; 1967.

44. Beck AT, Rush AJ, Shaw BF, Emery G. *Cognitive Therapy of Depression*. New York, NY: Guilford Press; 1979.

45. Haaga DA, Dyck MJ, Ernst D. Empirical status of cognitive theory of depression. *Psychol Bull*. 1991;110:215-236.

46. Jensen TS, Krebs B, Nielsen J, Rasmussen P. Immediate and long-term phantom limb pain in amputees: incidence, clinical characteristics, and relationship to preamputation limb pain. *Pain*. 1985;21:267-278.

47. Romano JM, Turner JA, Jensen MP, et al. Chronic pain patient-spouse behavioral interactions predict patient disability. *Pain*. 1995;63:353-360.

48. Buchanan DC, Mandel AR. The prevalence of phantom limb experiences in amputees. *Rehabilitation Psychology*. 1986;31:183-188.

49. Sherman R, Sherman C. Prevalence and characteristics of chronic phantom limb pain among American veterans: results of a trial survey. *Am J Phys Med*. 1983;62:227-238.

50. Winchell E. *Coping with Limb Loss*. Garden City Park, NY: Avery; 1995.

51. Krane EJ, Heller LB. The prevalence of phantom sensation and pain in pediatric amputees. *J Pain Symptom Manage*. 1995;10:21-29.

52. Caudill M. *Managing Pain Before It Manages You*. New York, NY: Guilford Press; 1999.

53. Craig KD, Weiss SM, eds. *Health Enhancement, Disease Prevention, and Early Intervention: Biobehavioral Strategies*. New York, NY: Springer; 1990.

54. McGarry J. Hypnotic interventions in psychological and physiological aspects of amputation. *Australian Journal of Clinical Hypnotherapy and Hypnosis*. 1993;14:7-12.

55. Fitchett G, Rybarczyk B, DeMarco G, Nicholas JJ. The role of religion in medical rehabilitation outcomes: a longitudinal study. *Rehabilitation Psychology*. 1999;44:333-353.

56. Gallagher P, MacLachlan M. Positive meaning in amputation and thoughts about the amputated limb. *Prosthet Orthot Int*. 2000;24:196-204.

Section II

Rehabilitation of Adults With Lower-Limb Amputations

Chapter 7

Partial Foot and Syme's Amputations and Prosthetic Designs

Lawrence R. Lange, CPO, FAAOP

OBJECTIVES

1. Discuss the benefits and detriments of partial foot and Syme's level amputations
2. Differentiate among the most common levels of partial foot and ankle disarticulation amputations
3. Discuss the loss of function at each amputation level and the most common types of prostheses for each level

INTRODUCTION

Recent advances in diagnostic methods for determining circulatory status, and improved vascular surgery, have increased the quantity and quality of distal limb amputations with fewer complications and greater survival. The rate of amputation in developed countries is 1.55 of every 1000 individuals.[1] In the United States, this amounts to approximately 387,500 patients. Lower-limb amputation accounts for nearly 92% of all procedures. An average 133,235 limb-loss–related hospital discharges occur each year. Although traumatic and malignancy-related amputations decreased from 1988 to 1996, dysvascular amputations rose 3% annually during the same period. Of this group, 97% underwent lower-limb amputations, and of these, 42.8% involved amputations from the toe(s) to the ankle. As the population of individuals over age 50 years increases, more people can be expected to undergo amputation. After age 50, the major cause of amputation is vascular disease with and without coexisting diabetes mellitus. With improvements in vascular disease treatment, transtibial and higher amputations have become less prevalent, whereas partial foot amputations have increased. Because of this, more health care professionals will treat patients with distal amputations. Knowing the advantages and disadvantages of various distal amputation levels and their prostheses will enable clinicians to provide optimum care.

BENEFITS AND DISADVANTAGES OF DISTAL AMPUTATIONS

The primary rationale for performing an amputation at any level is to provide the patient with a residual limb that will allow the best function. As compared with higher amputations, distal levels are generally associated with improved appearance, energy conservation, and better function. Preservation of joints and their accompanying muscular, ligamentous, and tendonous attachments contributes to more normal gait and therefore fewer pathomechanical aberrations.

Healthy individuals with traumatic amputations generally perform better than those with vascular or other systemic disease. Adequate soft tissue coverage over the distal end of the limb, overall condition of the residual limb, and appropriate prosthetic or orthotic devices are requisite in achieving reasonable recovery of function. Surgery performed without consideration to muscular balance will result in a suboptimal outcome. Concern must also include the patient's housing, finances, family support, and occupation. The individual's cognitive and physical ability also contributes to the success of rehabilitation. It serves no purpose to provide a patient with a device that he or she can not don or will not wear.

Although retaining some portion of the foot creates a residual limb that does not require a prosthesis for minimum ambulation, such ambulation is less than optimal. Bare limb ambulation can suffice for short distances. Distal amputations are easily disguised both by the prosthesis and the more normal gait associated with increased function and less energy consumption.

The most common detriment to distal amputation involves the risk of skin breakdown on the altered foot, particularly among patients with vascular disease. Ulceration also occurs among some otherwise healthy individuals. The manifold causes of ulceration include sensory deficits, dysvascular status, lack of adequate soft tissue coverage, and muscular imbalance. The rehabilitation team should anticipate the risk of breakdown when considering prosthetic treatment for each individual.

Foot length discrepancy in unilateral distal amputation reduces prosthetic options. Footwear modifications may be cosmetically unacceptable to the patient. Consequently, the plantar portion of the prosthesis should be as thin as possible. Components, especially prosthetic feet, suitable for more proximal levels of amputation can not be used at distal levels. Compromises between function and appearance are common.

DIGIT OR PARTIAL DIGIT AMPUTATIONS

Prior to determining the amputation level for a patient, the medical team will use instruments and tests including the Doppler ultrasound flow meter to determine the tissue viability.[2] The surgical credo is to retain as much length as possible. Thus, single digit amputations are frequently seen. Although the amputation of any small toe usually has little effect on gait, loss of the great toe interferes appreciably with terminal stance. Nevertheless, most people who have single digit amputation forego the use of a prosthesis (Figure 7-1). If abnormal gait is a concern, a rigid footplate with a rocker bottom shoe sole substitutes adequately for loss of late stance function.[3] The footplate should also have a longitudinal arch support to compensate for the loss of one or more insertions of the plantar fascia, which normally supports the arch. If the amputation resulted from neuropathy, a custom-molded foot orthosis/prosthesis with a resilient top layer reduces plantar pressure and distributes weight-bearing force over the maximum area. Amputation of two or more digits diminishes the weight-bearing area, making the use of a footplate with resilient top surface essential. The shoe insert includes a toe filler, which is a soft material sculpted to replace the length and width of the missing digits. With the insert,

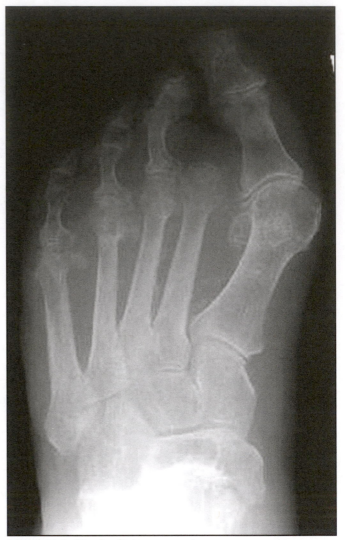

Figure 7-1. Single digit amputation.

the patient can wear most types of footwear. In the absence of neuropathy, the patient can ambulate with or without shoes. If the foot has poor tactile sensation, however, wearing properly fitted shoes is essential to protect the foot from plantar trauma and stubbing the forefoot. The insensate foot is at higher risk of recurrent ulceration; the rate of reoperation reaches 53.8% of adults with partial foot amputations.[4]

SINGLE AND MULTIPLE RAY AMPUTATIONS

Although trauma contributes to this level of amputation, it is most commonly seen in dysvascular feet. A ray amputation is the removal of both the toe and its metatarsal. It is possible to use a custom-molded foot orthosis/prosthesis with filler to recreate the missing volume of the foot. Whether the missing ray is in the

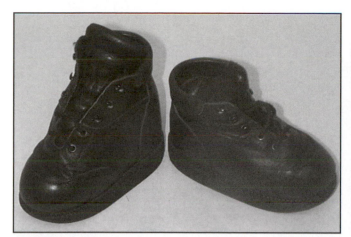

Figure 7-2. Custom molded shoes.

center of the foot or on the medial or lateral borders, the critical issue is mediolateral balance of the forefoot. Single first or fifth ray amputations usually function best with a reported 80% success in diabetic patients.[5,6] In contrast, multiple central ray amputations do not function as well[7]; they increase pressure on the borders of the foot and are usually accommodated by the patient's adoption of a wide stance base. Shoes with flexible soles, such as canvas tennis shoes, are undesirable because they do not support the narrow foot well. Sometimes, custom-molded shoes (Figure 7-2) are prescribed. Patients with ray amputation are more difficult to treat than those with other partial foot amputations.

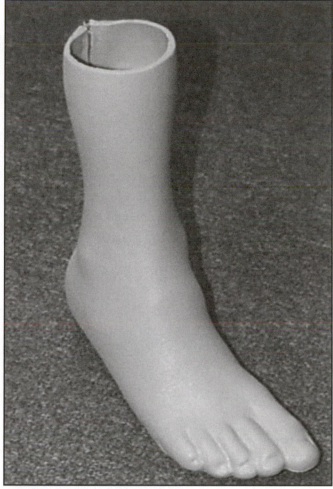

Figure 7-3. Foot prosthesis.

TRANSMETATARSAL AMPUTATIONS

Transmetatarsal amputation involves diaphyseal amputation through the five metatarsals. The relatively thin bony fragments apply considerable force against the distal skin closure during the late stance phase of gait. The suture is usually on the anterodorsal aspect of the amputation limb with little soft tissue padding. A healed transmetatarsal amputation, nevertheless, provides the prosthetist/orthotist with the opportunity to provide a device that is both functional and cosmetic.

Prostheses are of two basic types: either an insert fitted to the shoe or a socket fitted to the patient. The former is the foundation of an ankle-foot orthosis that may or may not be custom molded and will include a toe filler. This modified orthosis requires that the patient use a shoe that closes high on the dorsum of the foot, with either laces or hook and pile straps; a high quarter shoe, which extends over the malleoli, is particularly suitable. The appliance is usually made of semi-rigid plastic, which extends the lever arm proximally beyond the missing portion of the foot. Because it is not physically attached to the foot, the patient is likely to slide

on the device. Sliding can cause discomfort and may lead to reulceration and further surgery. The high shoe reduces motion between the foot and the appliance. Because of the type of footwear and the appliance, this type of transmetatarsal fitting is not as cosmetic as the alternative treatment.

The other type of transmetatarsal device is a socket fitted to the foot. Several designs[8-10] (Figures 7-3 and 7-4) are fabricated from a plaster mold of the residual limb. The socket can be made of silicone, polyurethane, thermosetting or thermoplastic plastics, leather, or a combination of these materials.[9] If the amputation is traumatic, the socket aligns the foot normally; if the insensate foot presents abnormal alignment, the socket accommodates the deformity. All sockets are made to fit intimately with the remaining foot while allowing full tibiotalar and some subtalar joint motion. The socket is attached to a semirigid foot plate with a toe filler. The prosthesis enables the patient to have good appearance, wear ordinary shoes, and have a virtually normal gait.

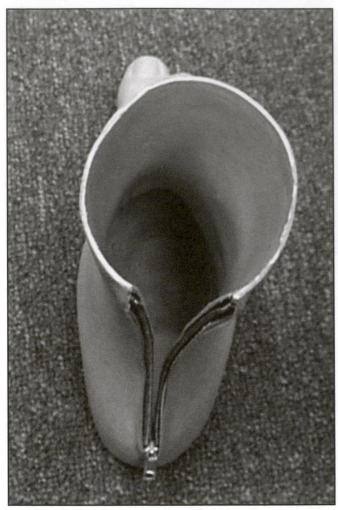

Figure 7-4. Foot prosthesis.

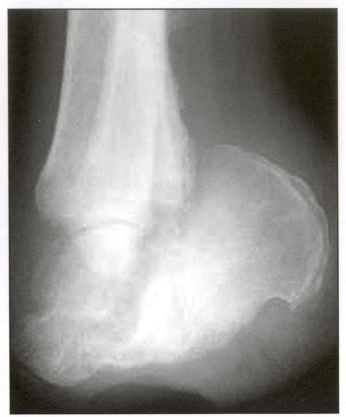

Figure 7-5. Chopart amputation.

LISFRANC AMPUTATION

First described by Jacques Lisfranc in 1815, this amputation is a disarticulation of the tarsometatarsal joints.[10] The operative site ordinarily has minimal bleeding; however, the foot is likely to develop equinus contracture because the normal insertions of the toe extensors and dorsiflexors are lost. Failed Lisfranc amputation is difficult to be salvaged to the Syme level amputation[11] and is usually revised to the transtibial level.

The moderately active patient would probably have to wear an appliance in a shoe that extends above the ankle to retain the prosthesis during swing phase and to distribute stance phase forces over an adequately large surface.[12,13] However, if activity is limited, a prosthesis with a more distal trimline may suffice.[14,15] The distal end of the socket should have a resilient liner to protect the amputation limb from high pressure concentration at this bony area. A rigid prosthesis enables the person to ambulate most effectively. Although one can bear

weight through the bare residual foot, provision for rollover in ambulation is lacking. It is difficult to produce a lightweight yet sufficiently sturdy prosthesis that restricts ankle motion to facilitate stance phase.[16,17] A carbon fiber reinforced footplate resists toe-off forces. The toe extension should be rigid to control dorsiflexion and plantarflexion during mid and late stance; otherwise, the limb would move against the socket, creating intolerable pressure with risk of skin breakdown. The shoe needs a rocker sole to improve mid and late stance.[18,19] Because the bare legs are the same length, adding a prosthesis to the amputated side creates a length discrepancy. Thus, the contralateral shoe should have a lift to equalize leg length. Patients with Lisfranc amputation should not walk in barefeet, particularly if the amputation was caused by vascular disease; the relatively small foot area subjects the remaining foot to high pressure.

CHOPART AMPUTATION

This procedure is named after Francois Chopart, a French physician. His disciple, Lafitteau, first described the procedure in 1792.[10] Chopart's amputation is a disarticulation at the midtarsal joint through the talonavicular and calcaneocuboid joints[20] (Figure 7-5). As with the Lisfranc amputation, muscular imbalance

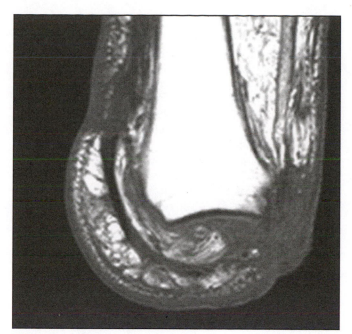

Figure 7-6. Syme's amputation.

causes the limb to develop equinus deformity and thus exposes the anterodistal end to excessive pressure. Achilles tendon lengthening prevents equinus from occurring.[21] The shoe insert with footplate and toe filler, shoe sole, and contralateral shoe sole resemble that recommended for Lisfranc amputation. Similarly, the patient should avoid barefoot walking.

SYME'S AMPUTATION

James Syme reported this level of amputation in 1842. Prior to the widespread use of anesthesia and antibiotics, foot disarticulation was preferred to diaphyseal amputation because mortality and morbidity were less if the cartilage was not disturbed and the surgery was swift.[2] Syme described a procedure for amputating the distal tibia and fibula through the distal cortical bone and retaining the heel fat pad to enhance end bearing. The heel pad must be secured to the distal end (Figure 7-6). Otherwise, distal end bearing is compromised and the major benefit of choosing this level over a transtibial amputation is nullified.

Although the amputation limb is appreciably shorter than the contralateral intact limb, the patient can ambulate without a prosthesis for short distances, assuming the absence of vascular disease, a healed amputation wound, distal bones sectioned parallel with the floor, and a well-secured fat pad. The leg-length discrepancy allows the prosthetist several choices in prosthetic feet, including a SACH (Solid Ankle Cushion Heel) foot, as well as a carbon reinforced foot with energy storing capabilities, which facilitates an excellent gait.[2] Feet

for Syme's prostheses are specifically designed for this purpose, and differ from feet intended for prostheses for more proximal amputation levels.

As with the Chopart prosthesis, the connection between the socket and the foot must be rigid.[2] The proximal trimline of the socket usually lies below the tibial tuberosity. If, however, the patient cannot tolerate full end bearing, the socket may extend more proximally, resembling a transtibial socket. Three basic designs for the mid and distal socket are used—the Canadian Syme, bladder-type Syme, and rigid socket with soft insert. The Canadian socket has a "window" used for donning and doffing purposes. The window is a rigid medial panel with hook and pile closures or zipper, which allows the bulbous end of the amputated limb to pass through to the bottom of the socket. The bulbous end provides suspension and rotational control of the prosthesis. The bladder-type socket usually does not have a window. It has a flexible silicone or polyurethane bladder with or without inflation, which aids suspension. A rigid socket with soft insert also does not have a window. It is shaped to conform to the contour of the malleoli to provide suspension.

The limb is difficult to fit if end bearing is intolerable. The range of alignment is limited. If the limb has a bulbous distal end, the prosthesis presents a rather thick ankle. The socket is difficult to adjust to accommodate soft tissue atrophy. Nevertheless, gait with a well-healed and properly fitted Syme's prosthesis is more satisfactory in appearance and efficiency than that with higher amputations.

REFERENCES

1. Dillingham TR, Pezzin LE, MacKenzie EJ. Limb amputation and limb deficiency: epidemiology and recent trends in the United States. *South Med J.* 2002;95:875-883.

2. Bowker JH. Amputations and disarticulations within the foot. In: Smith DG, Michaels JW, Bowker JH, eds. *Atlas of Limb Prosthetics: Surgical, Prosthetic, and Rehabilitation Principles.* 3rd ed. Rosemont, Ill: American Academy of Orthopaedic Surgeons; 2004:429-448.

3. Tang SF, Chen CP, Chen MJ, et al. Transmetatarsal amputation prosthesis with carbon-fiber plate: enhanced gait function. *Am J Phys Med Rehabil.* 2004;83:124-130.

4. Santi MD, Thomas BJ, Chambers RB. Survivorship of healed partial foot amputations in dysvascular patients. *Clin Orthop.* 1993;292:245-249.

5. Duke Orthopaedics. Foot and ankle amputation. In: *Wheeless' Textbook of Orthopaedics*; 1996. Available at http://www.wheellessonline.com/o13/50.htm

6. Dalla Paola L, Faglia E, Caminiti M, et al. Ulcer recurrences following first ray amputation in diabetic patients: a cohort prospective study. *Diabetes Care.* 2003;26:1874-1878.

7. Orthoteers. Amputation about the foot and ankle. Fellow of the Royal College of Surgeons, Trauma and Orthopedic Examination; 2004. Available at: http://www.orthoteers.co.uk/Nrupj~ij33lm/Orthfootamput.htm.

8. Lange LR. The Lange silicone partial foot prosthesis. *Journal of Prosthetics and Orthotics.* 1995;7:619-625.

9. Soderberg B, Wykman A, Schaarschuch R, Persson BM. Partial foot amputations, guidelines to prosthetic and surgical techniques. *Swedish Orthopaedic Association's Publication Series.* 2001;13:35-42.

10. Soderberg B, Wykman A, Schaarschuch R, Persson BM. Partial foot amputations, guidelines to prosthetic and surgical techniques. *Swedish Orthopaedic Association's Publication Series.* 2001;13:12-15.

12. Soderberg B, Wykman A, Schaarschuch R, Persson BM. Partial foot amputations, guidelines to prosthetic and surgical techniques. *Swedish Orthopaedic Association's Publication Series.* 2001;13:43-49.

13. Michael JW. Forefoot, toe amputations and prostheses: the quest to restore normal ambulation. *O&P Business News.* May 1, 2003.

14. Fillauer K. A prosthesis for foot amputation near the tarsal-metatarsal junction. *Journal of American Orthotic and Prosthetic Association.* 1980; 87-89.

15. Clark MW, Rosenberger R. Low-profile partial foot prosthesis. *J Assoc Children's Prosthet-Orthot Clin.* 1986;21:27.

17. Soderberg B, Wykman A, Schaarschuch R, Persson BM. Partial Foot Amputations, Guidelines to Prosthetic and Surgical Techniques. *Swedish Orthopaedic Association's Publication Series.* 2001;13:51-59.

18. Cohen-Sobel E, Caselli MA, Rizzuto J. Prosthetic management of a Chopart amputation variant. *J Am Podiatr Med Assoc.* 1994;84:505-510.

19. Sobel E, Japour CJ, Giorgini RJ, et al. Use of prostheses and footwear in 110 inner-city partial-foot amputees. *J Am Podiatr Med Assoc.* 2001;91:34-49.

21. Taranto M. Forefoot amputations. In: *Podiatry Encyclopedia.* Department of Podiatry, Curtin University of Technology; 2001. Available at: http://podiatry.curtin.edu.au/encyclopedia/amputation/content.html.

Chapter 8

Transtibial Prosthetic Designs

Kevin Carroll, MS, CP, FAAOP and Katherine Binder, CP

OBJECTIVES

1. Contrast immediate, temporary, and definitive prostheses
2. Discuss the different kinds of transtibial socket designs and modes of prosthetic suspension
3. Identify other components for the transtibial prosthesis
4. Describe the functional levels defined by Medicare applicable to all levels of unilateral lower-limb amputation

INTRODUCTION

The loss of a limb is a devastating experience under any circumstance. Patients must endure the emotional process of loss, grief, depression, and acceptance as described in Chapter 6. Some people feel they are now less than a "whole" person. Functionally, the person with transtibial (TT) amputation retains the all-important knee joint. The bones and muscles that extend below the knee provide good support for the prosthetic socket. The journey from new patient to active prosthetic user takes many months of healing and strengthening the body and opening the mind to a new way of living.

More than two-thirds of the those who experience a lower-extremity amputation this year will be older adults.[1] Peripheral vascular disease, with or without diabetes, is the primary cause; the second most common cause is trauma. Older adults usually face more challenges as they recover from amputation and learn to use a prosthesis. They often have complicated health problems, are physically weaker, and have reduced cardiac function. The skin on the residual limb is more delicate than that of a younger person and can be injured more easily, particularly in the presence of the relatively bony TT residual limb. If the older patient sustains trauma to the skin, it takes considerably longer for the wound to heal (Figure 8-1).

IMMEDIATE AND TEMPORARY PROSTHESES

An immediate postoperative prosthesis (IPOP) is a prosthesis applied in the operating room or during the first few days after surgery. Immediate postoperative prostheses have a socket that is either hand-molded from plaster bandages or fiberglass, or is a prefabricated plastic socket. Both types have a suspension belt, pylon, and foot. Patients who have IPOPs tend to be more optimistic and can focus on rehabilitation sooner. As early as the day after surgery, many with an IPOP can begin touch-down weight-bearing. Immediate postoperative prostheses protect the healing limb and reduce pain and joint contractures.[2] With an IPOP, the initial hospital stay is shorter, the length of time in a skilled nursing facility is reduced, and the incidence of return hospitalization is minimized.[3]

A temporary (preparatory) prosthesis consists of a socket, suspension belt, pylon, and foot. The prosthetist alters the socket to conform to changes in shape of the amputation limb. The patient is likely to need several sockets as the volume of the limb changes and activity level increases. The suspension belt may also be modified. The pylon and foot of the IPOP are the same as for the temporary prosthesis. Early ambulation encourages healing and can be tremendously beneficial to the patient's mental outlook. Use of a temporary prosthesis for an extended period of time is advantageous to the new patient. It allows for the continued process of residual limb maturation, which can take 6 months and sometimes longer.[4]

The pylon usually has an adjustment mechanism so that the prosthetist can alter the alignment as the patient's ability to walk improves. While wearing the preparatory prosthesis, the patient progresses to full weight bearing and begins gait training. The prosthetist, physical therapist, and patient must work together to monitor the residual limb for pressure spots, abrasions, and blisters. Chapter 11 details balance and gait training.

A prosthetic sock or cushioning gel liner worn between the socket and the residual limb protects the sensitive skin. Prosthetic socks are measured by their thickness or "ply," from 1-ply to 6-ply. As the volume of the residual limb decreases over the course of each day, the user can add additional socks to keep the socket fitting snugly.[5] Sock thickness that is too great can reduce the user's ability to feel the limb in the socket, which in turn reduces the sense of control over the prosthesis. Therefore, it is advisable to wear no more than 8-ply of sock. Clean prosthetic socks must be worn every day to prevent skin irritation.

Prosthetic socks are made from wool, cotton, and synthetic fibers. Wool is a cushioning fiber that conforms smoothly to the residual limb. Wool is resilient and absorbs perspiration without feeling wet. Cotton offers the advantage of being least allergenic; however, it offers minimal cushioning and absorbency. Synthetic socks wick moisture away from the skin and often include Lycra to improve elasticity. Some socks combine synthetic and natural fibers. For example, wool on the outside provides resiliency and cushioning, and synthetic fibers with Lycra on the inside so the sock conforms to limb contours while wicking perspiration away.[5] Wool socks are more expensive and have a tendency to shrink when dried in high heat. As the residual limb heals, individuals should try different socks and liners to determine what is most comfortable. Some patients combine a sock and a gel liner. Gel liners are discussed later in this chapter.

When is it time to move to a definitive prosthesis? This varies considerably from one person to the next and is usually appropriate when residual limb volume has stabilized, the patient has established a consistent activity level, and the physician, prosthetist, and physical therapist agree that the patient is ready.[4]

SOCKET DESIGNS

The definitive TT prosthesis consists of a custom-made socket, a pylon, and a foot; sometimes an additional suspension component is included. The socket is

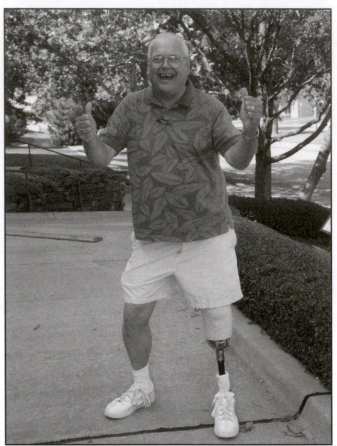

Figure 8-1. More than two-thirds of the people who experience a lower-limb amputation this year are older adults. (Courtesy of Hanger Prosthetics and Orthotics.)

the most critical component. It is the part of the prosthesis that touches the person's residual limb. The dramatic improvement in socket systems in recent years is due mainly to the introduction of new materials such as urethanes, mineral-based liners, and silicones. Much more flexible than the previously used rigid plastics, newer materials bend, expand, and contract with the residual limb, allowing the user greater control of the prosthesis without damage to the underlying skin. When a person walks, contracting the muscles in the residual limb, the socket contracts. When the muscles relax in the swing phase of gait, the socket instantly expands, retaining contact with the residual limb. In this prosthetic application, the responsive quality of the socket material is known as "memory."

Older TT socket designs tended to concentrate pressure points and often required additional leather and metal components. Contemporary sockets have total surface contact with the residual limb. Mapping the muscles, bony prominences, and vascular structures of the residual limb allows uniform distribution of force over the surface of the residual limb. As the user walks, muscles contract into channels in the socket providing

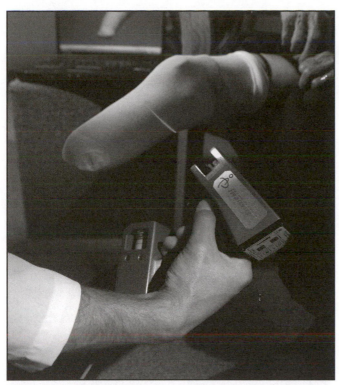

Figure 8-2. Computer scanning. The advent of computer scanning devices have improved the fitting process for prosthetic users. (Courtesy of Hanger Prosthetics and Orthotics.)

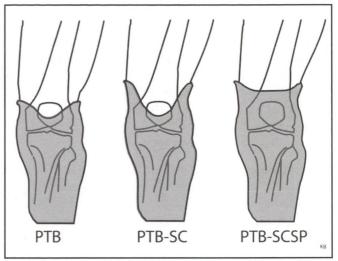

Figure 8-3. Prosthetic sockets are custom designed for each patient by their prosthetist and play the most critical role in the comfort and function of the prosthesis. Shown from left to right the PTB, PTB-SC, and PTB-SCSP socket designs. (Courtesy of Kevin Carroll, MS, CP, FAAOP, and Katherine Binder, CP.)

for comfortable function. The flexible socket fits into a semi-rigid carbon fiber frame. The frame has open areas over pressure-sensitive areas, for heat dissipation and flexibility, thus increasing comfort. The frame contributes to the stability of the prosthesis.

A key area of research and development in TT socket design involves analysis of the vascularity of the limb and the location of the nerve endings. Some people experience numbness in their residual limb after wearing a prosthesis for a few hours. Others become excessively tired. These symptoms may result if the socket presses a nerve or restricts blood circulation. To improve socket design and fitting, new computer scanning systems are increasingly used. With a hand-held laser scanner or wand, the prosthetist can capture and store a precise three-dimensional image of the residual limb (Figure 8-2). Information from the computer scan is transmitted to an automated carver that precisely shapes the model for the socket. These improvements in socket design result in what users say is the most important aspect of any prosthesis: comfort. An ill-fitting socket is uncomfortable; the user will stop wearing the prosthesis. Formerly, patients were conditioned to accept pain as a part of wearing a prosthesis. A socket that fits well does not cause pain. Pain indicates poor fit or a medical or psychological problem that needs to be examined and hopefully corrected.

Dysvascular patients benefit from the massaging action of total contact sockets. This increases venous return and reduces swelling and pain, particularly throbbing sensations. A total contact socket gives the user substantial sensory feedback because it is in direct contact with the skin throughout the amputation limb. These sockets also allow the older adult greater control of the prosthesis without surface damage to the fragile skin of the residual limb.

For users with short residual limbs, a modified socket with higher medial, lateral and anterior walls may be a good choice. This style of socket, known as supracondylar/suprapatellar, extends over the entire patella and femoral epicondyles.[5] Weight bearing is spread over a larger area, knee stability is improved, and the shape of the socket allows for self-suspension (Figure 8-3).

The silicone suction socket features a silicone liner that reduces shear forces against the skin when the user is ambulating. The low modulus elastomeric liner is more elastic than older liners made from polyethylene foam with or without leather. The direct contact of the silicone against the skin creates the suction that is the key to this socket's suspension. Sometimes a pin lock at the distal end of the liner locks the socket to the remainder of the prosthesis.

A few older TT socket designs are still in use. The patellar tendon-bearing (PTB) socket has an anterior wall that extends over a portion of the patella.[5] The PTB socket has an indentation below the patella that allows the patellar ligament to serve as a major weight-bearing surface. The posterior wall applies a counterforce that helps maintain the patellar ligament against the inden-tation. This design sometimes causes skin breakdown at the patellar ligament. Other socket designs include the total surface bearing, which does not have as pro-nounced a patellar ligament bulge as the PTB, and the hydrostatic, which involves drawing the soft tissues distalward to increase distal cushioning.

SUSPENSIONS

Many prosthesis users wear elastic sleeves as either a primary or secondary means of suspension. The sleeve is rolled on over the prosthesis, extending for several inches above the knee. It makes direct contact with the skin on the thigh, sealing the top of the socket to prevent air from entering or exiting. Sleeves are easy and effective to use; however, because the material is vulnerable to punctures, they must be replaced regu-larly. Suspension sleeves are meant to be airtight, and as such, can cause perspiration to accumulate, creat-ing discomfort for people who live in hot or humid climates. Prescription and over-the-counter antiperspi-rants help reduce perspiration.

The latest generation of suspension sleeve incorpo-rates a simple valve. Any air that pushes out of the top of the socket during ambulation, or when the user sits or stands, is released through the valve.

In recent years, gel liners have become popular accessories. They can provide an auxiliary means of suspension as well as enhance the user's comfort[5]; if the residual limb has scar tissue, skin grafts, or sharp bony prominences, a gel liner also serves as a protective layer. Some people wear a gel liner with a metal pin extending from the bottom for secure suspension (Figure 8-4). The liner is rolled onto the residual limb. The pin snaps into a lock in the bottom of the socket. New users may find it takes some practice to learn to position the liner so the pin hits the pin lock. The suction and tackiness between the skin and the gel liner serve as the primary means of suspension for the prosthesis. Sometimes suction also occurs between the gel liner and the socket, creating a secondary source of suction that improves overall sus-pension. The combination of the pin lock and the suction reduces the chances of losing suction in the prosthesis as the person stands, sits, and moves. Although gel liners with pins have many benefits, they tend to pull heavily on the distal end of the residual limb and thus should not be used if there are invaginated areas on the end of the limb.

Gel liners are also available with a lanyard system instead of a pin. A cord extends from the bottom of the gel liner and threads through a hole at the end of the socket. The residual limb is pulled into the socket with the lanyard cord; the cord is then secured on the exte-rior side of the socket .

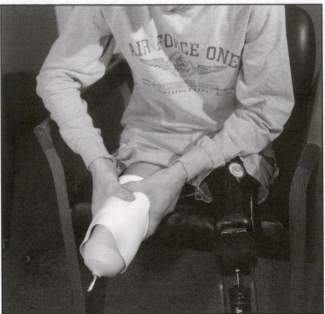

Figure 8-4. Donning the liner. Gel liners enhance the user's comfort and provide an auxiliary means of sus-pension. Gel liners are rolled onto the residual limb and often have a metal pin extending from the bottom. The pin snaps into a lock in the bottom of the socket. (Courtesy of Hanger Prosthetics and Orthotics.)

The newest gel liners do not have a pin or lanyard; instead they are worn with a socket that has a valve on the distal end. The user rolls the liner onto the residual limb then inserts the residual limb in the socket. Air inside the socket is pushed out the valve. A sleeve that extends over the knee seals the top of the socket to make it airtight. As the person walks, air continues to be pushed through the valve.

Gel liners that incorporate a hypobaric silicone ring also allow for suction suspension. A raised ring within the liner near the proximal end conforms to the shape of the socket wall to provide an airtight seal. When the user dons the prosthesis, air is pushed through the dis-tal valve, creating suction below the seal. This system eliminates the need for an external sleeve.

Although gel liners bring comfort for many users, it is important to remember that anything that comes between the residual limb and the socket reduces proprioception, and thus the user's control over the prosthesis. If gel liners are used, they should be as thin as possible while still providing adequate protective cushioning.

The Vacuum Assisted Suspension System (VASS) is a new approach to suspension. It consists of a gel liner, suspension sleeve and an air evacuation pump. The VASS creates a vacuum between the liner and the socket wall that promotes fluid exchange within the residual limb. This system appears to regulate volume

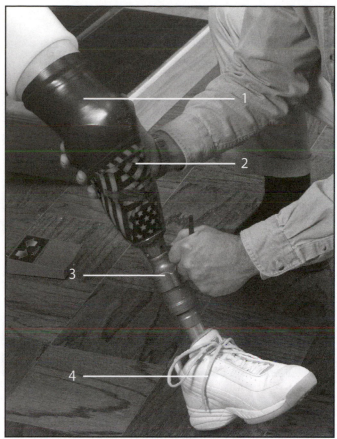

Figure 8-5. Components such as suspensions sleeves (1), custom-designed sockets (2), Vacuum Assisted Suspension System (VASS) (3), and feet (4) are recommended by the prosthetist on the basis of the user's functional level as defined by Medicare. (Courtesy of Hanger Prosthetics and Orthotics.)

fluctuations in the residual limb, making suspension more secure and reducing shear forces.[6] The VASS also reduces the accumulation of perspiration (Figure 8-5).

Finally, some patients wear older suspension systems, such as a cuff strap encircling the distal thigh just above the epicondyles. Others have a plastic or leather thigh corset with metal side joints that attach to the socket, or a leather waist belt with a fork strap that buckles onto the socket. If the patient is accustomed to any of these systems, it may be acceptable to duplicate the suspension in a replacement prosthesis. Nevertheless, the newer modes of suspension are usually preferable because they avoid thigh atrophy as is caused by the corset, provide more secure suspension, and create a more streamlined silhouette when the wearer sits.

DISTAL COMPONENTS

Components such as pylons and foot and ankle units are prescribed on the basis of the user's functional level as defined by Medicare.[7]

Medicare Functional Levels

The five functional levels are also known as "K codes." Level 0 (K0) states that the person does not have the ability or potential to ambulate or transfer safely with or without assistance, and a prosthesis does not enhance the quality of life or mobility. Level 1 (K1) states that the person has the ability or potential to use a prosthesis for transfers or ambulation on level surfaces at a fixed cadence, typical of the limited or unlimited household ambulator. Level 2 (K2) includes people who are community ambulators with the ability or potential to traverse low level barriers such as curbs, stairs, and uneven surfaces. Level 3 (K3) includes those who are community ambulators with the ability or potential to walk at a variable cadence, traverse most environmental barriers, and participate in more demanding vocational and recreational activities beyond simple locomotion. They could benefit from the use of more complex prosthetic components. Finally, level 4 (K4) refers to people who exceed basic ambulation skills and exhibit high impact, stress, or energy levels typical of the prosthetic demands of a child, active adult, or athlete.[8] Ideally, the patient would try two or three different components and select the one that feels best. In usual practice, however, the patient receives the one component that the prosthetic team believes is most suitable.

Prosthesis users have access to abundant information on components, particularly through the Internet. Even so, clinicians must remind consumers that not every new item suits everyone. The unique amputation level, skin condition, extent of bony prominences, age, lifestyle, functional level, and general health influence prosthetic prescription.

Pylons

The pylon is the component between the socket and foot. An exoskeletal pylon has a rigid exterior and is also known as a crustacean shank. Endoskeletal, modular, pylons have a central support and may have a shock-absorbing mechanism, which can emulate the mechanics of the anatomic leg.[2] In early stance phase, shock-absorbing pylons compress to absorb vertical shock; at push-off they rebound to improve propulsion, allowing for higher levels of activity. This action also helps protect the residual limb from injury, particularly if the skin is fragile skin and the joints are arthritic.

Torque absorption is another feature built into many pylons. Activities such as golf, tennis, aerobic exercise, and dancing require significant rotation of the foot. If the pylon does not absorb transverse stress, rotational force can apply damaging shear forces to the residual limb. Torque absorbers allow for rotation of up to 45 degrees in either direction; the amount of resistance usually can be adjusted to suit the activity. Alignment of the socket relative to the pylon and foot determines the comfort and ease of walking on the prosthesis (Figure 8-6.).

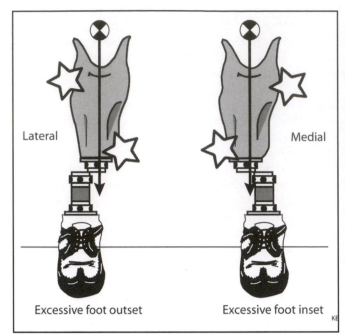

Figure 8-6. Alignment. The fixed spatial relationship between the various components of the prosthetic devices plays an important role in the function, comfort, and appearance of the device while the patient is sitting, standing, and walking. When the foot is excessively outset the patient will feel pain and pressure in the lateral-proximal and medial distal portions of the socket. Likewise, when the foot is excessively inset, the patient will experience high pressure on the medial-proximal and lateral-distal portions of the socket. (Courtesy of Kevin Carroll, MS, CP, FAAOP, and Katherine Binder, CP.)

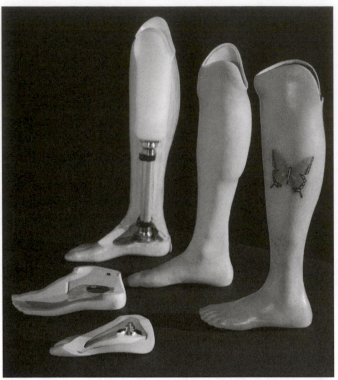

Figure 8-7. Custom cosmetic finishing of prosthetic limbs has evolved into an art form. Fabricated from stain resistant silicone elastomers, prosthetic legs and feet have lifelike contouring and shaping, as well as realistic toenails and skin shading. Some users prefer the high-tech look of their limb without a cosmetic covering. (Courtesy of Hanger Prosthetics and Orthotics.)

A final consideration regarding pylons relates to the finished appearance of the prosthesis. Some users like the high-tech look of their prostheses without a cosmetic cover on the pylon. Others want their prostheses to have a life-like appearance that matches the sound limb. Cosmesis is an art form, which may involve applying stain resistant silicone elastomers covers with flesh tones and characteristics such as veins, freckles, and body hair (Figure 8-7).

Foot and Ankle Units

A vast, increasing array of foot ankle units is available. Lightweight, energy-storing, and dynamic are some terms applied to prosthetic feet. Although some units incorporate wood and rubber, materials such as lightweight urethanes, graphite, and titanium are common in higher performance feet. Other designs increase stability on uneven terrain and have adjustable heels that allow users to wear shoes of various heel heights. (Figure 8-8).

All feet have a natural appearance to fit shoes and provide passive plantar flexion in early stance, toe hyperextension in late stance, and neutral position in swing phase. Five types of prosthetic feet include: Solid Ankle Cushioned Heel (SACH), single-axis, multiple-axis, dynamic response, and multiple-axis with dynamic response. For users with a functional level of K1 or K2, the standard foot is the SACH foot. This foot has an internal wood, aluminum, or plastic keel surrounded by a foam shell and has no moving parts. The SACH foot has good shock absorption at heel strike, is durable, inexpensive, and requires minimal maintenance.

Single-axis feet are a less frequent choice for level K1 and K2 TT users; however, more active users sometimes prefer the motion of this design. Limited ankle plantar flexion and dorsiflexion increases knee stability when the person walks and also improves the user's ability to walk up and down inclines. The embedded single-axis joint at the ankle and plantar flexion bumper at the heel both require regular maintenance. Multiple-axis feet allow for rotation of the foot, inversion/eversion, and dorsiflexion/plantar flexion. These feet increase both stability and comfort for users who regularly walk on uneven surfaces such as grass.[10] Both single- and multiple-axis feet have a space between the top of the

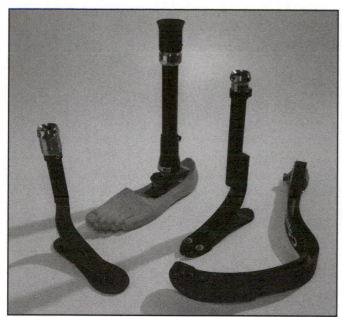

Figure 8-8. Prosthetic feet are recommended by the prosthetist on the basis of the user's functional level as defined by Medicare. (Courtesy of Hanger Prosthetics and Orthotics.)

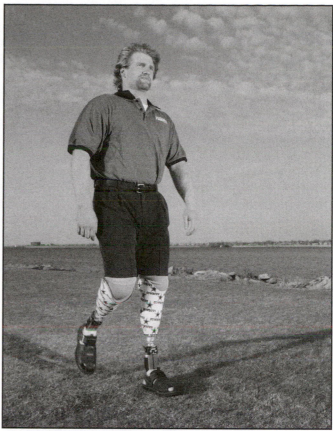

Figure 8-9. TT prosthetic users are often people who want to continue participating in recreational activities. Sports are usually pursued, over time, by people who have become very comfortable using prostheses and have accepted the devices as integral parts of their body. (Courtesy of Hanger Prosthetics and Orthotics.)

foot and the bottom of the shank. Although this gap is covered with leather it may detract from the natural appearance of the ankle. Some single- and multiple-axis feet have a mechanism that permits the user to adjust the foot angle to accommodate shoes with various heel heights. The mechanisms usually provide tilt for heels within a 2-inch range.

Feet categorized as "dynamic response" enable users to be more active for longer periods of time by providing good energy return.[9-11] Some of the energy the person expends when stepping forward is stored within the foot and then used to move the wearer through the next step. When wearing a dynamic foot, TT prosthetic users spend 50% of the time on the sound foot and 50% on the prosthetic foot.[10] Symmetrical loading balances the stress on the residual limb and the sound foot, especially important considerations for patients with diabetes. With a SACH foot, approximately 61% of the time is spent on the sound foot, placing more weight-bearing stress on the sound foot. Individuals with functional levels of K3 or K4—especially children, young adults, and athletes—benefit from dynamic response feet that absorb and release energy while the user is in motion[12] (Figure 8-9).

Although most feet attach directly to the pylon, an ankle unit between the foot and pylon can be helpful on inclines and rough terrain. Transtibial prosthetic users with a functional level of K2 or greater should consider an adjustable ankle unit. Some units can only be adjusted by a prosthetist, whereas others allow the user to

make adjustments. User-adjustable ankles are popular with people who wish to change shoes frequently, such as women who go from flats to moderately high heels or men who may want to change from regular shoes to cowboy boots. An adjustable ankle combined with a dynamic response foot offers extra cushioning, which should make walking easier.

FINAL THOUGHTS

High quality prosthetic care combined with comprehensive physical therapy leads most TT users to recover a fulfilling lifestyle. Unfortunately, some people have unresolved problems such as severe trauma, infection, and diabetes or vascular concerns that detract from optimum rehabilitation. Even those who face challenging circumstances can continue to improve function if they work with their care team on a long-term basis.

Transtibial prosthetic users are often active people who want to continue participating in recreational activities, some of them quite physically intense. Many people enjoy downhill and cross-country snow skiing, jogging, hiking, camping, and mountain climbing. Some adaptive prosthetic designs are waterproof and were developed for use in water skiing, swimming, and scuba diving.[13] Chapter 17 provides detailed information regarding adaptive prostheses for many activities. Advanced activities are usually pursued by people who, over time, have become very comfortable using a prosthesis and accept it completely as an integral part of their body. With a good physical therapy program, TT users can be very active with their prosthesis.

Some transtibial and transfemoral prosthesis users are professional athletes engaged in high-level competitions. They require specialized prostheses and the continual support of physical therapists and trainers who focus on competitive sports (Figure 8-10).

Finally, clinicians should maintain a positive outlook when working with older adults and avoid projecting negative stereotypes related to age. People over the age of 50 comprise the largest group of TT users. As with all patients, they deserve the utmost in comfort and physical therapy support to thrive.

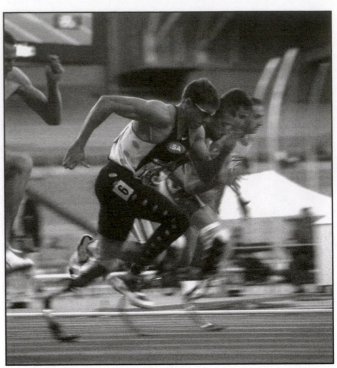

Figure 8-10. A small but growing group of TT and TF prosthesis users are professional athletes engaged in high-level athletic competitions such as the Paralympic Games. (Courtesy of Hanger Prosthetics and Orthotics.)

REFERENCES

1. Carroll K. Limb loss in older adults: Improving outcomes while reducing costs. *Orthopedic Technology Review*. 1999; 1:36.

2. Webber P. Great expectations. *Orthopedic Technology Review*. 2001;3:32.

3. Pinzur MS, Littooy F, Osterman H, Wafer D. Early post-surgical prosthetic limb fitting in dysvascular below-knee amputees with pre-fabricated temporary limb. *Orthopedics*. 1988;11:1051-1053.

4. Kapp S, Cummings D. Transtibial amputation: prosthetic management. In: Bowker JH, Michael JW, eds. *Atlas of Limb Prosthetics*. 2nd ed. St Louis, Mo: CV Mosby; 1992:453-478.

5. Uellendahl J. Prosthetic socks and liners. In: *First Step: A Guide for Adapting to Limb Loss*. Knoxville, Tenn: Amputee Coalition of America; 2001:56-58.

6. American Orthotic and Prosthetic Association. *Prosthetic vacuum technology. Buyer's Guide: Prostheses and Components*. 2002. Available at: http://www.aopanet.com. Accessed December 2003.

7. Rosenberger B. Medicare O & P Reimbursement. *inMotion*. 2000;10:53-54.

8. Western Amputee Support Alliance. Functional levels and lower extremity prostheses. Available at: http://www.usinter.net/wasa. Accessed March 2004.

9. Alaranta H, Kinnunen A, Karkkainen M, et al. Practical benefits of Flex-Foot™ in below-knee amputees. *Journal of Prosthetics and Orthotics*. 1991;3:179-181.

10. Snyder RD, Powers M, Fontaine C, Perry J. The effect of five prosthetic feet on the gait and loading of the sound limb in dysvascular below-knee amputees. *J Rehabil Res Dev*. 1995;32:309-315.

11. Lehman JF, Price R, Boswell-Bessette S, Dralle A, Questad K, deLateur BJ. Comprehensive analysis of energy storing prosthetic feet: Flex Foot and Seattle Foot versus Standard SACH foot. *Arch Phys Med Rehabil*. 1993;74:1225-1231.

12. Trost F. Energy storing feet. *J Assoc Children's Prosthetic-Orthotic Clinics*. 1989;24:82-85.

13. Carroll K. Adaptive prosthetics for the lower extremity. *Foot Ankle Clin*. 2001;6:371-386.

Chapter 9

Transfemoral Prosthetic Designs

Kevin Carroll, MS, CP, FAAOP; James C. Baird, CPO; Katherine Binder, CP

OBJECTIVES

1. Trace the history of transfemoral socket designs
2. Describe dynamic transfemoral sockets and the use of test sockets
3. Identify socket suspension designs
4. Delineate the qualities of various knee units including microprocessor units
5. Discuss ankle/foot combinations and endoskeletal and exoskeletal systems

INTRODUCTION

New technology has revolutionized the art and science of prosthetics with improvements in materials and components. Perhaps no single prosthesis has advanced more dramatically than the transfemoral (TF) prosthesis. Bulky, squared-off sockets have been eclipsed by sleekly contoured designs that give users a new level of comfort and mobility. Components such as knees, pylons, and feet now emulate the function of the human leg to a greater extent, especially with the addition of microprocessors. All of this translates into a vastly improved experience for most TF users, particularly when they follow a comprehensive plan of physical therapy with the close cooperation of family members, professional case manager, occupational therapist, and psychologist.[1,2] Individuals can expect comfort when walking for extended periods of time and can enjoy an ever broader range of activities including dancing, cycling, golfing, and tennis.

EVOLUTION OF TRANSFEMORAL SOCKET DESIGNS

Prostheses have existed since ancient time. A 3000-year-old functional prosthesis found on an Egyptian mummy had toe nails fashioned on the foot, indicating a concern with the cosmetic aspect of prosthesis. In the nineteenth century, prostheses were usually built from leather with sockets that wrapped around the thigh. In 1912, the Desoutter brothers of England introduced an aluminum TF socket with a rounded plug shape. The ischial tuberosity sat on the edge of the socket; daily volume changes in the residual limb caused the tuberosity to drift up and down in the socket. Thus began the central debate in TF socket design: Should the ischial tuberosity be contained within the socket or positioned outside of it?

In the 1950s, English prosthetists introduced the "H" socket. It was an attempt to prevent the tuberosity from slipping into the socket. Another development was the European Quadrilateral Socket (EQ) featuring a rectangular shape and an open distal end. Engineers James Foort and C.W. Radcliffe, PhD, at the University of California, Berkeley, brought this socket to the United States in the mid-1950s and modified it to include distal contact and renamed it as the quadrilateral socket. Their exploration of the biomechanics of alignment during ambulation remains the basis of contemporary prosthetic alignment (Figure 9-1).

The quadrilateral socket remained the socket of choice through the 1970s. The ischial tuberosity sat on the posterior brim of the socket and did not slip into the socket. However, in working with thousands of patients from across the world, the coauthor (K.C.) observed many situations where the tuberosity had slipped into the socket, resulting in a much better fit. With the tuberosity on the brim, the socket tended to shift laterally when the user was in the mid-stance phase of gait. When the tuberosity was inside the socket, lateral drift was eliminated; however, the medial socket wall tended to press on the pubic ramus. One solution was to lower the proximomedial wall to take pressure off the ramus. The snug anterior/posterior contour of the socket prevented the user from completely sinking into the socket. The resulting modified quadrilateral socket accommodates the ischial tuberosity, while keeping the ramus outside the socket without pressure.

The first major shift away from the quadrilateral socket was introduced in the late 1970s by prosthetist Ivan Long. His Normal Shape-Normal Alignment (NSNA) socket was based on the idea of a tight medial-to-lateral fit without causing intolerable pressure on the soft tissues.[3] The user had excellent medial-lateral control, resulting in more symmetry when walking. The femur was held in the position that matched the alignment of the sound femur.[4] Long claimed that if the medial-lateral dimension was correct, the ischial tuberosity or ramus did not need to be inside the socket for lateral support. Some people who wore the NSNA socket complained that they lost suction suspension when seated because the anterior aspect of the socket would sometimes protrude considerably above the thigh.

John Sabolich, CPO, analyzed the NSNA socket, and in the early 1980s, introduced a socket called Contoured Adducted Trochanteric-Controlled Alignment Method (CAT-CAM). The CAT-CAM socket was an attempt to lock the ischial tuberosity in the socket to prevent lateral shifting.[3] Enclosing the tuberosity, and sometimes the ischial ramus, in the socket came to be known as ischial containment and remains a primary option in TF socket design. Weight bearing in the ischial containment socket is concentrated mainly through the medial aspect of the ischial ramus.[5] The socket contours vary according to the patient's soft and bony tissues.[6,7] Counterforce within the socket is intended to keep the tuberosity and ramus firmly centered against the posteromedial aspect of the socket.[8] Supplemental weight-bearing support is derived from the gluteal muscles and the uniform distribution of pressure across the surface of the residual limb.[4,6] Sabolich also introduced a flexible posterior wall to reduce the likelihood of anterior gapping when the person sat. The medial wall was trimmed low enough to reduce any painful pressure that often occurred as the residual limb gradually lost volume over the course of a day, causing the user to sink farther into the socket. Eventually, Sabolich collaborated with another prosthetist, Thomas Guth, and in 1984, introduced a totally flexible version of the CAT-CAM

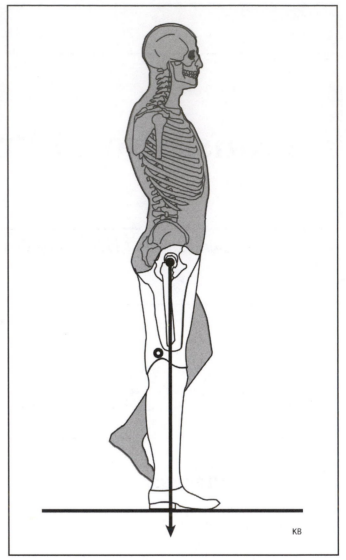

Figure 9-1. By aligning the knee axis posterior to a line between the hip joint and the ankle joint, the patient's weight forces the knee joint into extension, thereby preventing knee buckling. The knee will be locked tightly in accordance to the weight applied. However, excessive knee stability will result if the knee axis is moved too far posterior to the ankle-hip line. This will result in difficulty in initial knee flexion at push off as well as poor gait and difficulty using stairs and ramps. Likewise, if the knee axis is moved too far anterior to the ankle-hip line, the knee will be unstable and buckle.

socket that accommodated bone and muscle contours. The Sabolich Socket was the next development, offering a flexible, contoured socket that fit higher on the lateral aspect of the pelvis for increased stability.

Throughout the 1980s, prosthetists and researchers were seeking a scientific basis for the socket design. The coauthor (K.C.), with Sabolich and prosthetists Ed

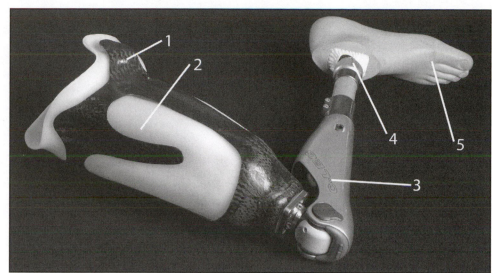

Figure 9-2. Components, such as rigid frames (1) and flexible inner sockets (2), are custom designed for each patient by the prosthetist and improve the comfort and function of the prosthesis. Knee joints (3), rotators (4), and feet (5) are recommended by the prosthetist on the basis of the user's functional level as defined by Medicare. (Courtesy of Hanger Prosthetics and Orthotics.)

Gormansen and Bill Copeland, initiated anatomical research to develop a greater understanding of muscle structure and function in the residual limb. Dissection on human cadavers at the University of Oklahoma and Oklahoma State University was performed to determine how to create pressure between the muscles to foster encouraging muscle hypertrophy throughout the residual limb. Fatty tissue of the ischial rectal fossa could cushion the tuberosity when enclosed within the socket and as such, would help distribute load more evenly over the tuberosity and ramus. The concept of using the fatty tissues was in direct opposition to ischial tuberosity and ramus containment sockets that displaced fatty tissue from the socket, causing pain where the ramus and tuberosity pressed against the socket. Measurements on 50 cadavers confirmed that the average distance from the tuberosity to the ischial spine was 1.75 inches. Consequently, the medial containment should not extend more than 1.75 inches, from where it presses on the sacral tuberous and sacral spinous ligaments, to avoid discomfort. Otherwise, the user may attempt to reduce discomfort by flexing the hip, leading to flexion contractures. This research demonstrated that ischial containment sockets should rarely exceed 1.75 inches of containment of the ischial ramus and are most effective with very short residual limbs. If the socket encases more than 1.75 inches of the ischial ramus, the socket will rotate away from the ligaments and the ischial ramus will be outside the wall.

The coauthor (K.C.) participated in additional research using magnetic resonance imaging and computed tomography scans of the thighs of people as they contracted their muscles. Analyzing how the muscles changed shape—expanding when contracted and narrowing when relaxed—formed the basis for designing the dynamic socket.

DYNAMIC TRANSFEMORAL SOCKET

The primary purpose of the dynamic TF socket is improved comfort. Made of flexible thermoplastic, the socket supports the muscles of the residual limb as the user walks. Muscles contracting freely and painlessly into compartments within the socket hypertrophy. In contrast, with rigid sockets, when the user contracts thigh muscles they press painfully against a socket wall. The natural reaction is to avoid pain by stopping muscle contraction; in just a few weeks, the muscles atrophy.

The design of the dynamic TF socket incorporates two components that work synergistically: a thin, flexible socket and a supportive frame reinforced with carbon fiber[9] (Figure 9-2). Cutouts in the frame enable it to accommodate extra girth when muscles contract, and then cling to the residual limb when muscles relax.

The use of test sockets and the advent of computerized scanning devices have improved the fitting process (see Figure 8-2). The test socket allows the prosthetist and patient to work together to determine such factors as contouring, trimlines, and the placement of cutouts in the frame.[10] Once the test socket is satisfactory, the final definitive socket can be made. For example, someone with a lot of soft tissue needs a socket that is relatively wide mediolaterally to accommodate the tissue as it spreads when the individual sits. A person with a muscular residual limb requires a narrower socket to conform to the firm tissue. Ideally, the residual limb contacts the socket directly, without liners or socks. This allows the user to feel the socket wall and perceive joint motion more keenly. Dynamic sockets are lightweight, and most importantly, comfortable. Comfort is the key ingredient.[9] Other components of the prosthesis will not matter if the socket is uncomfortable because the person will not wear the prosthesis.

Figure 9-3. Gel liners can enhance the user's comfort and provide an auxiliary means of suspension. Left: Lanyard system. A cord extends from the bottom of the liner and threads out through a hole at the end of the socket and then is locked on the proximal portion of the socket. Right: Pin System. The liner with a metal pin extending from the bottom is rolled onto the thigh. The pin snaps into a lock in the bottom of the socket. (Courtesy of Otto Bock Healthcare.)

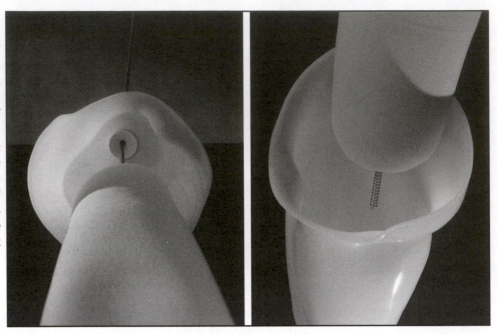

Socket comfort is associated mostly with standing, walking, and sitting. The average person spends more time sitting than standing, so comfort when the wearer sits is essential. The posterior portion of the frame has a cutout enabling the back of the dynamic socket to be completely flexible. It yields under the weight of the residual limb without pinching or pressing soft tissue.

Aside from comfort, sitting and standing are also intertwined with socket suspension. A typical suction socket features total contact between the thigh and the socket while the user stands. When the person sits, the socket is apt to gap. A poorly contoured socket allows air to enter through the brim of the socket, causing it to lose suction and possibly slip off. Muscles should be contracted whenever the user stands, gets in or out of a car, plays a sport, or walks. Instead of adjusting the socket or adding layers of socks to compensate for volume changes, users should focus on flexing thigh muscles to control the fit of the socket.[4] Muscular control promotes optimum health of the residual limb.

SUSPENSION

Although suction suspension is common, not all TF users can tolerate total suction. Some older adults, people with very short residual limbs, those with significant bony prominences, skin problems, or diabetes may do better with other types of suspension.

A suspension belt can be a primary or secondary means of suspension. An elastic neoprene band wraps around the proximal 8 inches of the socket and extends up the front of the hip to form a belt that circles the waist and fastens with hook and pile tape.[11] Constructed from porous materials, these belts offer good support while allowing air to circulate on the skin. Another popular option is the Silesian belt. It is Dacron webbing that attaches to the socket on the lateral and anteromedial walls and circles the waist. This simple, effective suspension can be removed and washed regularly. An older option is the steel or nylon hip joint with pelvic band and waist belt. This bulky suspension system works best for users who need maximum stability (eg, people who are obese or have weak hip abductors).[11]

As is the case with TT prostheses, gel liners used in TF prostheses can enhance comfort and provide auxiliary suspension.[12,13] The liner can have a pin lock system, as shown in Figure 8-4, a lanyard (Figure 9-3), or a 2-inch band incorporated into the midsection of the liner just below the ischium to seal the top of the socket to make it airtight. A few TF prostheses have a Vacuum Assisted Suspension System (VASS) comparable tot hat described for TT prostheses.[14]

KNEE UNITS

The knee unit should complement the user's functional level as defined by Medicare "K codes."[15] (For more information on Medicare functional levels, refer to Chapter 8, Transtibial Prosthetic Designs.) Designs of prosthetic knees range from simple hinges to sophisticated electronic devices.

Microprocessor control of computerized knees is based on biomechanical studies. Most units respond 50 times per second to information from sensors that detect the amount of force borne on the foot, the angle of the knee, and the speed of shank swing. An internal microprocessor automatically adjusts the response of the knee to the walking surface encountered by the

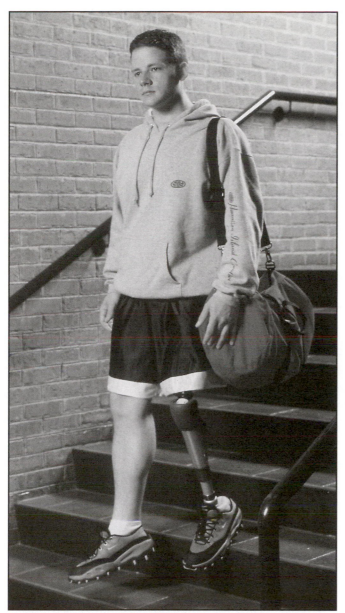

Figure 9-4. Computerized microprocessors integrated into prosthetic knees automatically adjust the response of the knee to the varying surface conditions encountered by the user. Users report that computerized knees improve their stability when walking and greatly reduce the likelihood of falling. The result is easier, more natural movement on level surfaces, and especially on ramps, stairs, and uneven terrain such as golf courses and hiking trails. (Courtesy of Hanger Prosthetics and Orthotics and Otto Bock Healthcare.)

user. The prosthetist uses a personal computer to adjust the knee to the individual's gait pattern. The knees are powered by a lithium-ion battery that provides 25 to 30 hours of use before needing to be recharged.

Prosthetic users report that electronic knee units improve their stability when walking, greatly reducing

the likelihood of falling.[16,17] The result is more natural movement on level floors, ramps, stairs, slopes, and uneven terrain such as golf courses and hiking trails (Figure 9-4). Hydraulic stance stability protects the user from inadvertent knee flexion. Comparison of the performance of adults fitted with a computerized knee to a basic hydraulic knee concluded that the computerized knee "was clearly superior at higher speeds during swing phase" and "users showed significantly lower flexion speeds at the beginning of swing phase"[18] The computerized knee also enabled wearers to walk with more symmetrical flexion angle, flexion speed, and extension speed, while consuming 4% to 7% less oxygen than those using older versions of hydraulic knee units.[19]

Medicare guidelines approve reimbursement for computerized knees for those with a functional level of K3 or K4. Several manufacturers do not recommend computerized knees for people who weigh more than 220 pounds. Some people with a functional level of K2, including new users, older adults, and people with balance problems, would also benefit from this technology, which increases stance stability. Long-time prosthetic users report that with computerized knees, their gait feels more natural and they participate in activities with an increased sense of confidence.[16,17]

Other types of prosthetic knees include the basic single-axis constant sliding friction knee unit, which is light-weight, durable, and less expensive. It is frequently used on temporary prostheses and on children's prostheses, which are usually replaced annually as the child grows. Although the basic sliding friction knee unit allows only one optimal walking speed, some versions have special features including friction mechanisms and weight-activated brakes.[20] The brake is often used with inexperienced walkers to help protect them from falling. This knee swings freely and has a friction brake that is activated when weight is applied in early stance phase when the knee is flexed less than approximately 15 degrees. Locking knees have a manual lock, which prevents any flexion throughout the gait cycle. They offer the greatest stability but produce an awkward gait, and are appropriate for a older adults who are unsteady on their feet or have poor muscle tone in the residual limb.

Polycentric knees are a good choice for active users who desire gait stability without the expense of a computerized knee unit. Polycentric knees, sometimes called "four bar" knees, are designed to be stable in early stance and to flex easily during preswing.[21] The polycentric knee varies its center of rotation during ambulation so that the weight line lies anterior to the instant axis of knee rotation for a longer period than with a single-axis unit.[22,23] Polycentric knees add weight to the prosthesis and have more moving parts that need to be serviced regularly.

Fluid-controlled knees are either pneumatic (air) or hydraulic (oil). They automatically increase or decrease swing phase resistance as users vary their walking speed. More active clients benefit from a single-axis or polycentric knee that incorporates a fluid-controlled unit. As the person walks faster, the piston inside the unit limits the flow of fluid, and thus, control of knee flexion. When the user walks slowly, the air or fluid flows easily, enabling the knee to move more slowly. In extremely cold weather, a fluid-controlled knee that uses silicone is a good choice.

Hydraulic systems are more durable than pneumatic ones, although some people prefer the bouncier gait offered by a pneumatic unit. As compared with sliding friction units, fluid units result in a more natural gait but add weight and maintenance to the prosthesis.

SHANKS

As described in Chapter 8, the shank transfers weight between the proximal portion of the prosthesis and the prosthetic foot, and is either exo- or endoskeletal. In the TF prosthesis, the endoskeletal shank (pylon) reduces the weight of the prosthesis appreciably and can help absorb the recurrent shocks of the heel striking the ground during ambulation. Many users prefer a dynamic pylon with shock- and torque-absorbing properties. Dynamic pylons act like a spring that compresses early in stance phase to absorb shock and releases late in stance phase to help propel the user forward. Units that also allow for axial rotation and torque absorption are especially appropriate for those who engage in sports such as golf or tennis.

A positional rotator is an accessory that increases the user's choice of posture. The rotator is placed above the knee unit. By pushing a button, the user enables the shank to be rotated in the transverse plane with respect to the knee. This feature is helpful when putting on shoes, sitting in tight spaces such as a car, and sitting on the floor tailor-fashion.

The endoskeletal shank usually has a one- or two-piece cover, which duplicates the shape and color of the sound leg. Covers are lightweight and fairly durable. One-piece covers are made of plastic foam with a skin-like finish. Although they allow for a smooth silhouette at the knee when the user sits, the portion of the cover in front of the knee stretches when the user sits or kneels. Covers are vulnerable to tearing and staining and usually need replacement every 12 to 24 months.

Two-piece covers are split at the knee and are less likely to deteriorate after repeated sitting. They are made of a firmer plastic and usually weigh a little more than one-piece foam covers. The finish may be a flesh-toned nylon stocking or a customized airbrushed urethane. The mid-range of finishes is made from durable, stain-resistant silicone, which will look good for several years. Airbrushed urethane or silicone finishes can be customized to give the appearance of body hair, freckles, veins, and even tattoos (see Figure 8-7).

Ankle-Foot Units

Prosthetic feet for the TF user are selected from the same array of designs discussed in Chapter 8. The absence of a natural knee joint, however, presents concerns regarding the relationship between the prosthetic foot and knee. Generally, ankle-foot units with a moving joint that allows rapid plantar flexion provide better shock absorption at heel strike than nonarticulated feet. Dampening shock allows the foot to plantar flex more quickly, decreasing the instability of the knee that might otherwise occur from heel strike to midstance. Single-axis, multiple-axis, and dynamic response feet that allow for substantial plantar flexion are better choices for TF users than SACH feet, which provide minimal plantar flexion[11] (see Figure 8-8).

LIFE WITH A TRANSFEMORAL PROSTHESIS

As technology moves forward, rehabilitation outcomes for TF users of all ages have improved dramatically. Key developments are: new materials that are lightweight, durable, and flexible; an increased understanding of the anatomy of the residual limb; comfortable socket designs; and improved components such as computerized knee units. Advanced technology is most effective when used by people with unilateral and bilateral amputation who are in good physical condition, which usually translates to a balanced diet, regular exercise, adequate rest, and good stress management. Willingness to adhere to a course of physical therapy, including a home exercise program, is critical (Figure 9-5). Some clinicians discourage people with TF amputation from expecting very much lifestyle recovery. Patients have been told they would never run, dance, or play sports. In working with thousands of TF users across the country, the co-authors have seen people who race, snow ski, skydive, scuba dive, rock climb, and are professional athletes in the international Paralympic Games.[19] Chapter 17 describes transtibial and TF prostheses designed for athletic use. Optimism and encouragement, balanced with an understanding of the individual's abilities, are powerful tools in the rehabilitation process. There will always be those who struggle and those who exceed all expectations.

REFERENCES

1. Otto JP. Total patient care: Just a dream? *The O&P Edge.* 2003;2. Available at: www.oandp.com/edge. Accessed June 2004.

2. Angelico J. Prosthetic primer: transfemoral prosthetics: above-knee. *inMotion.* 1999;9:40-47.

3. Long I. Normal shape-normal alignment (NS-NA). *Clin Prosthet Orthot.* 1985;9:9-14.

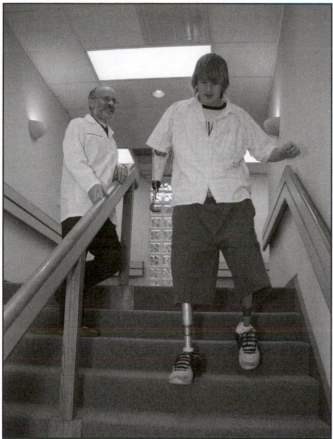

Figure 9-5. Bilateral TF users expend significantly more energy when walking. Therefore, they must be in excellent physical condition. Shown: The first documented case of a bilateral TF prosthesis user walking naturally, step-over-step down stairs without using the handrail. This was accomplished through intensive training and exceptional physical strength and determination on the part of the patient. First, the patient was trained to pick things up off the floor by bending the knees. This was accomplished by externally rotating both knees and firing all of the muscles contained in the socket as well as the gluteal and abdominal muscles. Because the knee is no longer in the line of progression, knee flexion resistance increases. This exercise not only helps to strengthen the patient but also helps build confidence. Next, the patient is taught to descend the stairs while holding the handrail by placing the prosthetic foot half way on the landing, initialing knee flexion and using the hydraulics' resistance to control descent. When the patient has enough confidence with this activity, he or she may begin practicing without the handrail. (Courtesy of Hanger Prosthetics and Orthotics and Otto Bock Healthcare.)

4. Long I. Walking normally with an above-knee prosthesis. *inMotion*. 2003;13:18-20.

5. Sabolich J. Contoured adducted trochanteric-controlled alignment method: introduction and basic principles. *Clin Prosthet Orthot*. 1985;9:15-26.

6. Radcliffe CW. Comments on new concepts for above knee sockets. In: Donovan R, Pritham C, Wilson AB Jr, eds. *Report of ISPO Workshops, International Workshop on Above-Knee Fitting and Alignment*. Copenhagen, Denmark: International Society for Prosthetics and Orthotics; 1989:31-37.

7. Hoyt C, Littig D, Lundt J, Staats T. The UCLA CAT-CAM above-knee socket. UCLA Prosthetics Education and Research Program, March 1987; Los Angeles, Calif.

8. Schuch CM. Modern above-knee fitting practice. *Prosthet Orthot Int*. 1988;12:77-90.

9. Carroll K. Adaptive prosthetics for the lower extremity. *Foot Ankle Clin*. 2001;6:371-386.

10. Carroll K. Prosthetics and aging: mobility for the long run. In: *First Step: A Guide for Adapting to Limb Loss*. Knoxville, Tenn: Amputee Coalition of America; 2001:43-45.

11. Schuch CM. Transfemoral amputation: prosthetic management. In: Bowker JH, Michael JW, eds. *Atlas of Limb Prosthetics*. 2nd ed. St Louis, Mo: CV Mosby; 1992:509-533.

12. Uellendahl J. Prosthetic socks and liners. In: *First Step: A Guide for Adapting to Limb Loss*. Knoxville, Tenn: Amputee Coalition of America; 2001:56-58.

13. Beil T, Street G, Covey S. Interface pressures during ambulation using suction and vacuum-assisted prosthetic sockets. *J Rehabil Res Dev*. 2002;39:693-700.

14. American Orthotic and Prosthetic Association. Prosthetic vacuum technology. *Buyer's Guide: Prostheses and Components, 2002*. Available at: http://www.oandp.com. Accessed December 2003.

15. Rosenberger B. Medicare O & P Reimbursement. *inMotion*. 2000;10:53-54.

16. Karoub J. Micro-electro-mechanical systems prosthesis helped save amputee on Sept. 11. *Smalltimes: Big News in Small Tech*. January 25, 2002. Available at: http://www.smalltimes.com. Accessed May 2004.

17. Rindfleisch T. Computerized knee gives city man a better artificial leg. June 22, 2003. Available at: http://www.lacrossetribune.com. Accessed May 2004.

18. Kastner J, Nimmervoll R, Kristen H, Wagner P. What are the benefits of the C-leg? A comparative gait analysis of the C-Leg, the 3R45 and the 3R80 prosthetic knee joints. Available at: http://www.ottobockus.com. Accessed January 2004.

19. Schmalz T, Blumentritt S, Tsukishiro K, et al. Energy efficiency of transfemoral amputees walking on computer-controlled prosthetic knee joint "C-leg." Available at: http://www.ottobockus.com. Accessed January 2004.

20. Wiest J. What's new in prosthetic knees? In: *First Step: A Guide for Adapting to Limb Loss*. Knoxville, Tenn: Amputee Coalition of America; 2003:91-94.

21. Michael JW. Prosthetic primer: prosthetic knees. *inMotion*. 1999;9:29-31.

22. Michael JW. Prosthetic knee mechanisms. *Phys Med Rehabil*. 1994;8:147-164.

23. Oberg KET, Kamwendo K. Knee components for the above-knee amputation. In: Murdoch G, Donovan RG, eds. *Amputation Surgery and Lower Limb Prosthetics*. Oxford, United Kingdom: Blackwell Scientific Publications; 1988:152-164.

Chapter 10

Hip Disarticulation and Transpelvic Prosthetic Designs

Kevin Carroll, MS, CP, FAAOP; Christina Skoski, MD; Katherine Binder, CP

OBJECTIVES

1. Outline the development of hip disarticulation/transpelvic (HD/TP) prosthetic design
2. Explore the attributes of HD/TP socket designs
3. Highlight the role that alignment plays in the function, comfort, and appearance of the prosthesis when the user sits, stands, and walks
4. Review HD/TP components, including hip joints, knee units, and ankle/foot combinations
5. Emphasize the importance of good physical conditioning and health for the HD/TP prosthetic user and identify the challenges confronting such patients

INTRODUCTION

People who experience hip disarticulation (HD) or transpelvic (TP)* amputation challenge health care professionals in terms of fitting a prosthesis and then teaching the person to use it successfully.[1-3] Many HD and TP patients walk on a prosthesis every day and attend school, work, drive, and play sports. Rehabilitation potential is determined by a variety of factors. First, the patient must have a prosthesis with a comfortable socket. This is most likely to occur when the person works with a prosthetist experienced in high-level amputations. Second, the HD/TP user must have an exceptional desire to wear a prosthesis, and third, must be physically fit and healthy. The client needs great patience with the fitting and the rehabilitation process. A strong support network of people who encourage the person is vital. The patient must be highly committed to long-term rehabilitation with a physical therapist who understands the individual's needs and believes in the person's potential for recovery. Several months of

physical therapy and day-to-day experience are usually required for the user to gain functional independence with a prosthesis.[4]

Rejection of a prosthesis is common among people with HD and TP amputation.[1] They have no foot, knee, or hip. Clearly, this level of loss greatly magnifies issues of comfort, energy expenditure, control, balance, and stability. Children are the most likely to accept and adapt to using an HD/TP prosthesis. Older adults, often already challenged by ill health, weakness, inactivity, balance problems, and cognitive decline, are likely to have a difficult time using a high level prosthesis. Walking with a HD/TP prosthesis requires up to 200% as much energy as normal ambulation.[5,6] Those who have tried a prosthesis and then rejected it generally state the primary reason is discomfort, a direct result of a socket that does not fit properly.[7] If a prosthesis feels uncomfortable and unstable most of the time, the person using it has little choice but to remove it and rely on crutches, a wheelchair, or other devices for mobility.

---

* *"Transpelvic" refers to amputations through any portion of the pelvis. Formerly, these amputations were referred to as partial or complete hemipelvectomy.*

EVOLUTION OF HIGH-LEVEL PROSTHETIC DESIGNS

It is now possible to achieve comfort and function at the HD/TP level because of advanced materials and designs.[8] In the 1940s, the tilting table prosthesis was standard. The inherent flaw of this system was positioning a mechanical hip joint in line with the patient's center of gravity. The prosthesis was so unstable that the hip joint had to be locked, making attempts at walking very stiff.

In 1954, Canadian rehabilitation engineer Colin McLaurin, DSc, introduced a HD prosthesis that featured an unlocked hip joint placed anterior to the acetabulum. This positioned the center of gravity behind the mechanical hip joint and anterior to the knee joint during weight bearing and prevented the prosthesis from collapsing at the knee and hip.[9,10] Gait was smoother than with the tilting table design. Eric Lynquist, a Danish prosthetist, designed a hip joint with 5 degrees of anterior pelvic tilt, making it possible to reposition the ankle laterally.[11] His design retained the stable anterior positioning of the hip joint. Lynquist extended his work to encompass the needs of TP patients, outlining a fitting process for a "Canadian-type plastic socket for hemi-pelvectomy."[12]

In 1957, engineer Charles Radcliffe validated the idea of shifting the center of gravity posterior to the hip unit and anterior to the knee.[13] This approach to alignment is still used.

In the early 1980s, the coauthor (K.C.) began fitting patients with an anatomically correct HD/TP socket. The hip joint was moved onto the lateral aspect of the socket close to the acetabulum, into the space where the natural hip joint had been.[14] Ongoing experience with approximately 40 HD users and 20 TP users indicates high acceptance.

SOCKET

Of the many components composing a prosthesis, the socket is the most critical. Its fit determines comfort. A 1984 study of 20 HD and TP users showed that only three wore their initial prosthesis full-time. All were then fitted with a new prosthesis that featured a silicone rubber socket, and their prosthetic usage was monitored for 3 years. Most individuals increased the time they wore their prostheses, with 90% of this group reporting that increased comfort was the primary reason. The number of full-time users rose from three to 13.[15]

The anatomically correct socket mimics the natural placement of the hip. This is accomplished by out-setting the mechanical hip joint in its own compartment lateral to the socket cavity, positioning it in the space once occupied by the natural hip.[14] The suprailiac region, around which the socket wraps completely, is markedly indented, thus improving suspension and reducing lateral pistoning. In an approach similar to the transfemoral (TF) suction socket, the HD prosthesis is suspended by containing the residual soft tissues within the socket.[16,17] Unlike previous designs, this socket has a solid floor that is parallel to the ground. This prevents the residual tissues from slipping out of the socket as the user walks (Figure 10-1). Prior to the advent of the anatomically correct socket, the coauthor (K.C.) had seen several patients, especially postmenopausal women, with fractured ribs each year. Users stated that they felt they were slipping through the socket and thus tightened the top of the socket, exerting undue pressure to the lower rib cage.

For HD users, ischial containment increases control by keeping the tuberosity inside the socket.[8] Ischial containment stabilizes the mediolateral and anteroposterior aspects of the prosthesis.[16,17] The medial trimline of the socket must not press on the pubic ramus. By fabricating the socket from thin thermoplastic, flexible areas can be incorporated in the socket to relieve potential pressure points.[18,19] Cushioning material placed underneath the ischial tuberosity relieves pressure.[8] Pressure on the ramus can be so painful that the prosthesis will not be worn.

The TP socket encompasses the sound buttock, including the ischial tuberosity to increase control. The gluteal ring, which wraps around the inferior border of the gluteal muscles, must be covered when casting the socket. From the front, the gluteal ring passes through the perineum, following the proximal area of the Scarpa's triangle on the sound side and then passing lateral and inferior to the trochanter, returning to the inferior border of the gluteal muscles. Gluteal muscles on the sound side are held within the socket during stance phase on the prosthesis, thereby absorbing pressure.

The upper and lower trimlines of the socket affect function and comfort. The HD socket is suspended by snug fit on the torso just above the iliac crests; the upper trimline is usually just above the crests.[14] By extending it an inch or so higher, weight bearing is distributed over a larger area, making it more comfortable. The TP prosthesis compresses soft tissues, because the patient lacks an iliac crest. The socket is shaped to achieve suspension with the upper trimline extending even higher above the waist. Bringing the trimline to the ribcage provides additional support for the back and may act as a brace to control postoperative scoliosis. Very high trimlines may need to be modified to allow for movement at the waist. Sockets fabricated from flexible plastic and silicone provide both support and comfort.[8] The lower anterior edge of the TP socket may push into the thigh when the user sits. This causes some discomfort, but maintains a counterforce in the direction of the tuberosity and gluteal muscles. Ultimately, the

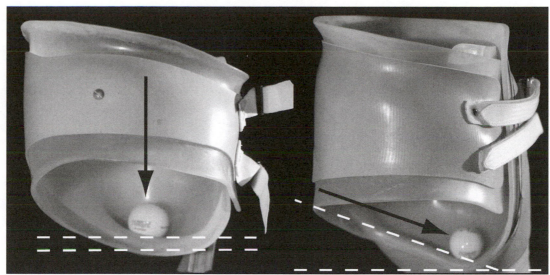

Figure 10-1. Unlike previous HD/TP designs (right), the anatomically correct socket (left) has a solid floor that is parallel to the ground. This prevents residual tissue from slipping out of the socket as the user walks, and prevents the pelvis from sliding forward, putting pressure on the ramus. As demonstrated in these photographs, the anatomically correct socket holds a golf ball in the weight-tolerant area of the ischial tuberosity, whereas in previous designs, the ball rolled forward to the pressure-sensitive ramus. In addition, containment of the ischial tuberosity increases control by keeping the tuberosity inside the socket, stabilizing the medial-lateral and anterior-posterior aspect of the prosthesis. (Courtesy of Hanger Prosthetics and Orthotics.)

patient must understand that trimming the socket is a compromise. What may be lost in terms of comfort will improve function, or some function may be sacrificed to improve comfort.

People with fragile skin should have a soft gel liner under the socket. The liner can have a hole cut for the sound leg.[14] The liner is then stretched around the trunk, adding a protective layer between the skin and the socket. Friction on the soft tissues is reduced and the material provides a more even distribution of pressure. The liner lessens the risk of abrasions and increases comfort, enabling people to wear their prostheses for longer periods of time.[7,20]

The anatomically correct HD/TP socket allows the thigh section to be the same length as the sound side. The sound knee is level with the prosthetic knee when the user sits. (Figures 10-2 and 10-3). Hip disarticulation and TP users report greater comfort when sitting with the anatomically correct socket because it provides a level sitting surface. Misplacing the hip component beneath the tuberosity causes the pelvis to tilt unnaturally when the person sits, pressing on the vertebrae and leading to back pain and scoliosis.

HIP, KNEE, AND FOOT-ANKLE UNITS

Distal components are recommended on the basis of the user's functional level as defined by Medicare. For more information on functional levels, refer to Chapter 8.

The simplest hip joint is a hinge that allows flexion and limited extension. Users who need extra stability may benefit from a locking hip joint with a stride limiter, or a hip flexion bias system. This is a spring-loaded mechanism that pushes the thigh forward as the toe leaves the ground, allowing the foot to clear the ground.[21] Strut hip systems are another option. The strut is a flat piece of carbon composite material that joins the hip to the knee. During stance phase, the strut compresses to store energy; at toe-off, the stored energy is released, flexing the hip and knee and accelerating the swing phase of the gait.[21] Regardless of hip joint, it is the anatomically correct placement of the joint that ensures optimal function and mobility. The joint should be attached anterior to the lateral aspect of the ischial tuberosity.

Although any type of knee unit, pylon, and foot-ankle unit can be used in a HD or TP prosthesis, the shank should be endoskeletal to minimize weight. For more information on prosthetic knees, feet, and other components, refer to Chapter 9 (Figure 10-4 and see Figure 8-8).

Every component added to the prosthesis increases weight. Because the HD and TP prosthesis must replace such a large portion of the body, it is much heavier than TF or TT prostheses, typically 10 pounds or more. This weight places a strain on the pelvic tissues and can be very tiring for the user. Therefore, it is important to select components to be certain the benefits they offer are worth any increase in weight. Shock and torque

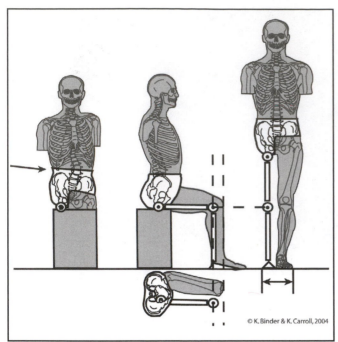

Figure 10-2. When the HD socket has the hip component beneath the ischial tuberosity, the base of support is narrow and less stable. With the hip joint in this position, when the patient is standing, the mechanical knee center is level with the anatomical knee center. However, when seated, the hip joint folds under the socket so that the mechanical knee center falls short of the anatomical knee center. In addition, while the wearer is seated, the pelvis will tilt unnaturally, pressing on the vertebrae and leading to back pain and possibly scoliosis. Also, this unnatural curvature of the spine causes the lower margin on the ipsilateral rib cage to impinge on the proximal socket brim. (Courtesy of Kevin Carroll and Katherine Binder.)

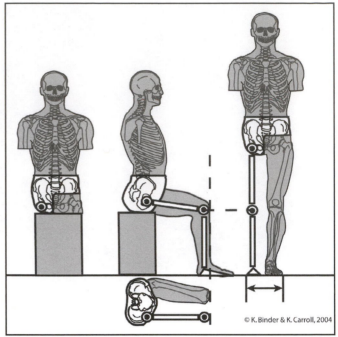

Figure 10-3. The anatomically correct socket mimics the natural placement of the hip. This is accomplished by outsetting the mechanical hip joint in its own compartment lateral to the socket cavity, positioning it in the space once occupied by the natural hip joint. This position allows for a wider, more stable base of support, as well as for the mechanical knee center to be level with the anatomical knee center whether the patient is standing or seated. In addition, because the hip compartment is not under the ischial tuberosity, there is no unnatural pelvic tilt and compensatory scoliosis; therefore, no impingement of the lower border of the rib cage occurs on the socket brim. (Courtesy of Kevin Carroll and Katherine Binder.)

absorbers should be placed above the knee; proximal placement eliminates the pendulum effect that occurs when these components are installed lower (Figure 10-5). For information on the cosmetic finish of the prosthesis, refer to Chapter 6 (see Figure 8-7).

Hip disarticulation and TP users should visit their prosthetist several times during the first year of using a prosthesis, ideally at 2 weeks, 1 month, 3 months, 6 months, and 1 year.[14] In subsequent years, a biannual visit usually suffices to allow for inspection of the prosthesis and residual tissues and monitoring of spinal alignment. If pain occurs, an office visit is indicated immediately.

HEALTH CONCERNS

For HD and TP prosthetic users, obesity is a serious problem. With a socket that wraps around the torso, excess girth makes it much more difficult to achieve a comfortable fit. Being overweight stresses the trunk muscles on the amputated side and the entire sound leg, particularly the joints. Walking on a HD or TP prosthesis is very challenging even for people who are in good shape. Gaining weight adversely affects socket fit, diminishing comfort and control of the prosthesis. Conversely, losing weight will cause the socket to fit too loosely. Therefore, more than at any other level of amputation, people with HD or TP prostheses need to maintain a healthy, stable weight. This is usually accomplished by eating a balanced diet and exercising daily. Those who struggle with weight control should be referred to a nutritionist.

Physical fitness has a positive effect on the health and mobility of HD and TP users. Fitness is a state of being that one gradually builds toward and maintains over the lifetime. New patients who are motivated towards fitness must understand the importance of not attempting to do too much too soon. Recuperating from surgery, chemotherapy, or radiation may take several months. For those who truly want to walk and enjoy a

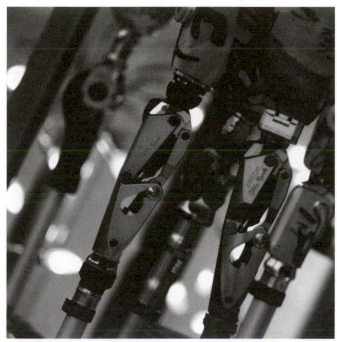

Figure 10-4. Prosthetic knees are recommended by the prosthetist on the basis of the user's functional level as defined by Medicare. (Courtesy of Hanger Prosthetics and Orthotics.)

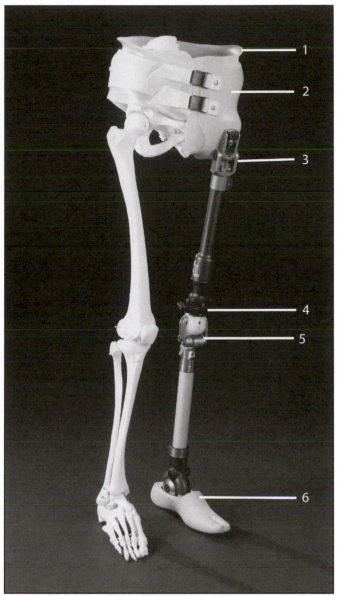

Figure 10-5. Components such as flexible inner sockets (1) and rigid frames (2) are custom designed by the prosthetist. Hip joints (3), rotators (4), knee joints (5), and feet (6) are recommended by the prosthetist on the basis of the user's anticipated function. (Courtesy of Hanger Prosthetics and Orthotics.)

fulfilling life style, physical fitness must become a priority. Swimming is an excellent exercise because it does not place additional stress on the joints. Many other recreational activities are suitable for people with high amputations. Specific exercises with illustrations are available at www.hdhphelp.org.

Maintaining the strength and stability of the skeleton is another important aspect of fitness. Older adults face a greater challenge due to the age-related loss of bone mass.[7] Weight-bearing exercise, weight lifting, and a low fat, high calcium diet are key. All new patients should be evaluated for osteoporosis, and appropriate interventions instituted.[22] Surgical disruption of musculoskeletal attachments, combined with the effects of gravity, often lead to the development of scoliosis. People with TP amputation have lost half the muscle and tendon attachments that held the lower back straight and are particularly vulnerable. Hip disarticulation users will be able to sit, stand, and walk in a reasonably symmetrical fashion, but often develop scoliosis. Although scoliosis cannot be completely corrected, if it is detected early it is possible to prevent it from progressing. Patients should be examined for scoliosis at least once a year. Sitting sockets can reduce the tendency towards back malalignment.[23] In some cases, it may be necessary to add a trunk orthosis, especially if the person uses a wheelchair most of the time. For those not willing to use a full sitting socket, the prosthetist can provide a pelvic leveler, a small foam cushion that contours to the sitting surface on the amputated side.[24] Sitting sockets are also recommended as a protective measure to prevent injury when people with HD and TP amputation participate in sports where a prosthesis is not worn. Those with bilateral HD or TP amputation need a sitting socket to provide a stable sitting surface.[14]

Women with HD or TP amputations may be cautioned about pregnancy.[4] Absence of one hip or half of the pelvis makes it difficult for a woman to tolerate the enlarging abdomen. A few HD and TP users have had normal pregnancies. Because HD patients retain the supportive bony structure of the pelvis and associated musculature, their bodies can support the weight of a pregnant uterus. As pregnancy progresses and the size of the abdomen increases, the socket can be modified to maintain adequate suspension.[25] Those with TP amputation may experience a tilted uterus, which may interfere with socket fit. Higher incidence of transverse lie, breech presentation, and prolapsed umbilical cords are associated with TP.[4] Because it is much more difficult to maintain adequate suspension in pregnant women who have TP amputation, we recommend that women forego use of the prosthesis at 20 weeks gestation to eliminate placing undue pressure on the growing fetus. A maternity sling that extends under the abdomen or has elastic wraps may be useful. The increased metabolic demands, cardiovascular changes, and oxygen consumption that normally occur during pregnancy may further add to the already high energy demands of walking with a HD or TP prosthesis.

When people relax at home it is very common for them not to wear a prosthesis. It is usually more comfortable to sit without the prosthesis. As noted, a sitting socket or pelvic leveler provides a level sitting surface. Patients should avoid hopping on the sound leg when not wearing a prosthesis. Hopping puts tremendous stress on lower limb joints and increases the chances of falling. Instead, people should use properly fitted crutches or crawl short distances.[4] Everyone with HD and TP amputation should be fitted with lightweight axillary or forearm crutches that have shock absorbing tips. A program of upper body strengthening can help individuals minimize injuries related to overuse of the wrists, elbows, and shoulders. Many HD and TP prosthesis users find a cane essential to stability when walking.[4]

FINAL THOUGHTS

Hip disarticulation and TP prostheses are rejected more than any other prosthesis.[1] Therefore, when working with these patients, clinicians must think in the long term. Ongoing communication between the patient and the rehabilitation team is essential to success. When frustrations run high, it may be necessary for the patient to take a break. This can make the difference between giving up on a prosthesis, and eventually moving forward. The recovery process is slower and the outcome less favorable than that of people with more distal amputations. A well fitting socket, carefully selected components, and precise alignment, combined with slowly paced physical therapy, can lead to the utmost level of lifestyle recovery for HD and TP prosthetic users (Figure 10-6).

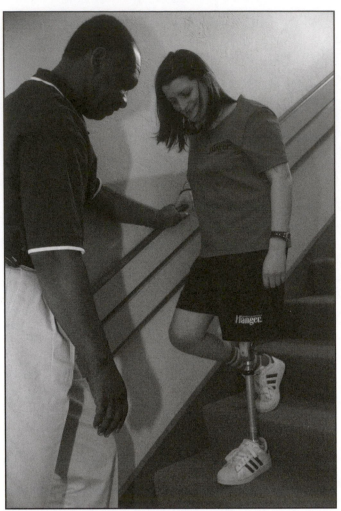

Figure 10-6. The successful rehabilitation of a person with a HD or TP amputation relies on many factors including an exceptional desire on behalf of the patient to wear a prosthesis and an experienced and committed rehabilitation team that includes a prosthetist, physical therapist, social worker, and physician. (Courtesy of Hanger Prosthetics and Orthotics.)

REFERENCES

1. Jensen S, Mandrup-Poulsen T. Success rate of prosthetic fitting after major amputations of the lower limb. *Prosthet Orthot Int.* 1983;7:119-122.

2. Robinson KM, Lackman RD, Donthineni-Roa R. Rehabilitation after hemipelvectomy. *Univ Penn Orthop J.* 2001;14:61-69.

3. Van der Waarde T, Michael J. Hip disarticulation and transpelvic amputation: prosthetic management. In: Bowker JH, Michael JW, eds. *Atlas of Limb Prosthetics.* 2nd ed. St Louis, Mo: CV Mosby; 1992:539-552.

4. Skoski C. HP/HD Help. Available at: http://www.hdh-phelp.org. Accessed January 29, 2004.

5. Huang CT. Energy cost of ambulation with Canadian hip disarticulation prosthesis. *J Med Assoc Alabama.* 1983; 52:47-48.

6. Waters RL, Perry J, Antonelli D, Hislop H. Energy cost of walking of amputees: the influence of level of amputation. *J Bone Joint Surg Am.* 1976;58:42-46.

7. Carroll K. Prosthetics and aging: mobility for the long run. In: *First Step: A Guide for Adapting to Limb Loss.* Knoxville, Tenn: Amputee Coalition of America; 2001:43-45.

8. Angelico J. Sockets for hip disarticulation and hemipelvectomy amputees. *inMotion.* 2001;11:19-20.

9. McLaurin CA. Hip disarticulation prosthesis. *Report No. 15.* Toronto, Canada, Prosthetic Services Center, Department of Veterans Affairs; 1954.

10. McLaurin CA, Hampton F. Diagonal type socket for hip disarticulation amputees. Chicago, Ill: Northwestern University Prosthetic Research Center, Publication V.A.V1005 M 1079; 1961.

11. Lynquist E. New hip joint for Canadian-type hip disarticulation prosthesis. *Artificial Limbs.* 1958;5(2):129-130.

12. Lynquist E. Canadian-type plastic socket for a hemi-pelvectomy. *Artificial Limbs.* 1958;5(2):130-132.

13. Radcliffe CW. The biomechanics of the Canadian-type hip disarticulation prosthesis. *Artificial Limbs.* 1957;4(2):29-38.

14. Carroll K. Hip disarticulation and transpelvic amputation: Prosthetic management. In: Smith DG, Michael, JW, Bowker JH, eds. *Atlas of Amputations and Limb Deficiencies: Surgical, Prosthetic, and Rehabilitation Principles.* 3rd ed. Rosemont, Ill: American Academy of Orthopaedic Surgeons; 2004:565-573.

15. Van der Waarde T. Ottawa experience with hip disarticulation prostheses. *Orthot Prosthet.* 1984;38:29-33.

16. Sabolich J. Contoured adducted trochanteric-controlled alignment method (CAT-CAM): introduction and basic principles. *Clin Prosthet Orthot.* 1985;9:15-26.

17. Sabolich J, Guth T. The CAT-CAM-HD: A new design for hip disarticulation patients. *Clin Prosthet Orthot.* 1988;12:119-122.

18. Imler C, Quigley M. A technique for thermoforming hip disarticulation prosthetic sockets. *Journal of Prosthetics and Orthotics.* 1990;3:34-37.

19. Madden M. The flexible socket system as applied to the hip disarticulation amputee. *Orthot Prosthet.* 1985;39:44-47.

20. Uellendahl J. Prosthetic socks and liners. In: *First Step: A Guide for Adapting to Limb Loss.* Knoxville, Tenn: Amputee Coalition of America; 2001:56-58.

21. Haslam T, Wilson M. Hip flexion bias. *Houston Medical Center Prosthetics* [company pamphlet]; 1980.

22. Kulkarni J, Adams J, Thomas E, Silman A. Association between amputation, arthritis and osteopenia in British male war veterans with major lower limb amputations. *Clin Rehabil.* 1998;12:348-353.

23. Stark G. Overview of hip disarticulation prostheses. *Journal of Orthotics and Prosthetics.* 2001;13:2:50-53.

24. Sugarbaker P, Malawer M. Rehabilitation of patient with extremity sarcoma. In: *Musculoskeletal Surgery for Cancer: Principles and Techniques.* New York, NY: Thieme Medical Publishers; 1992.

25. McFarlen JM. Modification for pregnancy of a hip disarticulation prosthesis. *Orthot Prosthet.* 1963;181-183.

Chapter 11

Basic Lower-Limb Prosthetic Training

Melissa Wolff-Burke, PT, EdD, MS, ATC; Elizabeth Smith Cole, PT; Mary Witt, PT

OBJECTIVES

1. Discuss physical examination, including assessing the patient's mobility status
2. Determine a physical therapy diagnosis and prognosis based on the examination
3. Plan interventions for prosthetic use, including care of the prosthesis and accessories, donning and doffing various types of prostheses, care of the skin and sound limb, and establishing a wear schedule
4. Instruct the patient in weight transfer, socket control, and balance
5. Outline a program for teaching the patient to ambulate with a prosthesis, including possible use of an assistive device
6. Explain techniques for accomplishing daily activities such as dressing, toileting, ambulating over various terrain, carrying objects, transferring into cars, as well as dealing with falling and rising from the floor
7. Suggest means of maneuvering in the community

INTRODUCTION

This chapter covers the examination, evaluation, development of a physical therapy diagnosis, and interventions for persons with lower-limb amputations. The overriding objective is to provide the reader with a framework for structuring efficient and comprehensive care in this patient population. From the time the referral is made for prosthetic training to discharge, the physical therapist will benefit from having a plan and the tools at hand to meet the multiple needs of the patient. This chapter will provide basic forms and guidelines to promote optimal outcomes.

PATIENT EXAMINATION

Prior to meeting the patient, the therapist should have the tools and information to expedite the examination process and insure the patient's confidence in the physical therapist. By having comprehensive information in advance, the physical therapist can anticipate

the needs of the patient. Obtaining information relating to the physical condition, physical and emotional health of the patient, and current limitations will assist with goal setting. The physical, medical, and psychological status of the patient plays an important role in the rehabilitation outcomes. Contacting the prosthetist will yield information about possible fitting difficulties, donning technique, as well as prosthetic components. Understanding the specific components for each patient allows the physical therapist to be adept and confident when teaching the patient how to use the prosthesis.

The examination is "the process of obtaining a history, performing a systems review, and selecting and administering tests and measures to gather data about the client/patient. The initial examination is a comprehensive screening and specific testing process that leads to a diagnostic classification."[1] An intake form that covers basic medical information should be sent to the patient prior to admission to the rehabilitation department (see Appendix A—Physical Therapy Intake). The patient should send this form to the clinic prior to the first appointment. Information about what to expect and what to wear to physical therapy should be included on the form. The patient should be told to bring loose, comfortable shorts (a bathing suit can be useful for persons with high level amputations), the shoes that were worn when the prosthesis was aligned (as changing shoes can alter the fit and alignment), extra residual limb socks, the shrinker, and appropriate assistive device. It is helpful to remind the patient to continue to work on the home exercise program if one was given prior to discharge from the hospital. If the patient has diabetes, a reminder to eat a regular meal 1½ to 2 hours prior to the appointment and not skip a meal is important. The patient can not exercise or be seen if blood glucose measures under 100 mg/dL or over 240 mg/dL at the time of the examination,[2] or has a blood pressure reading with the diastolic over 110 mmHg or systolic over 220 mm Hg (see Appendix B—Pain Questionnaire). Most patients sustained amputation because of peripheral vascular disease.[3-5] As pain impacts the ability to put weight through the prosthesis,[6,7] efforts at decreasing pain will improve weight bearing, velocity, and safety in ambulation.[8]

Mobility Status

Once the intake information has been gathered the physical therapist can progress to an assessment of the patient's mobility status. This chapter will cover mobility assessment as it relates to using the prosthesis. Mobility independent of a prosthesis was covered in Chapter 3 on postoperative management and would of course be part of the intake examination. Extensive instruction in donning and doffing the prosthesis is necessary and will be covered in this chapter under Interventions.

The authors have developed an intake form that includes the use of standardized tests that have been shown to have reliability and validity for persons with amputations. This form includes questions about the functional ability of the patient (transfers, activities of daily living [ADL], self-care), environmental considerations (housing, transportation), limb condition (residual and sound), cardiovascular status, the prosthesis, equipment needs (assistive devices for ambulation, transportation, home or work environment), and the patient's goals (see Appendix C—PT Initial Evaluation Form). During the initial examination, or later in rehabilitation, it is appropriate to assess the functional ability of the patient. The 2-minute walk test was found to be reliable in a study of 33 individuals with transtibial (TT) amputations.[9] It was also found to have construct validity in a retrospective study of 290 individuals with TT, transfemoral (TF), or bilateral amputations.[10] The Lower Extremity Functional Scale (LEFS) has been shown to be reliable and have construct validity when tested in 107 patients with lower extremity musculosk-

eletal dysfunction[11]; however, it was not reported if any of the patients had amputations.

The examination process is dynamic; the physical therapist is not obligated to use a rigid protocol of tests and measures. The physical therapist should use the tools that will meet and challenge the mobility of the particular patient for an accurate evaluation. Other tools can be used to examine the functional abilities of persons with amputations. The Amputee Mobility Predictor has demonstrated reliability and validity for assessment of functional ability when a patient receives a prosthesis or to assess ambulation potential prior to receiving a prosthesis.[12] The Activities-specific Balance Confidence Scale has been shown to be reliable and have construct validity for elderly persons[13] and persons with lower-limb amputations.[14,15] The reliability and validity of the Houghton Scale, the Prosthetic Profile of the Amputee Locomotor Capabilities Index (PPA-LCI), and the Prosthesis Evaluation Questionnaire were established using samples of 55 to 329 persons with amputations.[16] The Prosthetic Profile of the Amputee demonstrated reliability, and face and construct validity when tested in 89 persons with lower-limb amputations.[17,18] The Locomotor Index has successfully identified the differences in functional ability of older and TF amputees from younger and unilateral amputees.[19] The Timed Get-Up-and-Go Test is an easy test to perform in the clinic and has identified elderly persons with balance deficits,[20] but has not been tested in persons with amputations. The frequently used Functional Independence Measure has not been shown to be a useful predictor of successful prosthetic use[21] or rehabilitation outcome in persons with amputations.[22]

Additional considerations when assessing mobility status using a prosthesis are specific to each level of amputation. Because the incidence of a second amputation is relatively high (10% per year for persons with vascular amputations),[23] the therapist should promote prosthetic fitting and rehabilitation while the person has a unilateral amputation. If the first amputation level was TF and the patient mastered prosthetic usage,[24,25] and/or at least one anatomic knee joint was preserved,[26] it is more likely that the patient will continue to be a successful ambulator. Ambulation at the bilateral TT level is easier than with one TT and one TF amputation or two TF amputations.[6] However, it is possible to ambulate with high level bilateral amputations if the person does not have other serious medical disorders. A person with a bilateral hip disarticulation (HD) was reported to ambulate 30 steps/minute, and 500 meters after 4 days of training with a reciprocating gait prosthesis.[27] For a person with a triple limb amputation, confidence and positive attitude appear to be the primary factors for success over early prosthetic fitting, training, and home modification.[28]

Other pathologies and impairments that can affect mobility and goal attainment include compromised cardiovascular status, poor preamputation fitness level and ambulation ability, irreducible knee or hip contractures, diabetes, peripheral vascular disease, morbid obesity, blindness, connective tissue disorders, faulty nutritional status, poor motivation, clinical depression, severe neurological impairment, and cognitive dysfunction.[21,23,29] In a study of 12 men who lost a limb over 25 years ago, a higher incidence of osteoarthritis was found in the nonamputated knee compared to able-bodied men without amputation of comparable age.[30]

Functional outcomes for the person with a unilateral amputation will need to include consideration of the health of the remaining limb. Limb loss creates problems with overheating, particularly for the person with multiple amputations.[31,32] These conditions are examples of the many considerations to be made when designing the rehabilitation program or developing a wearing and walking schedule for a person with an amputation, but they should not be used to discourage a patient from obtaining a prosthesis or be used as an excuse for failure to succeed at using a prosthesis. Age has not been shown to be a significant factor in relation to predicting prosthetic ability.[21,33] In a review of 23 persons over 90 years of age with an amputation, 74% were successfully fitted for a prosthesis, and 56% wore the prosthesis full time.[34]

Goal Setting

The goal-setting component of the examination must involve the patient.[32,35] "Seventy-three percent of the elderly reached their rehabilitation goals (most frequently ambulating with the aid of a walker) which is only slightly less than the younger amputation group."[36] It is imperative that the patient and the physical therapist identify and work toward the same goals. Ideally, goals are determined by the patient. It is the task of the physical therapist to determine the feasibility of the goals and design appropriate strategies and interventions to meet the patient's goals. Goals should be precise and include a target date, such as, "I want to be able to walk while holding my grandson's hand at his birthday" or "I want to play nine holes of golf this June."[35] With the patient's permission, it is reasonable to include the caregiver in the discussion about goal setting as this person may have an idea about the patient's previous activities, hobbies, and abilities that would be helpful for realistic goal setting.

EVALUATION

The evaluation is "a dynamic process in which the physical therapist makes clinical judgments based on data gathered during the examination. This process may identify possible problems that require consultation with, or referral to, another provider."[1] Using the data gathered during the examination (the intake information, the performance of the patient, the results of specific mobility tests and measures, and the patient's goals), the therapist is able to make judgments about the current and future mobility impairments and abilities of the patient. The physical therapist may identify the need for a referral to occupational therapy, orthopedics, internal medicine, social work, mental health, or other health care specialists. The physical therapist should contact the referring physician to report the evaluation findings, and when necessary, make referrals to the appropriate health care practitioner.

DETERMINING A PHYSICAL THERAPY DIAGNOSIS AND PROGNOSIS

The processes of examination and evaluation lead directly to the diagnosis. "The objective of the physical therapist's diagnostic process is the identification of discrepancies that exist between the level of function that is desired by the patient and the capacity of the client/patient to achieve that level."[1] The Musculoskeletal Practice Pattern for a person with an amputation is, "Impaired Motor Function, Muscle Performance, Range of Motion, Gait, Locomotion and Balance Associated with Amputation."[1] The physical therapy diagnosis will direct the prognosis, plan of care, and interventions needed to achieve the highest level of function.

The prognosis "is the determination of the predicted optimal level of improvement in function and the amount of time needed to reach that level."[1] The difficulty persons with unilateral and bilateral amputations may experience in various ADL is identified in Table 11-1. This table may assist the physical therapist in determining possible levels of function related to the level of amputation. Changes in prosthetic technology are pushing the boundaries of what has traditionally been considered possible for a person with an amputation. The table should be used as a guide and not as the final statement of goal attainment. This information can be shared with the patient and used to establish expectations that will vary with the abilities of the individual.

Ambulating with a prosthesis is similar to an athletic event because of the high energy demands of both endeavors. The extra energy used to ambulate and cope with balance challenges will play a large role in the outcomes of rehabilitation.[24,25,37] The added energy costs of ambulation for the person with an amputation can be as low as 9% for a person with a unilateral TT amputation and as high as 125% for a person with a transpelvic (TP) amputation (hemipelvectomy).[37] A person with a bilateral amputation (TT and TF) may use 280% more energy for prosthetic ambulation.[38]

Table 11-1

ADL Difficulty

	Unilateral TT	Unilateral TF	Bilateral TT	TT to TF	Bilateral TF	Bilateral HD	Unilateral HD and TP
Sit	No limitation	No limitation	No limitation	No limitation	No limitation	No limitation	No limitation
Stand	No limitation	No limitation	No limitation	No limitation	No limitation	No limitation	No limitation
Walk	No limitation	No limitation	Slight limitation	Some limitation	Some limitation	Some limitation	Some limitation
Stairs with rail	No limitation	No limitation	No limitation	No limitation	No limitation	Difficult	Some limitation
Curbs	No limitation	No limitation	Some limitation	Some limitation	Difficult	Difficult	Difficult
Public Transportation	No limitation	Some limitation	Some limitation	Difficult	Not advised	Not advised	Some difficulty
Stairs without rails	No limitation	Some limitation	Some limitation	Difficult	Not advised	Not advised	Some difficulty
Carry	No limitation	Some limitation	Unlimited with some objects	Limited	Not advised	No	Some difficulty
Push	No limitation	Some limitation	Some limitation	Difficult	Not advised	No	Some limitation
Lift	No limitation	Some limitation	Some limitation	Difficult	Difficult	No	Difficult
Kneel	No limitation	Some limitation	Difficult	Difficult	Difficult	No	Some limitation
Pull	No limitation	Some limitation	Some limitation	Difficult	Not advised	No	Some limitation
Get up and down from floor	No limitation	No limitation	Unlimited	No limitation	Difficult	Difficult	No limitation
Step over objects	No limitation	Difficulty increase with the height of the object	Unlimited	Difficult	Very difficult	Difficulty increases with the height of the object	Difficult
Assistance device(s) usually necessary	Often no device	Sometimes a cane	Sometimes a cane (Wheelchair for night or if prostheses are in repair)	One or two canes (Wheelchair for night or if prostheses are in repair)	Usually two forearm crutches (Wheelchair for night or if prostheses are in repair)	Two forearm crutches (Wheelchair for night or if prostheses are in repair)	Sometimes a cane (Wheelchair for night or if prostheses are in repair)

Adapted from Karacoloff L. *Lower Extremity Amputation*. 2nd ed. Pro-Ed: Austin, Tex; 2005:162,165.

Because the average physical and cardiac condition is poor in persons with an amputation due to vascular disease,[39] patients should participate in daily aerobic activities, stretching as well as strengthening exercises.

As the level of the amputation moves higher, the patient will decrease gait velocity so as not to exceed tolerable oxygen cost.[40] In addition, amputations due to dysvascular conditions result in higher energy consumption and slower walking speeds when compared to those with a traumatic amputation.[40] The importance of considering cardiovascular status relates to reintegration in the home and community as persons with an amputation will physically be unable to move as quickly or for as long as prior to the amputation.

A VO_2max of 50% was identified as the minimum necessary for a person with a unilateral amputation to be a functional ambulator.[41] As it is unlikely that the physical therapist has access to the equipment to assess %VO_2max, the Rating of Perceived Exertion Scale (RPE) can be used, but its reliability and validity for use as a generalized psychophysiological measure of relative exercise intensity has been questioned when tested in persons who are healthy, have a cardiac history, or have chronic pain.[42-45] Although the RPE has not been tested in persons with amputations, it is possible to use the RPE, a pre- and postexercise heart rate, and the result of a 2-minute walk test, to demonstrate changes in endurance, but the reliability or validity of these combined measures has not been published.

The time for meeting the functional goals for persons with amputations has not been established. *The Guide to Physical Therapy Practice* gives a range of 15 to 45 visits with a caveat that any of the following could alter the number of visits or duration of care: accessibility and availability of resources; adherence to the intervention program; age; anatomical and physiological changes related to growth and development; caregiver consistency or expertise; chronicity or severity of the current condition, comorbidities, complications, or secondary impairments; concurrent medical, surgical, and therapeutic interventions; decline in functional independence; level of impairment; level of physical functions; living environment; multisite or multisystem involvement; nutritional status; overall health status; potential discharge destinations; premorbid conditions; probability of prolonged impairment; functional limitations or disability; psychological and socioeconomic factors; social support; and stability of the condition.[1]

BASIC PROSTHETIC USE

Function and Care of the Prosthesis

The interventions for basic prosthetic training begin with patient education about the prosthesis and how to care for it. The prosthetist and physical therapist should explain to the patient how the prosthesis works and, if there is a knee or hip unit, precautions to avoid getting the fingers pinched in the unit. A review will assure that both the physical therapist and the patient are familiar with the function and limitations of the prosthesis. Chapters 7, 8, 9, and 10 describe the various prosthetic devices. Table 11-2 gives instructions for the care of the prosthesis, liners, and socks.

Sock Management

Sock management prepares the patient for donning the prosthesis and providing education on frequent volume changes. For many prostheses, socks will be used to maintain the fit and comfort of the socket. Socks are made from wool, cotton, polyester, and blends, and vary in thickness. The condition of the residual limb should be documented prior to donning socks or the prosthesis. As the volume of the residual limb changes during a treatment session, during a single day, and over time, the patient will need to adjust the number of socks worn to maintain the fit of the prosthesis. The person with a new amputation should be encouraged to keep a variety of socks at hand for adjustments in fit that will need to be made frequently. New pain in the residual limb is often related to wearing too few or too many socks. Determining the number of socks is a trial and error process. When donning the socket, the patient should meet resistance from the socket and should not slide in too easily.

A nylon sheath, similar to a lady's knee-hi stocking, is often applied as the first layer to decrease friction, and to help prevent allergic reactions, followed by the thickest sock or a roll-on silicon or urethane liner. A nylon sheath can be worn under the roll-on liner if 3 to 4 inches at the top of the liner are in contact with the skin. Socks come in thicknesses of 1-ply, 3-ply, and 5-ply. The patient can add socks up to a combined thickness of 5- to 15-ply before a new socket, socket adjustment, or a soft insert is needed due to loss of fit. Socks that are used over a roll-on liner with a suspension pin have a hole in the bottom. The sock should clear the pin to not interfere the locking mechanism free (Figure 11-1).

Socks should be applied with care to avoid wrinkles, which can create high pressure areas. Socks can be cut to various lengths. Roll-on liners can also be cut to size by the prosthetist. If the limb has a conical shape and is not filling the distal portion of the socket, the patient will perceive excess distal movement. A very short cap sock can be applied over the distal residual limb. This cap sock should be covered by a 1-ply sock to prevent the cap from slipping into the bottom of the prosthesis. Another way to prevent socks from slipping to the bottom of the socket is to use the outer sock as a sling. By folding the edge over the entire proximal brim and fixing the edge to pressure sensitive tape (Velcro [Velcro USA, Manchester, NH] hook side) that has been attached to the outer wall of the proximal socket, the socks will be prevented from slipping down during ambulation.[46]

The sock for a person with a hip disarticulation/transpelvic amputation (HD/TP) is a fabric liner, which differs from other socks, in that there is not as much concern with volume changes and the patient will not typically be adding or subtracting socks throughout

Table 11-2

CARE OF THE PROSTHESIS, LINERS, & SOCKS

GENERAL CARE: Your prosthesis requires proper care and maintenance to provide good performance. The following general guidelines and suggestions that will help you care for your prosthesis. Please refer to the instructions that should come with your prosthesis or contact your prosthetist.

Prosthesis	*Gel Liners*	*Socks*
Cleaning		
Wipe the socket daily with mild soap and warm water. Pat dry. Clean the leather parts of your prosthesis with saddle soap weekly. If your prosthesis has a valve, clean the threads with a damp toothbrush. Check with your prosthetist regarding the water-resistant nature of the prosthesis. Unless the prosthesis is designed for the shower, do not shower in it. Always dry any part of the leg that becomes wet.	Wash daily. Turn inside out. Holding it over the sink, use warm water and a mild soap to gently clean the gel side of the liner. Do not scrub. Be sure to rinse with plenty of water and wipe dry with a lint-free towel.	Change socks daily or more often if moist with perspiration. Wash socks in mild soap and warm water. Rinse thoroughly. Do not put wool socks in the dryer; dry them flat and thoroughly.
Doffing		
When you take your prosthesis off, lay it on the floor so that it does not fall and possibly crack.	The liner can be placed over a large bottle or similar upright support to dry.	To maintain the shape of the sock, dry with a rubber ball in the closed end of the sock.
Wear & Tear		
If your prosthesis shows dark discolored areas in the finish, or no longer fits well, inform your prosthetist. Inspect the prosthetic foot by removing your shoe weekly. If the covering is torn, have it repaired. If sand or dirt accumulates in the shoe, remove it and clean the foot with a damp cloth. You might not be able to vary the height of the heel of your shoes. Shoes should be kept in good repair, particularly the heels.	If your liner becomes torn or frayed, consult your prosthetist.	Replace socks that are torn or worn thin.
Do not take the valve apart. Avoid using excessive powder when putting the prosthesis on as powder can clog the valve.		
If there should be any malfunction of the prosthesis, take it to your prosthetist. Do not repair it yourself. Never use abrasive or sharp objects on your prosthesis.		

the day. A small pad may be added to the amputated side; alternatively, snug Lycra (Invista, Wichita, Kan) shorts or a panty girdle, appropriately modified, may provide enough pressure to be used as an interface to accommodate any small volume changes that may occur. The liner may simply be the patient's underwear, cotton exercise shorts, or a leotard with the ipsilateral leg hole sewn closed. Any exposed skin can be protected with powder to prevent sticking to the socket. Undergarments with seams will be more comfortable worn inside out to prevent the seam from pressing into tender skin. The garment should be long enough to allow the top to fold over (sling-type) the top edge of the prosthesis to secure it. A full-body leotard is

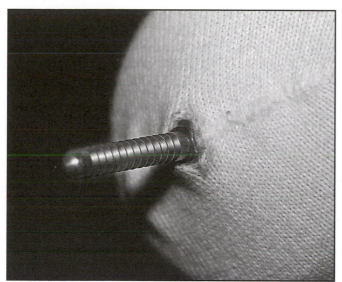

Figure 11-1. Pin and sock: Showing proper amount of sock clearance for pin.

comfortable and cannot slip into the socket. The disadvantage is the added step of removing the leotard when using the toilet. A garment can be custom-made specifically for the person with a HD/TP that provides the same interface, padding, moisture absorption, and functions as underwear (Knit-Rite Inc, Kansas City, Kan; Royal-Knit, Lee Summit, Mo,).

Donning and Doffing the Nonsuction Socket

Positioning the socket is the next step in donning the prosthesis. It requires patience, dexterity, and endurance to learn this skill. Prior to standing on the prosthesis, the patient should be given an idea of the normal pressures and sensations of snugness felt within the socket. Skin tension is a sensation that can be simulated by taking both hands and encircling the limb and pulling proximally. Skin tension occurs when the weight is borne into the socket. Because pain will limit function, the patient must be able to distinguish between pain and the new sensation of skin tension being produced by bearing weight in the socket.

Donning

Transtibial

While seated, the person with a TT amputation will align the tibial tubercle with the relief for the tubercle in the socket, and smooth wrinkles from the liners/socks. The patient may remain seated or may stand with support, and shift weight onto the prosthesis, pull wrinkles from the socks, and apply and tighten the suspension system (neoprene sleeve or cuff strap if one is being used), being careful to not rotate the prosthesis during this process.

Transfemoral

While sitting, the person with a TF amputation will align the adductor longus tendon with its channel in the socket and loosely don the suspension belt if one is present. While standing, the patient adjusts the prosthesis to match the toe-out of the sound side and tightens the suspension belt.[47] Adjustments are made to the liner/socks to decrease wrinkles, and the socks are pulled over the brim of the prosthesis. To ensure that the socket does not internally rotate on the residual limb when the suspension belt is tightened, the patient should bear weight on the prosthesis while tightening the belt. Another way to prevent excessive toe-in is to stabilize the prosthetic toe on the base of stable furniture or the parallel bars, while tightening the suspension belt. Early in the training process, the patient may choose to don the prosthesis while supine. With assistance, the patient can come to standing and final adjustments to fit are made at that time.

Hip Disarticulation and Transpelvic

The patient stands and leans against a chair, wall, or bed for stability. The socket is opened and slid onto the torso, and the straps are fastened loosely. Once the torso is inside the socket, the patient aligns bony prominences with the relief areas of the socket. Straps are tightened to provide snug, yet tolerable, containment within the socket. The socket fit is intimate and must be snug against the abdomen to allow use of the abdominal muscles during ambulation. Patients should be advised that the tightness of the socket needed for ambulation may initially result in discomfort especially after eating, and can interfere with bending. As with all prostheses, tolerance will improve over time.

Doffing

Doffing the nonsuction socket is not usually a problem. While sitting, the patient loosens the suspension strap, slides a thumb into the top 2 to 3 inches of the socket and pulls off the prosthesis. Doffing the HD/TP socket consists of unfastening the straps and sliding the residual torso out of the socket. Once the prosthesis is removed and the skin checked (see following section), the patient reapplies the shrinker. A shrinker or another appropriately fitting compressive garment is worn continuously unless the prosthesis is on or the patient is bathing.

Donning and Doffing the Suction Socket

Several ways to don a suction socket are described in Table 11-3. The roll-on liners are in the suction category as they create a negative atmospheric pressure as well as being somewhat adherent to the skin.[46] To doff the socket, the patient loosens the valve and pulls out of the socket. It is occasionally necessary for the patient

Table 11-3

DONNING THE SUCTION SOCKET

Method	Technique
Elastic Bandage	Remove the valve. Use a 4- or 6-inch width elastic bandage. Loosely apply the bandage, starting at the groin and wrap in a spiral manner around the thigh, leaving 6 inches at the end of the residual limb. Thread the end of the bandage through the valve hole. Place the thigh in the socket. Shift weight on/off the prosthesis; during weight bearing on the prosthesis pull a portion of the bandage gently through the valve opening. After several bouts of weight shifting, the bandage will be completely off. Apply the valve and remove excess air by pushing or pulling the valve while weight bearing. Adjust skin tension at the socket brim.
Stockinet	Remove the valve. Use an open-ended Stockinet, usually 4 to 6 inches wide, and 36 inches long. Apply stockinet up to the groin and leave 2 to 3 inches at the end of the residual limb. Thread the end of the stockinet through the valve opening. Place the thigh in the socket. Using the up and down motion described above, pull the entire stockinet out. Apply the valve and remove excess air by pushing or pulling the valve while weight bearing. Adjust skin tension at the socket brim.
Easy Prosth	Remove the valve. Apply talcum powder to the residual limb and inside the socket. Apply Easy Prosth to the residual limb. Place the thigh in the socket. Pull the loop through the valve opening. Bear weight into the socket and slide Easy Prosth out through valve opening using the pumping motion described above. Apply the valve and remove excess air as above. Adjust skin tension at the socket brim. Easy Prosth: Bauerfeind Prosthetics USA, 55 Chastain Rd, Suite 112 Kennesaw, GA 30144.
Lotion	Remove the valve. Apply a small amount of nonviscous lotion, such as an over-the-counter moisturizer, to the residual limb and socket. Place the thigh in the socket. Wipe excess lotion at the valve opening and apply the valve. Remove excess air as above. Adjust skin tension at the socket brim.
Roll-on liner (with lanyard or pin)	Turn the liner inside out and roll it onto the residual limb. If the liner has a lanyard, attach it to the distal end of the liner. Don socks over liner as needed. Ensure that the socks are not impeding the locking mechanism. Place the thigh in the socket. Secure the lanyard in the lock or click the pin into the locking mechanism.
TEC	Apply petroleum jelly, vitamin E, bacitracin, or vitamin A and D ointment to the residual limb. Pull the liner on. Wipe any excess lubricant off the liner and hands. TEC liner: Otto Bock, North American Headquarters, Two Carlson Parkway, Suite 100, Minneapolis, MN 55447-4467.

to slide the hand into the top of the prosthesis to break the suction.

Quick Assessment of Socket Fit

After the patient dons the prosthesis, the therapist should perform a quick assessment of socket fit. While the patient stands within the parallel bars, bearing weight through both the upper and lower extremities, the levels of the anterosuperior iliac spine (ASIS), iliac crests, and shoulders are checked visually and manually. The shoe on the prosthesis should be flat on the floor.[46] The patient should attempt symmetrical weight bearing and report sensations of pressure or pain. As the feelings generated by the socket and weight bearing on the amputated limb are new to the patient it is unlikely that any socket will "feel right" in the early stages of rehabilitation.

The prosthesis is often slightly shorter than the sound side, to allow for easier swing during the early gait-training period. Within a few weeks, the prosthesis can be lengthened. The fit of a socket can be assessed by the Pen, Powder, Ball of clay, or Lipstick test[46] as described in Table 11-4. The person with a TF, HD, or TP socket should sit for 10 to 15 minutes to test the comfort of the socket.

Transfemoral Socket

For the person with a TF amputation wearing a quadrilateral socket, the therapist should palpate the placement of the ischial tuberosity while wearing a glove to determine whether the socket fits properly. The therapist asks the patient to flex forward at the hip and locates the ischial tuberosity. Once the patient is stand-

Table 11-4

TESTS TO ASSESS SOCKET CONTACT

Test	Used to Determine If:	Technique	Assessment
Pen or chalk	Residual limb is pistoning in the socket.	Mark the posterior or anterior trim line of the socket with a ball pen or colored chalk. Observe the line during swing phase.	If a space between the line and the brim of the socket is more visible, the contact is inadequate. More socks may be needed or the socket adjusted.
Powder	Residual limb is in contact with the bottom of the socket.	Sprinkle powder into the bottom of the socket. Carefully don the socket, walk 15 steps, then carefully remove the socket.	*Proper contact*: Powder is transferred to sock. *Improper contact*: Powder is on bottom or around the sides of the socket
Ball of clay	Residual limb has appropriate contact with the bottom of the socket.	Place a pea-sized ball of clay in the bottom of the socket. Carefully don the socket, walk 15 steps, then carefully remove the socket.	*Proper contact*: Clay has flattened to 1/8- to ¼-inch thick. *Too much contact*: Clay is thinner. *Too little contact*: Clay is not deformed.
Lipstick	A sensitive area is in contact with the socket.	Apply lipstick to the outermost sock over the sensitive site. Carefully don the socket, walk 15 steps, then carefully remove the socket.	*Proper contact*: Lipstick mark is transferred to the bony relief area of socket. *Improper contact*: Lipstick mark is above or below the bony relief area.

Reprinted from *Orthotics and Prosthetics in Rehabilitation*. Lusardi MM, Nielsen C, p 463, Copyright ©2000, with permission from Elsevier..

ing erect, the therapist should feel pressure between the ischial tuberosity and the posterior shelf of the socket. Persons with a TF amputation may feel intense pressure over the ischial tuberosity. For the ischial containment socket, the therapist passively flexes the hip on the prosthetic side while the patient stands, nonweight bearing on the prosthesis, to locate the ischial tuberosity. The limb and prosthesis are passively returned to the standing position. The ischial tuberosity should lie within the socket, resting in a relief area.

If the socket has a valve, it is removed and a small bulging of tissue should be apparent in the opening, with the distal portion of the residual limb resting in the bottom of the socket. (Figure 11-2). It is important to note that for proper alignment, the pylon may not be perpendicular to the floor.[46]

Hip Disarticulation and Transpelvic Sockets

After the patient has sat for a few moments, and again at 15 minutes, the therapist manually checks for signs of excess pressure at the lower ribs (especially posterior) and at the femoral triangle. The distal aspects of the lowest ribs are vulnerable to excessive pressure and subsequent tenderness. Question the patient about numbness at the anterior proximal aspect of the contralateral thigh and manually determine that the edge of the socket is adequately flared away from the femoral triangle and anterior thigh.

Skin Checks

Immediately after the patient ambulates, the therapist should check the skin for areas of increased redness, changes in contour, or sites of pain. The patient should be instructed regarding pressure-sensitive and pressure-tolerant areas of the residual limb. The patient and the therapist should look for areas of reactive hyperemia (redness), abrasion, bruising, or undue warmth, which may indicate a potential problem area. Reactive hyperemia will occur over pressure-tolerant areas. The patient and the therapist will save themselves and the prosthetist from worry if redness over pressure-tolerant areas is distinguished from redness over pressure-intolerant areas. "If a pressure-tolerant area shows evidence of excessive pressure, socket fit and alignment may be appropriate, but the amount of weight bearing or duration of wearing time may need to be decreased. If pressure-sensitive areas are showing signs of too much pressure, it is more likely that socket fit or alignment needs to be adjusted."[46] Figures 11-3 and 11-4 for pressure-tolerant and intolerant areas on the TT limb.[46] Pressure-sensitive areas to be assessed in the person with a HD/TP are the coccyx, sacrum, anterior superior iliac spine (ASIS), lower ribs, and femoral triangle. The femoral nerve, artery, and vein can be compromised by the TF or HD/TP prosthesis when the patient is sitting. Skin at the waist is subject to friction and abrasion due to an overly snug suspension belt or pistoning of the prosthesis.

To assess the health of the tissue, the skin should blanch with firm pressure and return to its normal color within 10 minutes.[46] If this does not occur, the area is a likely site for skin breakdown. For persons with dark skin, color changes may not be apparent, so visual inspection should not be the only means of assessing fit. Attention to warmth, edema, resting pain, and pain upon palpation may provide additional clues about potential areas of skin breakdown.

If the patient has particularly sensitive or insensitive skin, previous systemic infections, or comorbidities that would impair healing, skin checks should be more frequent. Change in climate, prosthetic use, or activity can affect the residual limb, so skin checks should be frequent whenever weight-bearing pressures are altered. Problem areas need to be assessed and addressed immediately by the prosthetist and the physical therapist. Repositioning the socket, changing the number of socks, and assessing socket fit manually may improve fit. In addition to teaching the patient the method and importance of skin checks, he/she is also able to practice donning/doffing techniques under the watchful eye of the physical therapist. See Chapter 5 for details regarding residual limb care.

Wearing Schedule

The patient should be given guidelines for a wearing schedule. Table 11-5 presents a wearing schedule flow chart. Periods of weight bearing in early prosthetic training should be in increments of no longer than 10 minutes.[46] The patient can increase the duration of wearing the prosthesis daily if no skin problems or pain are evident. "Wearing" the prosthesis and "weight bearing" in the prosthesis are different skills. The patient needs to increase both slowly, but may be able to sit comfortably in the prosthesis, nonweight bearing, for longer amounts of time. Either way, skin checks in the early stages of prosthetic rehabilitation should be frequent, at least every hour. Supervised practice during the doffing/redonning process will uncover problems or concerns of the patient, which can be addressed early and will encourage the individual's responsibility for self-care.

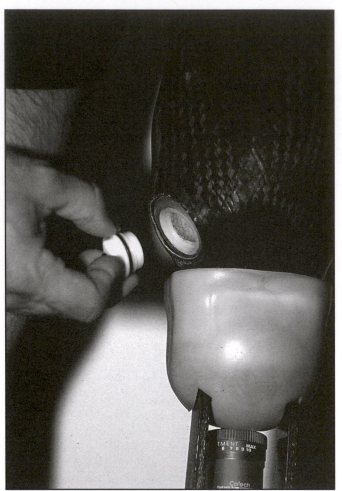

Figure 11-2. Socket and valve: Observation of tissue through socket valve as part of the process to assess fit.

If there are no complications, the patient may move quickly to full-time daily wearing. A study of function and prosthetic use found that 94% of unilateral prosthesis users wore the limb daily and 76% wore it at least 9 hours/day.[48] Persons with the physical ability to tolerate a well-fitting prosthesis usually put it on early in the morning and remove it at bedtime or at a time analogous to when a person without an amputation would remove his/her shoes. The authors have noted that elderly patients with TF amputations often wear the prosthesis only for several hours a day and remove it when at home.

Table 11-6 provides a list of common problems that can arise early in rehabilitation. If there are no significant problems, the patient is ready to begin ambulation training.

INITIAL PROSTHETIC TRAINING

The patient is now ready to begin weight bearing, weight shifting, balance, foot placement, and pelvic and trunk rotation exercises all within the safe confines

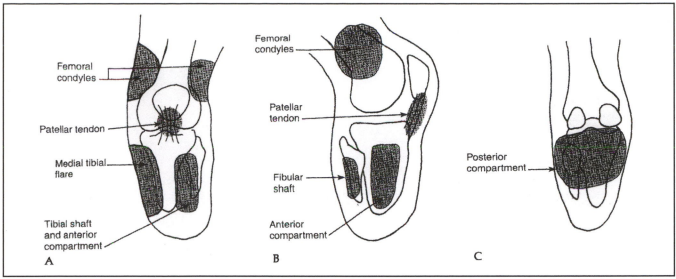

Figure 11-3. Pressure-tolerant areas of the residual limb. (A) On the anterior surface, pressure-tolerant surfaces include the patellar tendon, the medial tibial flare, along both sides of the tibial shaft, and the medial and lateral femoral condyles. (B) On the lateral view, pressure tolerant areas include the patellar tendon, anterolateral compartment, and the shaft of the fibula. (C) On the posterior surface, most structures within the popliteal fossa are pressure tolerant. (Reprinted from *Orthotics and Prosthetics in Rehabilitation*, Lusardi MM, Nielsen C, pp 439-441, © Copyright 2000 with permission from Elsevier.)

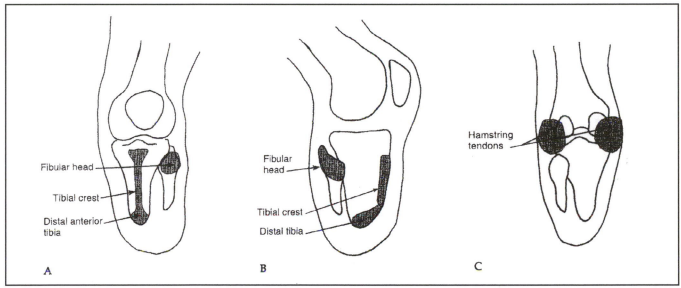

Figure 11-4. Pressure-intolerant areas of the residual limb. (A) From anterior view, areas that are pressure intolerant include the head of the fibula, crest of the tibia, and distal anterior tibia. (B) Laterally, the fiular head must be relieved of pressure. (C) On the posterior surface, tendons of the hamstring muscles need to be protected. (Reprinted from *Orthotics and Prosthetics in Rehabilitation*, Lusardi MM, Nielsen C, pp 439-441, © Copyright 2000 with permission from Elsevier.)

of the parallel bars. It is often difficult to maintain the emphasis on these basic activities as the patient is focused on walking. The time spent in the parallel bars with these activities will decrease the time needed to correct poor habits that might develop in a hurried rehabilitation process or when the patient is allowed to walk back and forth in the parallel bars unsupervised. The ability to control the prosthesis, "feel" the floor, and balance on the prosthesis are critical skills for safe, effective ambulation.

Although little objective evidence supports the interventions recommended, experience and the writings and presentations of others in rehabilitation form the basis of the proposed interventions.[6,46,49-52] Abundant anecdotal evidence, patient feedback, and clinical experience are the foundations upon which evidence-based

> ## Table 11-5
> ## WEARING SCHEDULE FLOW CHART
>
> Instructions: Please record the time you are in your prosthesis (total wearing time) and the time you are bearing weight in your prosthesis (walking time) three times/day. Record other information in the Comments area.
> Recommended wearing time: _____ minutes/day in _____ periods.
> Increase wearing time by _____ minutes/day if you do not have pain or problems with your skin.
>
> | | Morning | | Afternoon | | Evening | | Comments | | | |
> |---|---|---|---|---|---|---|---|---|---|---|
> | Date | Total Wearing | Walking Time | Total Wearing | Walking Time | Total Wearing | Walking time | Redness | Pain Score* | # of Socks | Assistive Device |
> | | | | | | | | | | | |
> | | | | | | | | | | | |
> | | | | | | | | | | | |
> | | | | | | | | | | | |
> | | | | | | | | | | | |
> | | | | | | | | | | | |
> | | | | | | | | | | | |
> | | | | | | | | | | | |
> | | | | | | | | | | | |
> | | | | | | | | | | | |
> | | | | | | | | | | | |
> | | | | | | | | | | | |
> | | | | | | | | | | | |
> | | | | | | | | | | | |
> | | | | | | | | | | | |
> | | | | | | | | | | | |
>
> *0 = No pain, 10 = Extreme pain
>
> Please follow these instructions as prescribed. Spending too much time in the prosthesis too soon can result in pain and skin breakdown. Check your skin frequently!

practice develops. Our experience complements research regarding motor learning, specifically whole versus part training, amount of practice, order of practice skills, the transfer of practice to using a new skill, the use of mental practice, and guidance versus discovery.[53]

Weight Transfer, Socket Control, and Balance

While standing within the parallel bars bearing weight through the upper and lower extremities, the patient progressively shifts more weight onto the prosthesis and over time should be able to bear full weight in single-limb stance without holding the bars. Skills such as shifting side-to-side, forward and backward, and from the front of one foot diagonally toward the heel of the opposite foot are introduced. These activi-

ties can be made more challenging by placing a foam pillow, rocker board, or other compliant surface under the patient's feet. (Figure 11-5) Early in rehabilitation, to emphasize weight bearing in the prosthesis, it is important that the patient avoid lateral or anterior/posterior trunk flexion and concentrate on moving the shoulders and pelvis as a unit to encourage adequate weight transfer into the socket. When shifting weight to the prosthetic side, the person with a HD/TP amputation should become aware of "a point of no return." This occurs when the body weight shifts too far laterally. Due to the fixed hip adduction/abduction of the prosthesis, the patient is not able to correct by cross-stepping with the sound limb laterally to the prosthesis; a fall to the prosthetic side may result if the patient cannot stabilize with hand gripping.

Table 11-6

TROUBLESHOOTING COMMON PROBLEMS WITH A PROSTHESIS

Pain

Pain problems often need to be addressed by the prosthetist. The physical therapist should obtain specific information about the pain and work with the patient and prosthetist to alleviate it. It may take some time to notice improvement after these changes are made, as the tissue may still be irritated. Where is the pain? At what point in the gait cycle does the pain occur? Does the pain persist after the prosthesis is removed? Does decreased weight bearing help? Does changing the number of socks help? Is the socket on correctly? Does doffing and redonning help? Has the limb changed shape, therefore altering pressures within the socket?

Skin Breakdown

A patient who has compromised circulation or delayed healing and develops any skin irritation or breakdown from prosthetic wearing should discontinue use of the prosthesis immediately. The prosthetist should be notified. In some cases, discontinuation of prosthetic use is not indicated if appropriate measures are taken to address the cause and protect the damaged area. See Chapter 5.

Length Discrepancy

When standing, verify that the patient is positioned properly in the socket, the shoe heel height has not changed, and a contracture or pain has not caused the altered position. Use a thickness of tile or magazines under the shoe on the lower side to achieve a level pelvis, then measure the height of the lift.

Pin Will Not Click Into Socket Mechanism

Re-don the liner. If this does not help, remove a sock and re-don the socket. If that does not help, ask the patient to stand, but not walk, and perform weight-shifting exercises. If the pin does not click into place, notify the prosthetist.

Inability to Remove Prosthesis

Sometimes this occurs for those using liners with pins, or if the patient perspires profusely, or the thigh has become edematous. Encourage the patient to relax, bear weight while sitting or standing, and push the release valve. Gently lift or pull the residual limb out of the socket. Alternatively, have the patient lie supine to relax tissue. A small amount of soapy warm water can be poured onto the skin between the limb and the silicon liner. Pull the liner away from the skin to allow the water to reach the bottom of the gel liner.

Pistoning

Tighten the suspension strap or add socks. If these techniques prove fruitless, notify the prosthetist.

Noises

If the noise is that of losing suction, the patient can try to expel air through the valve while bearing weight. If that does not help, reapply the prosthesis. Encourage the patient to "walk actively" by contracting the muscles of the residual limb, especially during the stance phase of gait. If the noise is mechanical (eg, squeak or groan), notify the prosthetist.

Damage

If the patient has fallen or has damaged the prosthesis in any way, discontinue prosthetic use and notify the prosthetist immediately.

Balance confidence in persons with unilateral TT and TF amputations is low whether the amputation was for vascular or nonvascular reasons, or if the person had or had not fallen in the past year.[14,54] Using an assistive device, the fear of falling, and the need to concentrate while walking are strongly related to balance confidence.[14] Standing with eyes closed against perturbations is an advanced skill that will challenge the patient to respond to unexpected movements. Responding to minimal perturbations will develop the balance response skills and perhaps decrease the likelihood of falling.[54]

Yigiter et al[55] reported that proprioceptive neuromuscular facilitation (PNF) resistive gait training techniques improved stride length and prosthetic weight bearing more than traditional treatment (weight shifting, balancing, stool-stepping, and gait exercises) among 50 patients with a TF amputation. The research evidence behind PNF is limited and controversial. Our clinical experience is that a combination of rehabilitation techniques, those with anecdotal and those with research evidence, can be used for successful rehabilitation. The physical therapist should work on basic balance skills to develop the patient's confidence, as this will have a great impact on the person's functional ability.[13]

Stepping forward and backward with the sound side limb should be a steady motion with evidence of trunk and sound side limb control. The emphasis is on contracting the muscles within and outside the socket while bearing weight on the prosthesis. Instruct the patient to become aware of the feel of contracting musculature within the socket, particularly at initial contact of the prosthesis and during the entire stance phase of gait. Placing a tennis ball under the sound foot, while bearing weight on the prosthesis, will further challenge the balance, single-limb stance, and coordination abilities of the patient.[12] (Figure 11-6).

Jaegers et al[56] studied 11 men with TF amputation and found that those with atrophied hip-stabilizing muscles walked with extreme lateral bend of the trunk towards the prosthetic side. Pain, prosthetic misalignment, and a femur that is positioned in abduction following surgery may also contribute to hip musculature weakness, pelvic instability, and truck side bending. To diminish the contralateral pelvic drop that often occurs with a TF amputation, the patient can place the prosthetic limb on a small step stool and practice hip hiking. This activity will encourage abductor strengthening in midstance when it is needed to stabilize the pelvis and prevent contralateral pelvic drop.

Next, the patient can step forward and backward in place with the prosthesis as the swing limb. Here the emphasis is on forward pelvic motion and controlling the prosthesis (specifically the swing speed, knee flexion, and placement of the prosthetic foot). For the person with a TT or TF amputation, the therapist may sit on the floor or a rolling stool to assist with prosthetic foot placement or tap the buttocks to encourage muscular control to attain hip extension at heel strike. The facilitation technique of tapping provides sensory feedback, which may promote muscle contraction.[57] With most knee units, it will be necessary to teach the patient to isometrically contract the muscles of the residual limb during ambulation, particularly at initial contact, loading response, and throughout stance. Knee units with stance flexion do not require this active control. Encouraging the patient to look ahead and "feel" the placement of the prosthetic foot is important. The bad habit of looking down while walking is a difficult one to overcome.

Gait training for the person with a HD or TP amputation begins with teaching a pelvic tilt in the supine position, then against a wall while standing, then with the prosthesis in place. To learn prosthetic foot placement, the patient practices propelling the prosthesis forward

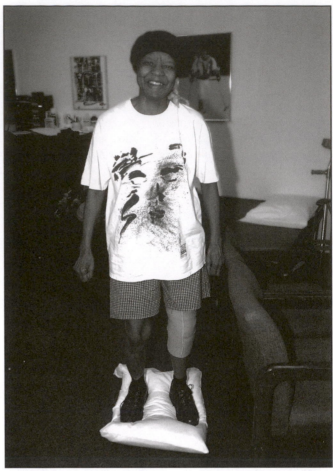

Figure 11-5. Balance on pillow. Balance challenge activity on a compliant surface.

in the parallel bars using only pelvic tilt. The verbal cue is a "gentle" tilt so as not to expend unnecessary energy. The tighter the fit of the socket, the easier it will be to perform the tilt. Due to lack of any musculature on the prosthetic side to assist ambulation, the sound limb will assist in prosthetic propulsion by using its hip extensors, quadriceps, and especially the gastroc-soleus complex. Vaulting (ie, exaggerated plantar flexion of the sound ankle) is acceptable, and may be unavoidable, as long as the shoulders of the patient are level and the momentum of the pelvis remains forward.

Forward pelvic motion is a critical skill. Clinical experience confirms that the loss of anterior pelvic translation is a source of gait deviation and increased cost of energy; a hip that is stationary or hiked during ambulation is less efficient in producing the forward motion of normal gait. "Even while patients who are learning to walk with a prosthesis are focused on conditions of the environment and prosthetic foot movement through space, they must move the pelvis on the amputated side forward so that the pelvis' trajectory is parallel to the floor."[46] Perry has identified 10 degrees of pelvic rotation as one component of efficient gait.[40]

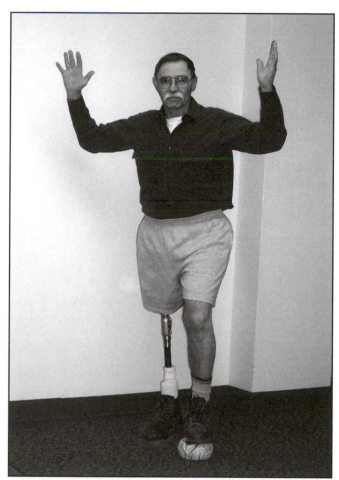

Figure 11-6. Advanced balance. Placing the nonprosthetic limb on a small ball and maintaining balance over prosthesis.

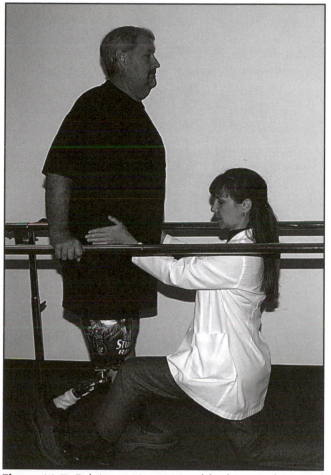

Figure 11-7. Pelvic rotation. Using blocking and manual contacts the therapist can assist initiation of pelvic rotation

The therapist can use manual pressure on the hips, trunk, or shoulders to emphasize desired movements by leading or resisting the movement. By blocking the prosthetic foot when the patient is in a position of terminal stance on the prosthetic side, the therapist can initiate and encourage the forward pelvic rotation needed to initiate knee flexion[51] (Figure 11-7) without having the patient resort to hip hiking, circumduction, or a posteriorly rotated pelvis. These are common compensations the individual may make when advancing the prosthetic limb in swing if the hip does not rotate forward.

Sidestepping and retroambulation within the parallel bars are important because we rarely walk in a straight line, particularly in a small kitchen and bathroom. Persons with a TF amputation often comment on the ease of walking backward. Unwanted knee flexion is avoided because of the hip hiking used to achieve rearward prosthetic foot placement and the fact that body weight is in front of the knee axis. Small steps will ensure that the prosthetic knee will not bend when weight is borne on the front of the prosthetic foot.

Computerized knee units have made many of these preambulation activities easier, as unwanted knee flexion is less likely to occur. It remains to be seen if the functional outcomes of persons using a computerized knee will significantly differ from those using non-computerized prostheses.

Standing on the prosthesis in single-limb stance is one of the most difficult early activities. A helpful exercise is stepping onto a low step with the sound side foot.[51] (Figures 11-8 and 11-9) The patient bears weight through the prosthesis and the arms while raising the sound foot onto a step. The prosthetic foot never leaves the floor. The lower the step, the easier it will be for the patient to perform this activity. As the patient demonstrates the ability to place the sound foot on a 2-inch step, with the eyes forward and with control, the activity can be made more challenging by gradually increasing the step height up to 8 inches, or lifting the hand on the side of the prosthesis. Lifting the sound side hand and finally performing this activity without handhold is the most challenging to the patient. The ability to perform this exercise slowly, with trunk and prosthetic control, is critical to ambulation without an

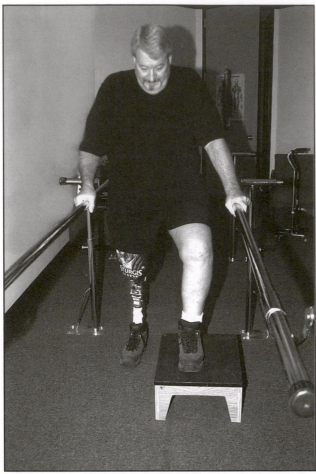

Figure 11-8. Step up. Beginning in the parallel bars or with any other stable surface the patient practices weight shifting onto the prosthesis.

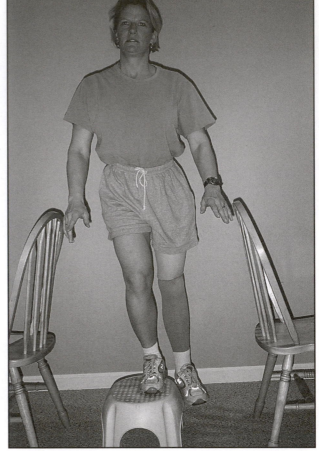

Figure 11-9. Step up. Beginning in the parallel bars or with another stable surface, the patient practices weight shifting onto the prosthesis.

assistive device. Using Perry's average cadence of 114 steps/minute,[40] this exercise simulates the 0.66 second needed for full body weight to be borne on the prosthesis for the single-limb support phase of gait.

Moving outside the safety of the parallel bars is the next step in challenging weight transfer, socket control, and balance. The exercises mentioned above should be repeated in this open environment, with attention directed toward safety (use of a gait belt, area clear of obstacles, assistance in guarding). This may also be the time to instruct the patient in getting up from the floor. Although often neglected, unsupported free standing while performing such functional tasks as reaching, tucking in a shirt, or holding a cup of coffee are worthwhile, nonambulatory activities that will challenge the patient and increase confidence in unassisted ambulation (Figure 11-10).

In addition to exercises that emphasize strength, coordination, and stability of the residual limb, exercises specific to the sound side should be included, as adequate force in these muscles helps improve functional gait abilities such as cadence and stride length.[58] Lateral

step-ups are excellent for strengthening the hip abductors on the sound side; the eyes should be forward and the hips level. With hands on hips, the patient performs the lateral step-up in front of a mirror to see hip heights. Begin with a 2-inch step and progress step height as strength and stability improve. (Figure 11-11).

The Total Gym (Total Gym Inc, San Diego, Calif), upright and recumbent stationary bicycles, upper extremity pulleys, and a treadmill can be used to help increase symmetry in strength and weight bearing on the amputated side. A treadmill with handrails allows weight-supported ambulation while the patient wears the prosthesis. This may in turn allow for increased duration of ambulation at varying speeds with less weight shifted to the upper extremities and the sound leg. At 3.0 mph with 40% body weight supported, treadmill ambulation has been shown to decrease energy expenditure for adults with TF and TT amputations.[37]

Although prosthetic knees do not provide assistance for stand-to-sit transfers, the patient using a TT or TF prosthesis should be instructed to use the prosthesis

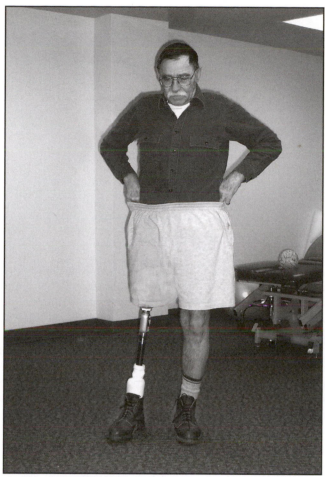

Figure 11-10. Balance. Practicing unassisted standing and balancing while tucking in a shirt.

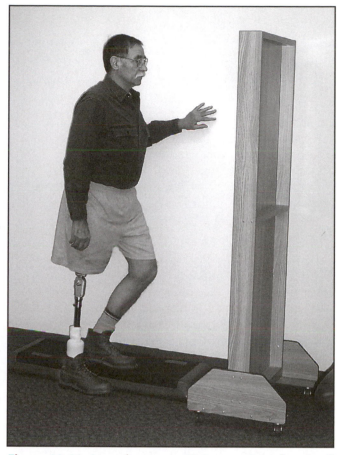

Figure 11-11. Lateral step up. Using a mirror for visual cueing, the patient steps up with the sound limb to develop awareness of pelvic position.

as much as possible during this activity. Teaching this important skill of nearly symmetrical weight bearing helps the patient to learn yet another way to use the muscles in the residual limb. Also, using the prosthesis helps alleviate some of the stress on the sound knee when performing the squat-like motion of standing to sitting. The following training hints are provided for specific knee units.

- *Polycentric knee.* The patient places the prosthetic foot slightly behind the unaffected foot and applies weight to the toe of the prosthesis. With slight pressure on the toe of the prosthesis and hip flexion, the knee will flex allowing the patient to sit. As the patient becomes more accustomed to using the prosthesis, slight prosthetic side anterior pelvic rotation, hip flexion, and weight shifting can cause the knee to flex for sitting, without placing the prosthetic foot behind the sound foot.

- *SNS knee.* This unit from Mauch Laboratories Inc (Dayton, Ohio) allows for two methods of sitting—with and without flexion resistance. To engage flexion resistance of the knee, slight knee flexion is performed, and the patient can sit

slowly, relying on the resistance of the knee unit.[59] To disengage flexion resistance, the patient hyperextends the prosthetic knee and sits.

- *Microchip knee.* With this device, the patient sits down using the flexion resistance of the knee unit throughout the entire motion.

Ambulation

The patient is now ready to begin walking. Walking within the parallel bars for the first time is an exciting event! The segmented activities described previously may have improved task performance and set the stage for ambulation, but it is the action of walking that will demonstrate that motor learning has occurred. With the aid of the therapist's verbal cues and manual contacts, the patient walks through the parallel bars demonstrating weight shifting, socket control, and pelvic and trunk rotation. Alternate hand placement on the bars simulates the reciprocal arm swing of normal gait. It is not desirable to provide constant manual or verbal feedback to the patient.[53] The patient must learn to develop a sense of the prosthesis, what needs to be done to control it, and how to create the desired action.[46]

Table 11-7
STABILIZING MUSCLES

Local Stabilizing system	Global Stabilizing System
Intertransversarii	Longissimus thoracis pars thoracis
Interspinales	Iliocostalis lumborum pars thoracis
Multifidus	Quadratus lumborum, lateral fibers
Longissimus thoracis pars lumborum	Rectus abdominis
Quadratus lumborum, medial fibers	Obliquus externus abdominis
Transversus abdominis	Obliquus internus abdominis
Obliquus internus abdominis (fiber insertion into thoraco-lumbar fascia)	

Reprinted from *Therapeutic Exercise for Spinal Segmental Stabilization in Low Back Pain*, Richardson C, Jull G, Hodges P, Hides J, page 14, © Copyright 1999, with permission from Elsevier.

Assistive Devices

When the patient exhibits satisfactory control of the prosthesis within the parallel bars, it is time to move out of the bars. Although some authors report that gait with a walker should be avoided,[6,46] our clinical experience finds that some patients fear ambulating with crutches because of previous falls or fear of falls. Practical limitations (insurance and schedule) may dictate that progression to a walker is needed. The two-wheeled walker allows for faster walking with less interruption than the four-footed walker, and is often preferred by patients.[60] Depending on balance and strength, various assistive devices and gait patterns can be used with the patient in the same manner used for people with other orthopedic diagnoses. Using the cane on the amputated side may assist weight shifting onto the prosthesis.[6] Perry concluded that, "...a well-fitted prosthesis that results in a satisfactory gait not requiring crutches significantly reduces the physiologic energy demand."[40] Though assistive devices do cost the patient energy, medical and physical conditions may not allow unassisted ambulation for some patients, especially elderly individuals.

Pelvic and Trunk Control

Control of the pelvis and trunk contributes to stability in ambulation. The lumbar multifidus and the transversus abdominis are muscles that provide the stability needed for controlled movement of the limbs and trunk.[61] A list of the local and global stabilization musculature needed for trunk and pelvic control in ambulation and ADL is in Table 11-7. If the trunk muscles do not contract or are delayed in contracting, the spine may not be prepared to stabilize against movement[61] generated by the arms, sound leg, and prosthesis, and may result in poor motion control, fatigue, and increased stress on other bodily structures. The physical therapist should not neglect trunk musculature as pelvic and trunk control are critical components of efficient ambulation. Deep

musculature cocontraction while walking is difficult and fatiguing,[61] but may be a critical area of rehabilitation that is missing from rehabilitation of persons with lower extremity amputations (Figure 11-12).

Trunk control is especially important for the person wearing a HD or TP prosthesis. Pelvic motion is needed to advance the prosthetic leg. Particular attention should be paid to the rectus abdominis for initiation of propulsion and for stabilizing the amputated side in the absence of functional long paraspinal musculature and the quadratus lumborum. Control of the ipsilateral deep paraspinal muscles needs to be maintained to prevent asymmetry at the lumbar spine and scoliosis with its associated respiratory consequences.

Activities of Daily Living

There is life beyond the parallel bars and the safety of the clinical environment. The physical therapist should be aware of environmental barriers that the patient will encounter on a daily basis and work to address these during rehabilitation. The following section gives techniques for practical activities for persons with a TF or higher amputation. The accommodations for the person with a TT amputation are minimal and any of the techniques described below can be used, in addition to accomplishing tasks just as they used to be done.

Dressing: Transfemoral and Hip Disarticulation/ Transpelvic

Generally it is easiest to dress the prosthesis prior to donning it. First, remove the shoe. then slide the pants onto the prosthesis (Figure 11-13). By applying a plastic bag onto the prosthetic foot, friction is decreased. To don a shoe, open the laces and tongue of the shoe fully. A shoe horn is generally necessary. The other leg of the pants can be slid onto the sound side. Finally, the prosthesis is donned. Personal ease and preference determine whether the patient wears the auxiliary suspension belts beneath or on top of undergarments. Wearing the belt

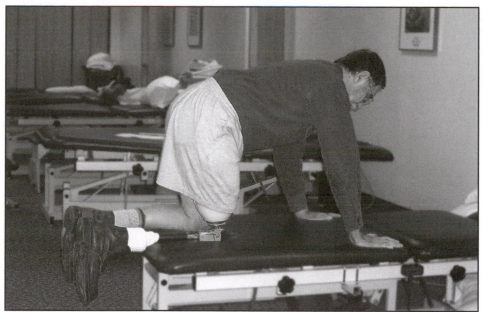

Figure 11-12. Core stability in quadruped. One of many exercise designed to improve core stability. Can be advanced by lifting one arm or leg and maintaining a neutral position of the spine.

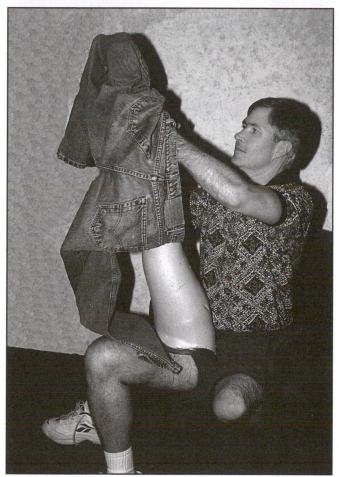

Figure 11-13. Dressing a prosthetic leg prior to putting it on.

modifications can include adding a zipper or hook and pile tape (Velcro [Velcro USA, Manchester, NH]) at the bottom inner seam. The seam may be split if the pant leg is narrow. When the patient is ready to wear boots, a zipper must be added to the inner side of the boots to allow for easy donning on the prosthetic foot.

Toileting: Transfemoral

Toileting skills should be practiced when there is no need to actually use the toilet. Skills include removing appropriate clothing, sitting on the toilet, re-donning the socket if necessary, and rearranging clothing if necessary. Suction socket wearers may lose suction because the vacuum is broken when the socket is pressed against the hard toilet seat. Although the therapist can teach basic skills, the patient must practice at home until a successful process is achieved.

Toileting: Hip Disarticulation/Transpelvic

The inferior portion of the socket generally crosses the midline of the torso of the person with a TP. Consequently, for women, it is necessary to remove the prosthesis and any protective garment for urination and defecation. Men do not need to doff the prosthesis for urination, but removal is necessary for defecation. Regarding the patient with a HD, the same rules typically apply even though the inferior aspect of the prosthesis does not cross the midline of the torso. Because there is a great variety of HD and TP designs, it is best to work with the patient and prosthetist to determine the most convenient and hygienic means of toileting.

Ramps, Curbs, and Stairs: Transfemoral

Ramp training should begin as soon as the patient can control the prosthesis on level surfaces with an assistive device. With most knee units, the patient should be instructed to descend the ramp with small

beneath is preferable to increase the ease of toileting. However, some patients find that wearing the belt on top of the undergarments is more comfortable. Clothing steps with active hip extension at prosthetic heel strike so that the prosthetic knee is locked into extension. (Picture 11-14) With a microchip knee, the patient is discouraged from achieving full knee extension because this will deactivate the flexion resistance mode of the knee unit. The patient should use the stance flexion feature of the microchip knee while descending the ramp. Ascending the ramp is easier. If the incline is too steep or if the patient is fearful, sidestepping with the prosthesis on the downhill side is helpful. Switch backing (going back and forth) up or down an incline, is also a useful way of decreasing the angle of the slope.

Ascending curbs and stairs is accomplished leading with the sound side. All patients begin descent leading with the prosthesis. The manually locked and sliding friction brake units do not permit step-over-step descent. Some individuals progress to the step-over-step method. Knee units with electronic or nonelectronic stance control (eg, C-Leg and SNS unit) allow a step-over-step approach for descending stairs more easily than with other units. The patient places the heel of the prosthetic foot on the lower step, and shifts weight onto the prosthesis. The patient should ensure that the knee is not hyperextended, as this will deactivate the stance flexion resistance. The patient relies on the resistance of the prosthetic knee as it flexes, and then places the sound side foot on the next lower step. Of course this skill should be practiced with the use of railings and a gait belt. Not all patients will be able or will want to learn how to descend stairs step-over-step. Descending stairs in this manner can be dangerous and takes a great deal of strength, concentration, and practice. Younger, more agile patients enjoy using their prostheses to the fullest of their capabilities and often use the step-over-step method or hop down stairs on the sound foot.

Ramps, Curbs, and Stairs: Hip Disarticulation/Transpelvic

Due to the lack of hip extensors on the prosthetic side, steep ramps are generally negotiated by sidestepping. Curbs and stairs are descended with the prosthetic side leading. Ascending stairs and curbs is done with the sound foot first. Microchip knees enable some patients to descend with a step-over-step pattern while still maintaining control and a constant speed.

Rising from the Floor: Transfemoral

- *Method 1*: The patient assumes the quadruped position and crawls to the nearest piece of stable furniture. Leading with the sound side, flexing the hip and placing the foot flat on the floor (one knee kneeling position), the patient leans forward onto the furniture, extends the sound hip, and brings the prosthesis forward to assume the standing position.

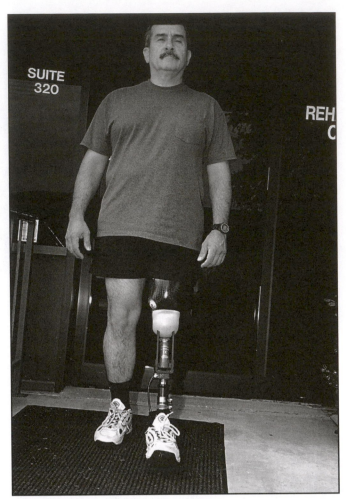

Figure 11-14. Declines. A patient descends with a slightly smaller prosthetic step.

- *Method 2*: "Walk" the hands back toward the knees while the hips and knees are extending. The patient shifts first onto the sound limb and then onto the prosthesis when the knee is completely extended.
- *Method 3*: Crawl toward furniture and pull up onto the furniture in prone then roll over to sit.

Rising from the Floor: Hip Disarticulation/Transpelvic

- *Method 1* (Easier): The patient rolls to the prone position and pushes with the hands to the quadruped position. The patient manually assists the prosthetic hip into flexion. The next position is kneeling on both knees, then leading with the sound side foot, placing that foot flat on the floor. With the use of a stable support, the patient pushes with the sound leg and both hands into standing (Figures 11-15).
- *Method 2* (Difficult; done without furniture—requires good hamstring flexibility): The patient

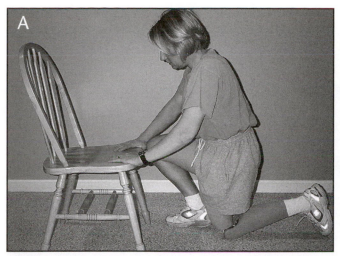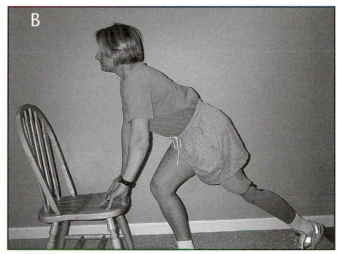

Figure 11-15. Getting up from the floor, Method 1. (A) The start of getting up from the floor shown using furniture for support from the kneeling position. (B) Progression of getting up from the floor for a person with a HD/TP. This technique also works for persons with lower level amputations.

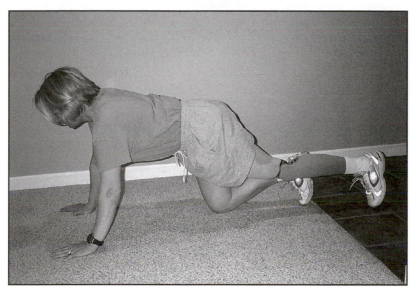

Figure 11-16. Getting up from the floor, Method 2. With the prosthesis in extension the patient is weight bearing on the remaining limbs.

begins in the prone position with the toes of the sound foot in contact with the floor. With the prosthesis fully extended, the patient pushes up to the quadruped position. The patient then "walks" the hands toward the feet until further movement is halted either by tightness of the sound side hamstrings or arm length. Then, with a very strong push from both arms, the patient balances on the sound side and then stands, allowing the prosthetic hip to flex until the limb is beneath the trunk and the person can bear weight (Figures 11-16 and 11-17).

- *Method 3* (Very difficult): The patient is in the long sitting position with hands slightly behind the buttocks. The sound side foot is placed beneath the buttock. With a strong push from the arms, the individual rocks forward onto the sound

foot, leaving the prosthesis flexed at the hip and extended at the knee. An extremely strong sound leg is needed to power the patient into the standing position (Figures 11-18 and 11-19).

Falling: All Levels

Many patients identify falling as their greatest fear. Persons with an amputation have a higher fall incidence (52.4%) than community-dwelling elders (30% to 40%) or institutionalized elders (50%).[62] The therapist should address falling and rising techniques and be aware that fear of falling will result in activity avoidance and a decreased quality of life.[54,62]

Other medical problems mitigate teaching this skill to many patients because of the potential for injury in the simple act of practicing it.[46] We believe that because patients with an amputation will fall, it is better to teach this skill than to leave the patient ignorant of the recom-

Figure 11-17. Getting up from the floor, Method 2. The patient uses the sound lower limb and both hands to walk backwards into an upright position.

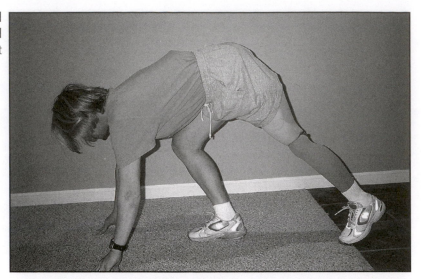

Figure 11-18. Getting up from the floor, Method 3. Beginning in long sitting with the prosthetic side leg in extension, the patient will push off hands and other leg to rise from the floor.

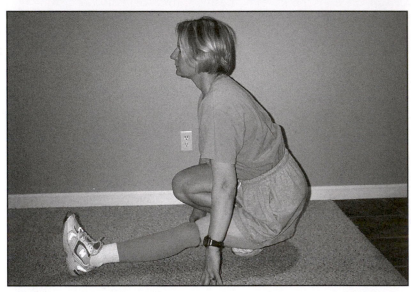

mended techniques for falling. To teach this skill safely, a mat, two pillows, two safety belts, and two helpers are necessary. The pillows are placed on the floor mat. The therapist should first demonstrate the technique. The two safety belts are placed on the patient, and two helpers stand diagonally behind the patient on each side, holding the belts. The patient is instructed to throw the assistive device out of the way, flex at the waist, and fall toward the unaffected side, landing laterally. The arms must be flexed at the shoulders, elbows, and wrists to land safely. The helpers allow the patient to fall onto the pillows gently (Figures 11-20, 11-21, and 11-22). The patient should never be pushed to start the fall but should be encouraged to initiate the simulated fall.

Kneeling and Crawling: Transfemoral, Hip Disarticulation, and Transpelvic

The patient should kneel onto the prosthesis first, and while holding on to a stable object, flex the sound hip and knee. One-knee kneeling and crawling are both possible although not particularly comfortable for long periods of time. One-knee kneeling on the prosthetic side for the person with a HD or TP is unstable due to lack of hip musculature. The person with a HD or TP drags the prosthesis behind; the toe of the prosthesis resists movement, limiting the patient to very short distances (Figures 11-23).

Turning: Transfemoral, Hip Disarticulation, and Transpelvic

As many patients have compromised circulation, teaching proper turning is imperative. When turning, the tendency is to pivot on the sound foot. The patient should be taught to avoid turning in this manner as it may be unsafe and can cause undue stress on both limbs. Pivoting can lead to increased socket internal rotation on the residual limb, particularly for those who wear a sock and waist belt. The patient should be taught to perform a series of small steps in a U-turn pattern towards the prosthesis as well as the sound side.

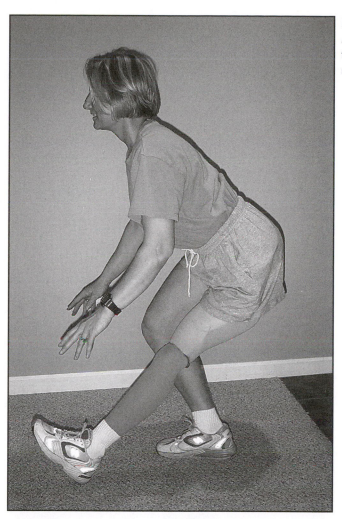

Figure 11-19. Getting up from the floor, Method 3. Maintaining forward momentum, and weight bearing on the nonprosthetic side, the patient is moving toward an upright position.

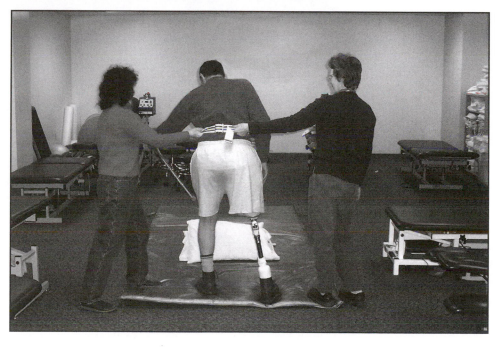

Figure 11-20. Falling. Using a gait belt and soft surfaces, the patient begins the falling sequence.

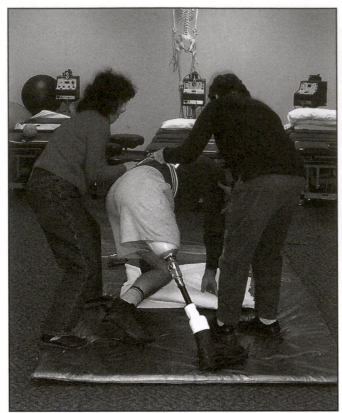

Figure 11-21. Falling sequence continued.

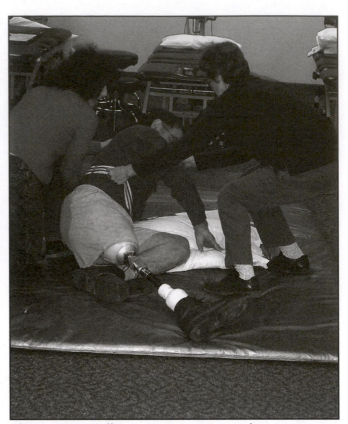

Figure 11-22. Falling sequence continued.

Figure 11-23. Kneeling onto the prosthetic knee first with the support of furniture. This position is necessary for crawling, getting up from or down to the floor.

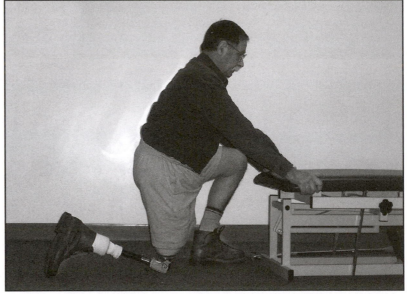

Carrying Objects: Transfemoral

Carrying objects should be practiced first in the controlled environment of the clinic for safety. Carrying challenges balance and confidence, and can be made more difficult by placing various obstacles in the patient's path as well as altering the environment with increasing forms of distraction. The patient can practice carrying a book, a cup of coffee, and eventually a heavy box.

Carrying Objects: Hip Disarticulation and Transpelvic

Obviously, the balance challenges are greater at these levels; the patient tends to favor carrying objects on the sound side and use the other arm for balance. When carrying objects that require two hands, such as large boxes or infants, the patient should maintain constant prosthetic knee extension and take small steps (Figure 11-24).

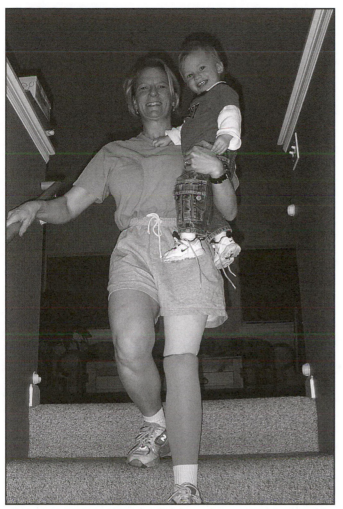

Figure 11-24. Carrying a child or objects. Keeping safety in mind, it is possible for a person with a lower extremity amputation to carry precious object.

Doors: All Levels

Doors vary in weight, width, resistance, and opening direction. For a door that opens away from the patient, the person should approach the door, push it open, place the assistive device or prosthetic foot to block the door, and step through. Halfway through the door, the patient may need to push the door further open and stabilize again with the assistive device or foot. To open a heavy door when no assistive device is used, extra leverage is needed. The patient may lean into the door to prevent the weight of the door from pushing the patient off-balance. For a door that opens towards the patient, the person should take short backward steps while holding the door handle.

Car Transfers: Transtibial and Transfemoral

The patient should move the car seat back as far as possible and sit on the seat leading with the hips. The patient then scoots the hips back into the seat and moves one leg at a time into the car. A patient who is very tall should scoot towards the middle of the front seat as far as possible, sometimes actually into the passenger seat, to allow for clearance for the prosthesis.

Car Transfers: Hip Disarticulation and Transpelvic

When entering a truck or a utility vehicle, it may be necessary to step onto the running board with the sound foot. Then the patient turns from the seat to avoid slipping off the edge, initiates prosthetic knee flexion, and sits. The prosthesis is lifted into the car. Tall patients may require a rotator on the femoral portion of the prosthesis to enable the limb to fit in the vehicle.

Community Mobility

"An amputee must be able to walk at least 600 steps a day to manage in a one-level house or apartment with moderate support provided by family or social agencies."[24] Nissen and Newman[63] identified factors affecting reintegration to normal living and found that poor reintegration occurred in community mobility, work, and recreation. In a study of 27 persons with a TT amputation, the ability to increase weight bearing in single-limb stance was a predictor of walking velocity.[8] Because walking velocity affects function,[8] all patients with amputations should be trained to vary their walking speed. In 11 patients with TF amputations due to trauma or cancer, comfortable walking speed was 29% slower than able-bodied individuals.[64] The elderly tend to have a slower self-selected walking speed. They increase their step frequency to increase their pace, whereas their younger counterparts increase their stride length.[65] Speed can be increased by asking the patient to take a longer step with the sound limb and a moderate step with the prosthetic limb.[51] More advanced skills needed for community ambulation include crossing the street and navigating escalators, elevators, and various types of terrain.

Hoxie and Rubenstein[66] showed that 27% of older pedestrians walked slower than the speed set at traffic lights and were unable to reach the opposite curb before the light changed. To simulate street crossing in the clinic, ask the patient to ambulate approximately 70 feet in 18 seconds. Treadmill training can assist learning various speeds for short distances. Actual on-road training is ideal. Walking speed at signalized intersections is correlated with self-reported activity level among elderly individuals.[67] The relationship between gait speed and function was assessed in persons who had suffered a stroke.[68] The following feet/minute are the minimum needed for safe community activity: 114 feet/minute for minimum community activity without a wheelchair and not crossing a street; 158 feet/minute for independent community activity and crossing narrow streets; and 236 feet/minute for community activity and to cross a broad street. These parameters appear to be realistic for community activity among persons with amputations.

Escalators

Using an escalator can be a daunting task for the person with an amputation. Before practicing this skill, find the emergency shut-off switch for the escalator. The sequencing for stepping onto an escalator is the same as for stairs, "Up with the good, down with the bad." Although it is usually easiest for the patient to step onto the up escalator in this manner some people feel more comfortable doing the opposite. Both methods should be practiced. For the person with a TF, HD, or TP amputation, escalators need to be approached cautiously. Extra time should be taken and initially another person should always accompany the patient. The assistant stands in front of the patient with the patient's hand on the helper's shoulder. To ascend, the sound foot steps first, followed quickly by the prosthetic foot. The patient should then hold both handrails. When stepping off the escalator, the sound foot steps first to obtain stable footing. Escalator descent is appreciably more difficult. Both hands are on the handrails as the prosthetic foot steps first, with the sound foot following quickly.

Elevators

Elevators are usually easy to enter and leave but should be practiced with a family member or the therapist the first few times. Stepping into the elevator can be done comfortably with either foot. This skill can be practiced in the clinic by using quick bursts of speed, especially if the patient exhibits fear of entering an elevator. The person with a HD or TP prosthesis needs to step into the elevator using the same pattern as for stairs, particularly if the gap between the elevator and the floor is uneven.

Uneven Surfaces

Grassy terrain is commonly part of most community ambulation. The patient with a TF, HD, or TP amputation often must vault or hip hike to clear the prosthetic foot. Forceful use of the hip extensors ensures that the prosthetic knee will be stable during stance phase. Knee units with stance flexion will not require this motion. The patient with a HD or TP may strike the prosthetic heel firmly to ensure full knee extension. It is difficult for the person with a HD or TP to ambulate on hilly terrain with the prosthesis, as uphill hip hiking is limited by the lack of active hip abduction to maintain a level pelvis and avoid side bending.

Care of the Sound Limb

Education regarding care of the sound foot is mandatory for every patient. The likelihood of bilateral amputation for persons with vascular disease increases 10% per year.[23,40] Although the patient may have been educated regarding proper foot care during the pre-prosthetic period, updating the information and reviewing procedures with the patient are prudent. Ascertaining who trims the patient's toenails is imperative, as this task is often neglected and should not be performed by patients with poor vision or diminished manual dexterity. Daily inspection of the remaining foot by the patient or a family member should be done in a well-lit area. When self-inspecting, a mirror should be used. The dorsum, sides, and plantar surface of the foot should be inspected, as well as between each toe. Hints on caring for the foot are presented in Table 11-8. Local hospitals or physicians may provide diabetic foot care clinics. Hopping should be discouraged because it imposes excessive pressure on the sound foot and increases the risk of falling.

HEALTH, WELLNESS, AND FITNESS

Lifetime fitness is critical for everyone. The person with an amputation can exercise by swimming, cycling, dancing, golfing, and propelling a wheelchair. Many public broadcast television stations offer seated exercise programs. A local YMCA or senior citizen center may have activity programs appropriate for the person with an amputation. The Amputee Coalition of America (ACA) is a national organization that provides various resources to people with amputations. The ACA (1-888-AMP-KNOW) has a resource catalog of videotapes, books, and pamphlets that address fitness. Several prosthetic manufacturers provide exercise or motivational videos free or for a nominal fee. The National Amputee Golf Association's magazine, *Amputee Golfer*, as well as First Swing—Learn to Golf seminars (1-800-633-NAGA) are informative.

SUPPORT SERVICES

Most metropolitan areas have a support group for persons with amputations. A hospital referral service, a social worker, or the Chamber of Commerce should be able to direct the patient and caregivers to the appropriate resources. The ACA publishes a bimonthly magazine *inMotion*, and holds an annual educational meeting. Other services include information for developing support groups and peer visitor training.

FOLLOW-UP VISITS

The patient should be seen regularly for follow-up visits. The purpose of these visits is to determine whether further physical therapy services or other services are necessary. Visits scheduled at 6 weeks, 3 months, and 6 months after discharge are helpful in determining if the patient is returning to maximal functional independence, thereby limiting the impact of the amputation and disability. Information obtained should include prosthetic wearing time, distances

Table 11-8

SOUND FOOT CARE TIPS

- Taking care of your foot every day will help maintain a healthier foot with fewer problems.
- Wash your foot every day. Avoid extremes of temperature. If you have decreased sensitivity or sensation in your foot, test the bath water with another part of your body or have a family member test the water temperature for you. After bathing, dry your foot completely, especially between your toes.
- In a room with good lighting, check your foot daily for sores, calluses, red spots, swelling, and blisters. Use a mirror to check all areas of your foot. Feel your foot for cold or hot spots. If your vision is impaired, ask another person to inspect your foot.
- Wear shoes (not slippers) at all times when out of bed. Never walk barefoot, including when getting up to use the bathroom at night and on the beach.
- Do not use chemical agents for the removal of corns or calluses. See your doctor.
- Use an emery board or pumice stone daily to smooth calluses. Do not cut calluses or corns yourself. See your doctor if calluses or corns are painful.
- Do not smoke. Smoking decreases circulation and will increase the risk for sores on your foot.
- Clean any wounds right away. Call your doctor, no matter how minor your wound. Remember that a small cut on your foot can quickly become bigger and infected. Always call your doctor if you get a blister on your foot, your skin cracks, or your foot hurts without reason.
- Use skin cream to decrease dry, scaly skin, but do not use cream between your toes.
- Check with your health care provider to determine if is safe for you to cut your toenails. If the answer is yes, cut toenails straight across. File the edges with an emery board so they are smooth, not sharp or jagged. Otherwise ask another person to cut your toenails.
- Make sure your diabetes doctor checks your foot at every visit.
- Keep your diabetes under control. High glucose levels are frequently the cause of foot problems.
- Do not buy shoes at self-service stores. Have shoes fitted by a shoe salesperson or a pedorthist. Ask your doctor or physical therapist for suggestions about where to purchase appropriate shoes.
- Buy and wear only comfortable, supportive shoes with a low heel and plenty of wiggle room for your toes. "Breaking-in" shoes may cause "breakdown" of your skin.
- Choose leather or canvas shoes. Do not wear sandals or plastic shoes.
- Check inside your shoes for foreign objects before putting them on.
- Wear socks without seams or tight elastic. Seams can rub your foot and cause blisters or sores.
- Put on a clean sock each day.
- A sock is the best remedy for a chilly foot. Do not use a heating pad or hot water bottle to warm your foot because, if you lack sensation, you may burn your foot.

walked, assistive device used, number of socks worn, types of activities performed, presence of pain, and any other problems or concerns. Annual check-ins with the physical therapist will support the patient's efforts to continue to use the prosthesis and work on advanced skills, such as running, if that is an appropriate goal. Visits can be coordinated via the office staff using a postcard reminder.

CONCLUSION

The principal goal of rehabilitation for people using a prosthesis is to allow as much independence as possible, thereby limiting the disabling effects of amputation. Using the examination process and interventions described in this chapter, the physical therapist and the patient should find success in achieving maximum function with minimal long-term disability.

The authors gratefully acknowledge Michelle Beamer, MPT, and G. Edward Jeffries, MD, for their editorial assistance, and Dennis Cole for his photographic assistance.

REFERENCES

1. APTA. *Guide to Physical Therapist Practice*. Alexandria, Va: American Physical Therapy Association; 2001.
2. Gordon N. *The Exercise Prescription*. Alexandria, Va: American Diabetes Association; 1995.
3. Pezzin LE, Dillingham TR, MacKenzie EJ. Rehabilitation and the long-term outcomes of persons with trauma-related amputations. *Arch Phys Med Rehabil*. 2000;81:292-300.
4. May B. *Amputations and Prosthetics: A Case Study Approach*. 2nd ed. Philadelphia, Pa: FA Davis; 1996.
5. Esquenazi A, Meier RH, 3rd. Rehabilitation in limb deficiency. 4. Limb amputation. *Arch Phys Med Rehabil*. 1996;77:S18-S28.

6. Ehde DM, Czerniecki JM, Smith DG, et al. Chronic phantom sensations, phantom pain, residual limb pain, and other regional pain after lower limb amputation. *Arch Phys Med Rehabil*. 2000;81:1039-1044.

7. Mersky H, ed. *Classification of Chronic Pain: Descriptions of Chronic Pain Syndromes and Definitions of Pain Terms*. 2nd ed. Seattle, Wash: IASP Press; 1994.

8. Jones ME, Bashford GM, Bliokas VV. Weight-bearing, pain and walking velocity during primary transtibial amputee rehabilitation. *Clin Rehabil*. 2001;15:172-176.

9. Brooks D, Hunter JP, Parsons J, et al. Reliability of the two-minute walk test in individuals with transtibial amputation. *Arch Phys Med Rehabil*. 2002; 83:1562-1565.

10. Brooks D, Parsons J, Hunter JP, et al. The 2-minute walk test as a measure of functional improvement in persons with lower limb amputation. *Arch Phys Med Rehabil*. 2001; 82:1478-1483.

11. Binkley JM, Stratford PW, Lott SA, Riddle DL. The Lower Extremity Functional Scale (LEFS): scale development, measurement properties, and clinical application. *Phys Ther*. 1999;79:371-383.

12. Gailey R. *Amputee Mobility and Performance Clinics Course Handout*. Reykjavik, Iceland: Ossur Corporation; 2002.

13. Hatch J, Gill-Body KM, Portney LG. Determinants of balance confidence in community-dwelling elderly people. *Phys Ther*. 2003;83:1072-1079.

14. Miller WC, Speechley M, Deathe AB. Balance confidence among people with lower-limb amputations. *Phys Ther*. 2002;82:856-865.

15. Miller WC, Deathe AB, Speechley M. Psychometric properties of the Activities-specific Balance Confidence Scale among individuals with a lower-limb amputation. *Arch Phys Med Rehabil*. 2003;84:656-661.

16. Miller WC, Deathe AB, Speechley M. Lower extremity prosthetic mobility: a comparison of 3 self-report scales. *Arch Phys Med Rehabil*. 2001;82:1432-1440.

17. Gauthier-Gagnon C, Grise MC. Prosthetic profile of the amputee questionnaire: validity and reliability. *Arch Phys Med Rehabil*. 1994;75:1309-1314.

18. Grise MC, Gauthier-Gagnon C, Martineau GG. Prosthetic profile of people with lower extremity amputation: conception and design of a follow-up questionnaire. *Arch Phys Med Rehabil*. 1993;74:862-870.

19. Treweek SP, Condie ME. Three measures of functional outcome for lower limb amputees: a retrospective review. *Prosthet Orthot Int*. 1998;22:178-185.

20. Wall JC, Bell C, Campbell S, Davis J. The Timed Get-up-and-Go test revisited: measurement of the component tasks. *J Rehabil Res Dev*. 2000;37:109-113.

21. Leung EC, Rush PJ, Devlin M. Predicting prosthetic rehabilitation outcome in lower limb amputee patients with the functional independence measure. *Arch Phys Med Rehabil*. 1996;77:605-608.

22. Muecke L, Shekar S, Dwyer D, Israel F, Flynn JP. Functional screening of lower-limb amputees: A role in predicting rehabilitation outcome? *Arch Phys Med Rehabil*. 1992;73:851-858.

23. Cutson TM, Bongiorni DR. Rehabilitation of the older lower limb amputee: a brief review. *J Am Geriatr Soc*. 1996;44:1388-1393.

24. Pernot HF, de Witte LP, Lindeman E, Cluitmans J. Daily functioning of the lower extremity amputee: an overview of the literature. *Clin Rehabil*. 1997;11:93-106.

25. Pandian G, Kowalske K. Daily functioning of patients with an amputated lower extremity. *Clin Orthop*. 1999;361:91-97.

26. Evans WE, Hayes JP, Vermilion BD. Rehabilitation of the bilateral amputee. J Vasc Surg. 1987;5:589-593.

27. Spence WD, Fowler NK, Nicol AC, Murray SJ. Reciprocating gait prosthesis for the bilateral hip disarticulation amputee. *Proc Inst Mech Eng* [H]. 2001;215:309-314.

28. Shin JC, Park CI, Kim YC, et al. Rehabilitation of a triple amputee including a hip disarticulation. *Prosthet Orthot Int*. 1998;22:251-253.

29. Andrews KL. Rehabilitation in limb deficiency. 3. The geriatric amputee. *Arch Phys Med Rehabil*. 1996;77:S14-S17.

30. Lemaire ED, Fisher FR. Osteoarthritis and elderly amputee gait. *Arch Phys Med Rehabil*. 1994;75:1094-1099.

31. Carlson JM. A flexible, air-permeable socket prosthesis for bilateral hip disarticulation and hemicorporectomy amputees. *J Prosthet Orthot*. 1998;10:110-117.

32. Davidson JH, Jones LE, Cornet J, Cittarelli T. Management of the multiple limb amputee. *Disabil Rehabil*. 2002;24:688-699.

33. Melchiorre PJ, Findley T, Boda W. Functional outcome and comorbidity indexes in the rehabilitation of the traumatic versus the vascular unilateral lower limb amputee. *Am J Phys Med Rehabil*. 1996;75:9-14.

34. Graham LA, Fyfe NC. Prosthetic rehabilitation of amputees aged over 90 is usually successful. *Disabil Rehabil*. 2002;24:700-701.

35. Cole E. Training elders with transfemoral amputations. In: Lewis CB, ed. *Geriatric Rehabilitation*. Vol 19. Philadelphia, Pa: Lippincott Williams & Wilkins; 2003:183-190.

36. Harris KA, van Schie L, Carroll SE, et al. Rehabilitation potential of elderly patients with major amputations. *J Cardiovasc Surg (Torino)*. 1991;32:463-467.

37. Hunter D, Smith Cole E, Murray JM, Murray TD. Energy expenditure of below-knee amputees during harness-supported treadmill ambulation. *J Orthop Sports Phys Ther*. 1995;21:268-276.

38. Steinberg FU, Sunwoo I, Roettger RF. Prosthetic rehabilitation of geriatric amputee patients: a follow-up study. *Arch Phys Med Rehabil*. 1985;66:742-745.

39. Cruts HE, de Vries J, Zilvold G, et al. Lower extremity amputees with peripheral vascular disease: graded exercise testing and results of prosthetic training. *Arch Phys Med Rehabil*. 1987;68:14-19.

40. Perry J. *Gait Analysis: Normal and Pathological Function*. Thorofare, NJ: SLACK Inc; 1992.

41. Chin T, Sawamura S, Fujita H, et al. %VO$_2$max as an indicator of prosthetic rehabilitation outcome after dysvascular amputation. *Prosthet Orthot Int*. 2002;26:44-49.

42. Whaley MH, Brubaker PH, Kaminsky LA, Miller CR. Validity of rating of perceived exertion during graded exercise testing in apparently healthy adults and cardiac patients. *J Cardiopulm Rehabil.* 1997;17:261-267.

43. Whaley MH, Woodall T, Kaminsky LA, Emmett JD. Reliability of perceived exertion during graded exercise testing in apparently healthy adults. *J Cardiopulm Rehabil.* 1997;17:37-42.

44. Chen MJ, Fan X, Moe ST. Criterion-related validity of the Borg ratings of perceived exertion scale in healthy individuals: a meta-analysis. *J Sports Sci.* 2002;20:873-899.

45. Wallbom AS, Geisser ME, Haig AJ, et al. Concordance between rating of perceived exertion and function in persons with chronic, disabling back pain. *J Occup Rehabil.* 2002;12:93-98.

46. Lusardi MM, Neilsen CC, eds. *Orthotics and Prosthetics in Rehabilitation.* Boston, Mass: Butterworth Heinemann; 2000.

47. Karacoloff L. *Lower Extremity Amputation: A Guide to Functional Outcomes in Physical Therapy Management.* 2nd ed. Gaithersburg, Md: Aspen; 1992.

48. Streppel KR, de Vries J, van Harten WH. Functional status and prosthesis use in amputees, measured with the Prosthetic Profile of the Amputee (PPA) and the short version of the Sickness Impact Profile (SIP68). *Int J Rehabil Res.* 2001;24:251-256.

49. Eisert O, Tester OW. Dynamic exercises for lower extremity amputees. *Arch Phys Med Rehabil.* 1954;35:695-704.

50. Engstrom B, Van de Ven C. *Physiotherapy for Amputees: The Roehampton Approach.* New York, NY: Churchill Livingston; 1993.

51. Gailey RS, Clark CR. *Physical Therapy Management of Adult Lower-Limb Amputees.* St Louis, Mo: Mosby Year Book; 1992.

52. Mensch G, Ellis P. *Physical Therapy Management of Lower Extremity Amputations.* Rockville, Md: Aspen Publishers; 1986.

53. Shumway-Cook A, Woolacott M. *Motor Control: Theory and Practical Application.* New York, NY: Williams & Wilkins; 2001.

54. Miller WC, Speechley M, Deathe B. The prevalence and risk factors of falling and fear of falling among lower extremity amputees. *Arch Phys Med Rehabil.* 2001;82:1031-1037.

55. Yigiter K, Sener G, Erbahceci F, et al. A comparison of traditional prosthetic training versus proprioceptive neuromuscular facilitation resistive gait training with transfemoral amputees. *Prosthet Orthot Int.* 2002;26:213-217.

56. Jaegers SM, Arendzen JH, de Jongh HJ. Prosthetic gait of unilateral transfemoral amputees: a kinematic study. *Arch Phys Med Rehabil.* 1995;76:736-743.

57. Voss D, Myers BJ. *Proprioceptive Neuromuscular Facilitation: Patterns and Techniques.* 3rd ed. Philadelphia, Pa: Harper and Row; 1985.

58. Powers CM, Boyd LA, Fontaine CA, Perry J. The influence of lower-extremity muscle force on gait characteristics in individuals with below-knee amputations secondary to vascular disease. *Phys Ther.* 1996;76:369-377.

59. *Mauch SNS Hydraulik Knee Control User's Manual.* Dayton, Ohio: Mauch Laboratories Incorporated; 1996.

60. Tsai HA, Kirby RL, MacLeod DA, Graham MM. Aided gait of people with lower-limb amputations: comparison of 4-footed and 2-wheeled walkers. *Arch Phys Med Rehabil.* 2003;84:584-591.

61. Richardson C JG, Hodges P, Hides J. *Therapeutic Exercise for Spinal Segmental Stabilization in Low Back Pain.* Edinburgh, Scotland: Churchill Livingston; 1999.

62. Miller WC, Deathe AB, Speechley M, Koval J. The influence of falling, fear of falling, and balance confidence on prosthetic mobility and social activity among individuals with a lower extremity amputation. *Arch Phys Med Rehabil.* 2001;82:1238-1244.

63. Nissen SJ, Newman WP. Factors influencing reintegration to normal living after amputation. *Arch Phys Med Rehabil.* 1992;73:548-551.

64. Jaegers SM, Vos LD, Rispens P, Hof AL. The relationship between comfortable and most metabolically efficient walking speed in persons with unilateral above-knee amputation. *Arch Phys Med Rehabil.* 1993;74:521-525.

65. Smidt G, ed. *Gait in Rehabilitation.* New York, NY: Churchill Livingston; 1990.

66. Hoxie RE, Rubenstein LZ. Are older pedestrians allowed enough time to cross intersections safely? *J Am Geriatr Soc.* 1994;42:241-244.

67. Keller P, Risiing AJ. Relationship between walking speed at signalized intersections and self-reported activity level of elderly individuals. *Issues on Aging.* 1998; 21:15-18.

68. Perry J, Garrett M, Gronley JK, Mulroy SJ. Classification of walking handicap in the stroke population. *Stroke.* 1995; 26:982-989.

Rehabilitation of Adults With Upper-Limb Amputation

Chapter 12

Body-Powered Upper-Limb Prosthetic Designs

Jack E. Uellendahl, CPO and Elaine N. Uellendahl, CP

OBJECTIVES

1. Contrast the characteristics of persons with upper-limb amputation with those who have lower-limb amputation
2. Calculate the functional length of transradial and transhumeral amputation limbs
3. Define prescription options, including passive, cable-operated, adaptive, electrically powered, and hybrid prostheses
4. Describe body-powered components of unilateral and bilateral transradial, transhumeral, and shoulder disarticulation prostheses, including terminal devices, wrist units, elbow units, shoulder joints, sockets, and harness and control systems
5. Discuss the physical prerequisites and motions for body-powered control

INTRODUCTION

In the highly specialized world of health care, upper-limb prosthetic rehabilitation occupies a small niche. Individuals with acquired amputations and those born with a major upper-limb deficiency belong to a small minority. Consequently, most prosthetists, therapists, physicians, and case managers never gain the practical experience necessary to optimize rehabilitation for this unique group of individuals. A few clinicians, however, do specialize in this ultrafocused area.

DEMOGRAPHICS

Acquired arm amputation is most commonly caused by trauma.[1] Men are more likely to experience limb loss. In recent years, an almost 50% decrease in traumatic and cancer-related upper- and lower-limb amputations is most likely due to improved occupational safety standards and advanced limb salvage procedures. Sophisticated vascular, orthopedic, plastic, and neurologic surgery has changed limb salvage markedly.[2-5] A dramatic example is replantation, reattachment of the patient's severed limb. Nevertheless, comparison of

people whose limbs were salvaged through reconstruction procedures and those who had amputation have shown (depending on level of amputation) little or no overall difference between the groups with regard to functional outcome. Those who underwent amputations had shorter hospital stays, fewer surgical procedures, fewer hospital readmissions, and fewer medical complications.[6] Incidence of congenital upper-limb deficiency has remained constant at 15.74 per 100,000 live births.[1]

DIFFERENCES BETWEEN UPPER- AND LOWER-LIMB AMPUTATIONS

Critical differences exist between the typical person with upper-limb amputation and someone with lower-limb amputation. Most upper-limb amputations are caused by trauma, whereas lower-limb amputation is overwhelmingly necessitated by vascular disease. When assessing the individual who has experienced trauma severe enough to result in limb loss, it is as important to treat the psychological problems of the individual as it is to focus on the prosthesis.[7] With trauma, no prolonged illness or preoperative stage is present prior to surgery.

Psychological differences between upper- and lower-limb amputation are evident. Self-image, self-esteem, and confidence are more commonly affected by upper-limb amputation. Compounding the problem, loss of the hand is more visible than leg absence, and the appearance of the amputated upper limb is usually less cosmetic than a lower amputated limb. Other psychological issues arise because the patient may initially have to rely on family and friends for basic daily needs, which can undermine self-esteem. The disparity between expectations of the capabilities of an upper-limb prosthesis and reality is due to several factors. Most people have never seen anyone who wears an upper-limb prosthesis; wishful thinking and media glamorization of ultra sophisticated appliances contribute to unrealistic expectations. It seems commonsensical that psychological "fragility" of traumatic patients, whether the amputation is upper or lower limb, must be managed carefully. Building rapport is essential, as is comprehensive patient education. Chapter 6 addresses psychological considerations and interventions.

The psychosocial perspective takes into account how the wearer interacts with others. A person operating an upper-limb prosthesis attracts more attention during social interactions because few people have ever seen a prosthesis, and hand absence is conspicuous. Communication often involves gestures. Unfortunately, both the static and dynamic appearance of a prosthesis is often poor or, at least, abnormal. The United States is one of a few countries where the hook terminal device (TD) is even considered for everyday use.[8] Even so, a teacher might initially frighten youngsters by wearing a hook. Society is better prepared for lower-limb disability with ramps and accessible restrooms becoming increasingly common, whereas few accommodations, such as lever-type faucet handles, are made for those with upper-limb deficiency.

Amputations at or proximal to the wrist deprive the patient of hand sensation and manipulative function. Individuals who are missing a portion of the hand are usually not treated prosthetically and thus will not be considered in this chapter. The discrepancy between upper-limb prosthetic function and the human limb is much greater than that between lower-limb prosthetic function and the anatomic leg. Dexterous prehension imposes different biomechanical requirements than balance and ambulation. Dominance is more significant in manipulative tasks than in ambulation.

Compounding the problem is the fact that the small number of people who are candidates for upper-limb prosthetic intervention accounts for relatively high component costs. Manufacturers are somewhat deterred by the modest potential market to devote funds to improve components and materials.

People with bilateral upper-limb absence, particularly in the presence of higher levels of loss, may prefer to rely on foot use rather than cope with prostheses, especially if the absence is congenital. In contrast, lower-limb loss still allows mobility in a socially acceptable manner if the individual uses a wheelchair or other assistive device.

In summary, the physical, psychological, and psychosocial distinctiveness of the individual with upper-limb loss must be factored into rehabilitation.

Upper-Limb Prosthetic Options

Prosthetic prescription is based on an assessment that should integrate psychological and psychosocial perspectives with the physical evaluation. Psychological issues deal with self-esteem and body image, whereas the psychosocial perspective looks at the individual's interaction with others and the physical environment and its challenges. Matching a prosthetic strategy to the full range of the patient's interests, rather than just basic activities, is essential for optimal outcome. The vocational and avocational circumstances of the patient must be considered, as well as the quality of family and peer support. All of these issues influence functional outcomes.

Physical assessment is often the only evaluation the patient receives, with attention paid to physiological and anatomical factors. Traumatic amputations are usually the result of a life-saving measure with surgery performed under emergency circumstances. The amputated limb may have considerable scarring and be painful. Pain can result from tissue and nerve damage incurred at the time of the accident, as well as the surgeon's having placed higher priority on saving the individual's life even at the expense of fashioning the amputated limb optimally. Etiologies and management of pain are considered in Chapter 4.

Length of the amputation limb is a major determinant in selecting prosthetic components. Classification of transradial (TR) and transhumeral (TH) amputations involves computing the length of the amputation limb as a percentage of the sound limb. On the amputated side, take a straight line measurement from the designated proximal bony prominence to the bony end of the amputation limb, with the distal soft tissue compressed proximally. On the sound side, measure from one designated bony prominence to the other.

Transradial amputations are measured from the medial humeral epicondyle to the end of the amputation limb; on the sound side, the distal prominence is the ulnar styloid. The standard percentages are:

- 100%   Wrist disarticulation
- 55% to 100%   Long transradial
- 35% to 55%   Short transradial
- 0% to 35%   Very short transradial

Transhumeral amputations are measured from the scapular acromion to the end of the amputation limb. On the sound side, the distal measurement point is the lateral humeral epicondyle. The percentages are:

- 90% to 100%   Elbow disarticulation
- 50% to 90%   Standard transhumeral
- 30% to 50%   Short transhumeral
- 0% to 30%   Humeral neck
- 0%   Shoulder disarticulation

With regard to adults with bilateral upper-limb amputation, upper limb length is calculated as a percentage of height. The forearm is 14% of height, and the upper arm is 19% of height. For example, an individual who is 5 feet, 10 inches tall with a TR amputation limb that measures 6 inches from the medial humeral epicondyle has an amputation that is 61% of the length of the preamputation forearm length, classified as a long TR amputation.

The patient and rehabilitation clinic have six prescription options. Not wearing or using a prosthesis is one choice. The other five classes of prosthetic control strategies are:

1. Passive (semi-prehensile)
2. Cable-driven (cable-controlled, body-powered)
3. Adaptive (activity-specific)
4. Electrically powered
5. Hybrid

A *passive* prosthesis is typically a cosmetic restoration lacking active prehension; often the wearer can shape the fingers of the artificial hand by bending their wire armatures. In addition to improving the patient's appearance, the passive TD can stabilize paper when the wearer writes and can assist in holding bulky bundles. Because the term "passive" is erroneously associated with a complete absence of function, many potential users of these devices either are not offered them or dismiss them.

A *cable-operated* control strategy entails a prosthesis powered and controlled by body movements transmitted to a harness and cable system. This is the most common type of contemporary prosthesis,[9] even though few fundamental improvements have been made in the last half century.

If the patient has worn a prosthesis previously, attention should also be given to prosthetic history, as well as current prosthetic usage and type, as these significantly affect acceptance of a proposed prosthesis or prostheses. An extended history with a particular control strategy, interface design, or TD can become a "security blanket" even in the presence of mechanically superior devices.

Electrically powered and hybrid prostheses are discussed in Chapter 13.

Transradial Prostheses

The prosthesis for the individual with TR amputation represents an individualized combination of a custom-made socket and harness and mass-produced wrist unit and TD. The TH prosthesis includes a TD, wrist unit, elbow unit, socket, and harness. For the individual with shoulder disarticulation, a humeral section and shoulder joint are added to the basic TH prosthesis. Key elements in rehabilitation success are the selection of components and the fitting of the prosthesis.

Terminal Devices

A TD is the component at the distal end of the prosthesis that is designed to function in place of the anatomic hand. Because the human hand is an incredibly complex instrument of manipulation, expression, and sensation, any mechanical replacement is a poor imitation.

Basic TDs are hands and hooks. Hands restore the general appearance of the absent body part; however, hand TDs are heavier, more expensive, and more vulnerable to mechanical and chemical damage than are hooks. Split hooks have two fingers, with one or both able to be moved, hooks are alternatives to hands. Many people find that hooks provide a higher level of dexterity than prosthetic hands because the more narrow fingers of the hook allow the user to see the object being manipulated more easily. Although hooks do not resemble the human hand, when a person uses a hook gracefully and efficiently, the hook takes on a more satisfactory appearance. Because hooks and hands have advantages and disadvantages, ideally the patient would be best served by having both types of TDs, which could be interchanged readily, with the aid of a quick disconnect wrist unit.

Terminal devices may be classified as being either active or passive. Active TDs open and close to enable the wearer to grasp and release objects. On a body-powered prosthesis, the harness system transmits force to operate an active TD, whether hand or hook. Shoulder and elbow motions provide the coordination for purposeful activity. For example, a person who wanted to use the prosthesis for writing would open the TD to grasp the pen and then close the TD to hold the pen and use proximal motions to move the prosthesis to form letters. Although a passive TD is not operated by a harness system, it may be used to stabilize objects. For example, a passive hand may prevent paper from sliding while the other hand writes. The wearer can use the sound hand to adjust the curvature of the fingers of the passive hand.

Voluntary-Opening vs Voluntary-Closing

A voluntary-opening (VO) TD has rubber bands or a spring holding the TD fingers closed. To open the fingers, the person applies tension through the harness.

Relaxing tension on the harness permits the rubber bands or spring to close the fingers. The rubber bands or spring hold the fingers closed whether for grasping or in the resting position. Grasp force depends on the VO mechanism (ie, the more rubber bands or the stiffer the spring, the greater the grasp force). Voluntary-opening TDs require no effort to maintain grasp on rigid objects. If the wearer is grasping a fragile object, such as a paper cup filled with water, the individual must maintain tension in the harness to prevent the fingers from snapping shut. A wide variety of VO TDs are manufactured, offering several finger shapes, textures, and materials.

To close the fingers of a voluntary-closing (VC) TD, the person applies tension through the harness to the cable attached to the TD (Figure 12-1). Maintaining tension on the cable allows one to continue holding the object; relaxing the tension on the cable opens the fingers. Alternatively, a locking mechanism can be used to maintain cable tension. Voluntary-closing TDs usually have the fingers open in the resting position, although some models permit the TD to remain closed when the wearer is not using it. Voluntary-closing TDs allow the wearer to grasp with a wide range of prehension force.

Shapes

Hooks are made in various shapes. The most common is the canted design. When the hook is pronated, the fingers slant toward the midline. The fingers differ in shape from one another, presenting a wide range of grasping surfaces. One alternative is the lyre-shaped hook, which has symmetrically shaped fingers; when this hook is pronated, the fingers point straight down. The lyre shape presents a less conspicuous contour.

Some TDs are designed for use with tools. For example, the Hosmer Dorrance #7 VO hook has a knife holder, nail holder, and chisel holder. Some models have a "back lock" feature that locks the opening size of the fingers around the object, preventing inadvertent finger opening until the person deliberately applies tension through the harnessing system. Other hooks have a plastic covering so that the TD bears some resemblance to a hand.

Hands are manufactured in passive and active designs. As compared with an active hand, the passive hand is lighter in weight, less expensive, and more durable. Passive hands have no mechanism permitting the wearer to open or close the fingers, although one may change the curvature of the fingers by bending them. Passive hands restore the appearance of the patient and serve as a stabilizer, as when the wearer signs a check, and as a gross holder, as when the individual holds a large package.

Active hands are manufactured with both VO and VC mechanisms.

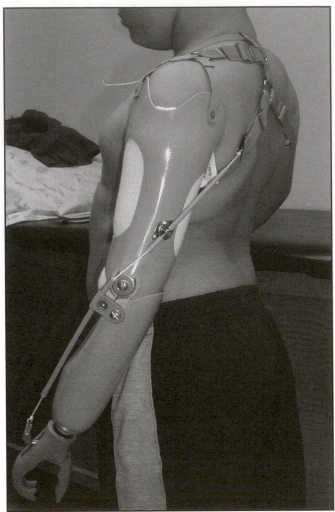

Figure 12-1. A voluntary closing terminal device is shown for this young boy with congenital limb absence at the level of the elbow. Note the open shoulder socket design used to retain maximum shoulder range of motion.

Materials

Hooks are made from aluminum, stainless steel, and titanium. Aluminum is lightweight but easily bent; thus it is suitable for light-duty usage and higher levels of limb loss. Stainless steel is more rigid but twice the weight of aluminum; therefore, such TDs are intended for heavy-duty use. Titanium is lightweight and rigid, but expensive. Most hooks have a neoprene lining. Lined surfaces provide greater friction for a more secure grip; the lining needs to be replaced when worn. Unlined hooks usually have a knurled surface to improve grasp security. The smallest hooks are covered with pink or brown plastic.

Prescription Considerations

When choosing between a hook and a hand, the clinic team and patient should consider both the patient's needs for a natural cosmetic effect and his or her func-

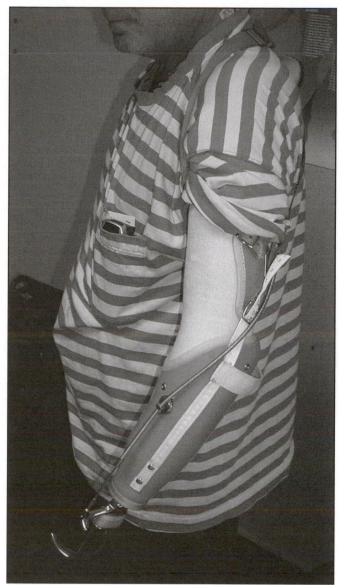

Figure 12-2. A transradial prosthesis using flexible hinges to allow retention of residual forearm rotation.

indicated. The slender hook fingers allow relatively good visual access to the objects being handled; in addition, hooks weigh less and are more durable than hand TDs.

Wrist Units

Supination and pronation are essential for effective orientation of the TD, whether hand or hook. The wrist unit is the component that enables the wearer to rotate the TD passively. Once the wrist unit is rotated, TD position is maintained either by friction in the wrist unit or by a lock. Friction wrist units are simpler in design and easier to use; however, if the wearer attempts to stabilize a heavy load, the friction unit may allow inadvertent rotation. If friction is adjusted to resist motion, it may be difficult or impossible for the wearer to rotate it. When the lock is engaged in a locking unit, a heavy object will not budge the TD. The drawback of a locking wrist unit is that it requires the added step of unlocking and relocking when a new position is desired.

If more than one TD is used, the quick disconnect wrist unit is practical. These wrists are manufactured in both friction and positive locking versions. Some units also allow two angles of wrist flexion plus the neutral position and should be considered for anyone who cannot reach the midline of the body in any other way. Wrist flexion is especially helpful for feeding, dressing, oral and facial hygiene, and toileting. Typical users are people with bilateral amputations, which include one or both TH amputations

Transradial Sockets

The TR socket is custom made of plastic, designed to enable the wearer to use the maximum amount of active elbow and forearm motion. The range of pronation and supination is associated with residual limb length; those who retain at least 50% of the forearm length usually have enough motion to effect usable rotation when wearing a prosthesis. The socket is typically trimmed below the humeral epicondyles with an oval "screwdriver" distal cross-sectional shape (Figure 12-2). The trimlines of the socket should not interfere with forearm rotation. Even with a well-fitted socket, the patient is apt to lose half of the physiological rotation range when wearing the prosthesis. Actively rotating the forearm reduces the need to rotate the wrist unit.

Limbs that are shorter than 50% of forearm length generally do not produce much active forearm rotation when encased in the prosthesis. This is because a smaller range of physiological rotation exists, and the cylindrical shape of the distal end makes transmitting natural forearm rotation to the prosthesis problematic.

A self-suspending TR socket encases the humeral epicondyles and the ulnar olecranon process. Anteroposterior and mediolateral snugness is essential to suspend the prosthesis throughout the range of

tional goals. Most new patients prefer a hand TD. This is plausible because lay people assume that technology can replace both the function and appearance of the anatomic hand. Unfortunately, this is not the case with the current state of the art. Most body-powered VO hands are mechanically inefficient, requiring much greater power input than the prehension force output. An electric-powered TD provides prehension forces three to six times the force possible with the three to six rubber bands worn by typical VO hook users.[10] If, however, the patient has a sound contralateral limb, the function expected from the TD is minimal and the cosmetic concern is paramount. Consequently, a hand TD may be the appropriate choice. However, for people with bilateral upper-limb loss, hook TDs are generally elbow motion. Generally sockets designed for short limbs extend to the antecubital fold, and those for long limbs are trimmed more distally. Most users don the self-suspending socket with tubular stockinet. First, the amputation limb is placed in the stockinet. Second, the amputation limb enters the socket. Third, the distal end of the fabric is pulled through a hole in the forearm of the prosthesis, and finally the patient pulls on the stockinet until the amputation limb is well lodged in the socket with soft tissue drawn inside the socket.

Tissue bunching above the trimline would impede elbow flexion. Self-suspending sockets block the wearer's ability to use active pronation and supination.

Self-suspending socket designs for body-powered prostheses are essentially the same as for the electrically powered prostheses.

Another option for the TR socket is the silicone suction socket. This method of fitting was originated for transtibial prostheses. The socket uses a liner made of soft flexible material such as silicon. The liner is stretched onto the limb and worn like a sock.[11] The material is airtight, providing suction suspension. Typically the silicon liner is secured to the socket via a locking mechanism; however, other means of attachment may be used.

Harnesses and Control Systems

Harnessing serves the dual roles of suspension and control of the body-powered prosthesis. In designing a harness system, the prosthetist should consider these roles separately. When the socket provides suspension, the harness requirements are altered, leading to simpler, looser, more comfortable harness designs.[12]

In the absence of any other suspension system, the harness must suspend the prosthesis securely from the upper torso to maintain the amputated limb securely within the socket. Therefore, the harness must be well anchored and its straps precisely positioned to resist the distraction forces of daily use. The axilla on the sound side affords a stable anchor point, used for most harness designs.

For control, the harness must transmit power through the cable system to the TD and elbow unit, if present. For the TR prosthesis where only the TD needs to be controlled, a single function "Bowden" cable is used. The cable passes through a continuous housing that runs from the harness to the TD, transmitting glenohumeral and scapular motion to the TD without affecting the elbow.

Cable efficiency is critical to the success of a body-powered fitting. Attention should be devoted to producing the straightest line of pull using materials that offer the least amount of friction such as Spectra cable in a Teflon-lined housing.[13]

The most common harness for TR and TH fittings is the figure-of-eight. It consists of several straps with specific functions and locations (Figure 12-3).

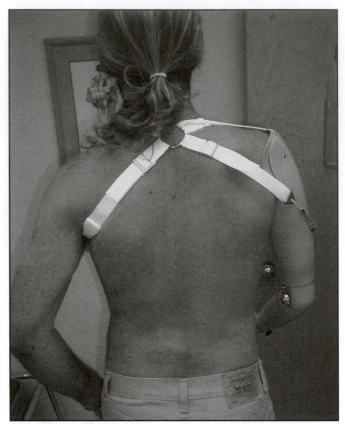

Figure 12-3. A transhumeral prosthesis harness using a conventional ring harness.

The cross point is located on the posterior side of the upper torso. Other straps radiate from the cross point, typically a ring that permits straps to move freely. It should be located below the 7th cervical vertebra to avoid discomfort caused by rubbing the prominent spinous process. The cross point should be slightly offset toward the sound side for people with unilateral amputation to afford the control attachment strap optimal excursion. For bilateral prostheses, the cross point is usually centered.

From the cross point moving toward the sound side is the axilla loop, which wraps around the axilla. It is the anchor, or stabilizer, of the harness system. The tighter the axilla loop, the more body motion the harness can transmit to the TD, but the more uncomfortable it is likely to be.

From the cross point moving superiorly toward the amputated limb and anteriorly across the shoulder is the anterior suspension strap, which lies in the deltopectoral groove. For the TR prosthesis, the anterior suspension strap is attached to the inverted Y strap, which anchors to the triceps pad or cuff on the posterior surface of the upper arm. It is responsible primarily for suspending the TR prosthesis.

When the TR socket is self-suspending, a figure-of-nine harness is indicated. It consists of an axilla loop leading to the control attachment strap. Because this harness is used only for control, the harness can be worn loosely and it thus generally well tolerated.

Regardless of harness design, the primary body motions used to control the TD are ipsilateral glenohumeral flexion and scapular abduction. A self-suspending TR socket may have a cross bar assembly tab attached to the posterior aspect of the socket to allow elbow flexion to contribute to TD control. Ipsilateral or biscapular abduction is used for tasks near the midline of the body. Glenohumeral flexion is used for TD operation when reaching with the prosthesis.

Elbow Hinges

Except for the self-suspending socket, the TR prosthesis includes a pair of elbow hinges, depending on the design of the socket and harness. Hinges extend from the proximal portion of the forearm shell to a cuff or pad on the upper arm and contribute to suspension of the prosthesis.

The flexible leather hinge is the most common type, used whenever forearm pronation and supination can be transmitted to TD. Flexible hinges do not stabilize the prosthesis. Rigid metal hinges stabilize and suspend the prosthesis. They are indicated for individuals with short or very short TR amputated limbs, especially when heavy use is anticipated. If the amputated limb is so fleshy that soft tissue would bunch in the antecubital fold during elbow flexion, polycentric hinges will accommodate this tissue.

A rarely used option for short and very short TR limbs is the step-up hinge. It has two pairs of distal straps and one pair of proximal straps. The distal straps are secured to the two portions of a split socket. Step-up hinges amplify elbow excursion, so that the patient can achieve acute flexion of the prosthetic forearm with moderate flexion of the anatomic elbow. Maximum flexion is useful for contacting the face with the TD, as when eating and performing facial hygiene. Step-up hinges are less durable than standard rigid hinges and require a split socket, which may cause the inner socket to protrude posteriorly when the forearm is fully flexed.

Transhumeral Prostheses

Elbow Units

Selecting the most appropriate elbow unit for the TH or shoulder disarticulation prosthesis should include evaluation of the patient's strength, control options, and compatibility with the other components of the prostheses. As compared with electric-powered elbow units, body-powered units weigh less and provide the proprioceptive feedback inherent in the cable control of body-powered elbow units; however, body-power offers less lifting force.[10]

All elbow units include a hinge to provide for elbow flexion and a locking mechanism to stabilize the forearm

at the desired angle. They require one control motion to activate the lock and another motion to flex the elbow. The locking mechanism is an alternator, ie, the first pull on the elbow lock cable locks the unit, the second pull unlocks it, the third pull locks it, and so forth.

Elbow disarticulation prostheses usually require outside locking hinges, which add relatively little bulk below the socket. Consequently, when the patient flexes both the anatomic and prosthetic elbows, the olecranon processes are at similar length. Outside locking hinges add more mediolateral bulk because they are positioned on the outside of the socket over the widest point of the epicondyles to match elbow centers. Most elbow disarticulation limbs have an oval shape distally, allowing the socket to capture physiological shoulder rotation, eliminating the need for a turntable mechanism to enable passive rotation.

Transhumeral amputations are fitted with internal locking elbows that have a hinge, lock, and turntable for passive rotation of the forearm. A friction turntable is simple and does not require a harness control source for operation. However, friction control may be inadequate for tasks exerting high force on the prosthesis. Therefore, locking humeral rotation may be beneficial. A locking humeral rotator has a control cable that can be actuated through a harness in parallel with the elbow lock or by chin-actuated nudge control.[10,14]

A spring lift assist or automatic forearm balance should be considered for all body-powered elbow units, especially the internal locking unit. Spring lift assists allow the prosthetist to optimize the force and excursion requirements of a particular component system with the abilities and needs of a particular user.

If insufficient excursion or force prohibits the use of both a body-powered TD and a body-powered elbow unit, a friction elbow unit may be beneficial. It allows the user to position the TD, usually with the sound hand, then operate the TD in the standard fashion. The friction elbow can not resist heavy loads held in the TD. A partial solution to this problem is the use of a ratchet elbow hinge. The ratchet permits forearm flexion to the desired angle while preventing inadvertent extension. Once the forearm is flexed from the fully extended position, the ratchet joint locks to extension but does not resist further flexion. It is unlocked by fully flexing the joint then allowing it to return to the fully extended position.

Transhumeral Sockets

Sockets for the TH prosthesis should provide a close coupling of the amputated limb and the prosthesis to maximize prosthetic function. Open shoulder designs[15] are preferable because they allow relatively unimpeded motion at the glenohumeral joint. Another option is the half-and-half socket.[16] It has a flexible silicon proximal section integrated with a rigid distal portion, extending below the axilla. The proximal section is fitted over the

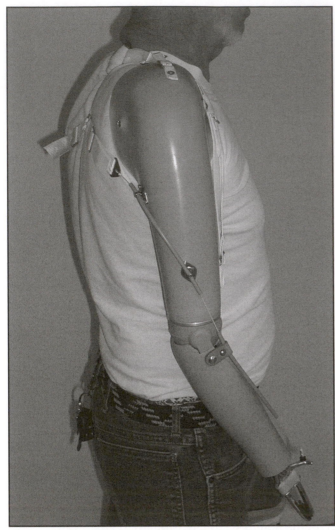

Figure 12-4. This humeral prosthesis is an example of a closed shoulder design used for this limb amputated at the proximal third of the humerus. The cable is made of Spectra. Along with the straight line of pull, this cable material offers excellent cable efficiency.

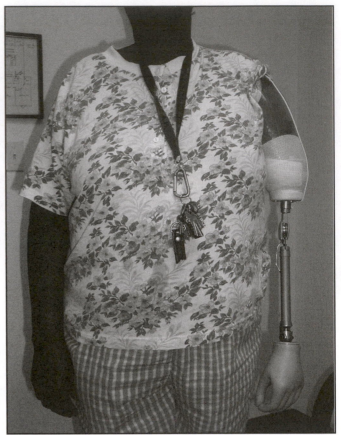

Figure 12-5. Primary suspension is achieved through the use of a 3S system for this endoskeletal passive prosthesis. No harness is required because no active components have been utilized. The prosthesis is shown in the prototype fitting stage and will be finished with a soft foam cover and prosthetic glove to match skin color as close as possible.

shoulder. The lateral deltoid area is cut away, improving flexibility and air circulation within the socket. A similar design is the flexible shoulder suspension system. A strip of Lycra-backed neoprene replaces the silicon proximal section and is attached to the anterior and posterior "wings" of the open shoulder socket.[10]

For short amputated limbs, closed shoulder sockets are usually necessary (Figure 12-4). The short lever arm prevents the individual from moving the prosthesis through a large range of motion. In this case, more extensive coverage of the shoulder area spreads the loading force over a larger area and provides convenient anchor points for the harness system. As with the TR level, silicone suction sockets (3S) have been used successfully for TH fittings if the amputated limb is reasonably long (Figure 12-5). If suction suspension is

used, the harness can be relatively loose; the harness changes from the dual purpose of suspension and control to one dedicated primarily to control.

Transhumeral Harnesses

As noted above, the most common harness for TH fittings is the figure-of-eight. For TH prostheses where both the elbow unit and the TD are to be controlled, a two-function "fair-lead" housing is used. Dual control design uses a housing proximal to the elbow and another housing distally. When the elbow unit is unlocked, tension on the cable causes the two housing pieces to be pulled together to flex the elbow. With the elbow locked, the same cable force is transmitted to the TD. Consequently, one cannot operate the TD while flexing or extending the elbow.

One solution to this problem is to design a control system where separate control cables are used for TD, elbow flexion, and elbow lock. This "triple control" system uses Bowden cables for each component; shoulder flexion causes elbow flexion, biscapular abduction operates the TD, and shoulder hyperextension locks and unlocks the elbow. The triple control harness can be operated most successfully by someone with wide, mobile shoulders. Many patients find it difficult to achieve proper separation of the controls in operating the harness system.[17] For these reasons it is rarely used in favor of other options such as a hybrid fitting combining an externally powered option for either the TD or elbow unit.

The TH harness has an anterior suspension strap made of Dacron webbing over the shoulder sewn to elastic webbing to help return the lock cable to its relaxed position. The lock billet attaches to the end of the Dacron strap and enables cycling the elbow lock using shoulder depression, extension, and abduction.

Although the anterior suspension strap aids suspension, the main suspensor of the TH prosthesis is the lateral suspension strap located on the superior surface of the shoulders. It attaches to the proximal portion of the axilla strap on the sound side, then to the anterior suspension strap, and finally to the socket at the acromion.

The final strap attached to the cross point is the control attachment strap. It extends inferiorly from the cross point to the control cable hanger and transmits the body motion to the TD. Ideally, the control attachment strap lies over the inferior third of the scapula. This strap needs to be snug to allow TD operation at all elbow angles.

One alternative to the figure-of-eight harness is the shoulder saddle or thoracic suspension system. The shoulder saddle has a pad over the shoulder of the amputated side, which is the starting point for an array of straps similar to that on the figure-of-eight harness. Because the suspension straps are mounted to the shoulder saddle, axial lifting is more comfortable than with the figure-of-eight harness. The shoulder saddle harness has a chest strap that stabilizes the harness against the sound side of the torso below the axilla, which avoids axillary impingement. The disadvantages of the shoulder saddle harness are that it is less cosmetic because the chest strap is visible in open neck clothing, it is less efficient in transmitting shoulder motion to the control cable due to the less secure anchorage on the torso, and it tends to be relatively bulky around the shoulder.

Shoulder Disarticulation Prostheses

Shoulder Disarticulation Sockets

The prosthetic interface for the shoulder disarticulation prosthesis is designed to spread loading over as large an area as possible to minimize pressure, yet cover as little area as possible to reduce heat and weight of the prosthesis. The large perimeter of the socket provides a stable foundation for positioning of the TD. Any por-

tion of the socket not needed for structural support, effective transmission of bodily movement, or harness anchor points can be cut away. A frame socket can be constructed of plastic or aluminum. The shoulder disarticulation socket is suspended by a simple chest strap.

Sockets may be worn with a sock (or a tailored short sleeve tee shirt), allowing for easy independent donning and doffing.

Shoulder Joint Units

The shoulder disarticulation prosthesis should have a shoulder joint that locks in the desired flexion angle and has a friction mechanism for abduction positioning.

The lock can be operated either by a cable nudge control or with an electric actuator. The rigidity of the locked shoulder joint allows the person to use the prosthesis as an extension of the body to transmit forces through the largest work area.[10] Additionally, the ability to operate the TD overhead is invaluable.

If a lower profile shoulder joint is required, as when fitting a prosthesis for the person with humeral neck amputation who is concerned with the appearance around the shoulder, a friction flexion/abduction joint is preferable.

BODY-POWERED CONTROL

Overview

Body-power refers to both the control method and the power source by which prosthetic components are operated through the use of the body's own force and excursion. This is the oldest control method for arm prostheses. Harnessing the force and excursion of proximal joint motions enables operating TD, wrist, elbow, and humeral rotation devices. Despite contemporary electronic technology, body power continues to be an effective and often-used form of prosthesis control. Atkins et al[18] reported that of 2477 individuals with upper-limb amputation responding to a survey, 63% indicated that they wore a body-powered prosthesis with a hook TD. These results compare favorably with our experience.

Several factors contribute to the continued popularity of body-powered control, namely lower initial cost, more robust construction, lower maintenance cost, lighter weight, and perhaps most important, greater proprioceptive feedback through the harness. Nevertheless, we strongly oppose any attempt to rate the various methods of fitting because all methods have merit, and the optimal option for a given individual is based on the unique needs of that particular person. Arm prostheses may best be thought of as tools rather than limb replacements. In this conceptual framework, it is easy to understand that each tool has specific functions and that several tools may be required to provide the desired scope of function. Therefore, a specific person may require several control methods to function with various prostheses. Electrically powered components offer options not possible with body-powered devices as discussed in Chapter 13.

Prerequisites

A fundamental requirement for the use of any body-powered component is the user's ability to produce adequate force and excursion. This means that the candidate must have sufficient shoulder strength to operate the TD and elbow, if present, as well as enough joint excursion to move the component through its full operating range. As a general rule, the patient needs to produce two to five times the prehension force realized at the TD. This is due to the mechanical inefficiencies of the devices themselves and the friction of the cable system. To operate a typical VO hook through its full range of opening, the wearer must pull the cable 2 inches, and to operate a conventional elbow, an additional 2.5 inches must be produced. The amputated limb must withstand these high forces to operate a body-powered prosthesis, especially a TH prosthesis.

In most cases the person with TR amputation will be able to operate any cable-operated TD easily. In the TR prosthesis, the cable attachment point is far from the center of rotation (shoulder joint) of the primary work sources, providing a good mechanical advantage. When the amputation level is above the elbow, the cable attachment is closer to the center of rotation, producing less force and excursion. For the individual with a long TH amputation this is generally not a problem because enough force and excursion can be produced to operate the TD and elbow unit. When the amputation level is higher, body-powered control of the elbow unit and TD are more difficult, or impossible, due to the lack of adequate force and excursion. The person with shoulder disarticulation usually will not be able to produce enough excursion to operate a fully body-powered prosthesis, and should be fitted either with an electric system or a hybrid system combining body-power and electric components.

Adequate force and excursion are related to other factors in addition to limb length. Other critical attributes include strength, range of motion, posture, and physical size. When force or excursion is insufficient, alternative power sources and control methods are indicated.

Motions Used for Prosthesis Control

Primary Work Sources (TD and elbow activation)

- Glenohumeral flexion
- Scapular/biscapular abduction
- Elbow flexion can be used to control a TD if the cable is anchored to the proximal edge of the TR

socket in a way that produces cable excursion with elbow flexion.

Secondary Work Sources (Generally used for lock activation in body-powered fittings)

- Glenohumeral extension, abduction/shoulder depression
- Shoulder elevation
- Chin nudge
- Chest expansion
- Abdominal expansion
- Glenohumeral adduction
- Other (any movable feature)
- Proprioceptive feedback

Cable actuation of body-powered prostheses provides users with a wealth of proprioceptive feedback through the physiological joints harnessed to the prosthetic components.[19] Users of these devices can readily perceive the position and speed of movement of the prosthetic components.[10] Body-powered cable-operated control offers many of the desirable characteristics of the theory of control proposed by Childress based on the work of Simpson referred to as Extended Physiological Proprioception (EPP),[20,21] which states:

The most natural and most subconscious control of a prosthesis can be achieved through use of the body's own joints as control inputs in which joint position corresponds (always in a one-to-one relationship) to prosthesis position, joint velocity corresponds to prosthesis velocity, and joint force corresponds to prosthesis force.[22]

Largely due to the inherent feedback provided via the cable and harness system, body-powered elbow control is generally well accepted and functional, assuming the patient has adequate force and excursion resources.[12,22]

BILATERAL PROSTHESES

Terminal Device Selection

It is generally advisable to use two different types of TDs to provide versatility. A commonly used combination is a canted-approach hook on the dominant side and a lyre-shaped hook contralaterally.[10] The canted hook allows good visual feedback of objects manipulated, whereas the lyre-shape provides better stability for large round objects. Another successful TD combination is a canted hook on the dominant side and an electrically powered TD on the nondominant side. This combination provides the fine manipulative capabilities of a hook with the superior gripping forces available with an electric TD, either hook or hand, and has been particularly well accepted by people with TH/shoulder disarticulation amputations. Voluntary-opening hooks

Case Studies: Transradial Amputation

A 40-year-old man presents with a right TR amputation due to a factory accident 2 months ago. The amputated limb measures 7 inches from the medial epicondyle to the distal bone end. The limb is well healed and does not appear edematous due to the excellent job he is doing wrapping with elastic bandage. There are no other injuries, and he is very eager to return to work. His job involves use of both hands in an environment that includes frequent exposure to water, heavy machinery, and dust. Physical evaluation reveals full range of motion at the elbow and shoulder with 60 degrees of pronation and 30 degrees of supination remaining. He is right-handed. After the clinic team and patient discussed prosthetic options, it was agreed that both a prosthetic hand and hook would best meet his vocational and avocational needs.

A prescription is formulated to address the heavy-duty nature of this man's work duties. One TD will be a Hosmer #7 work hook, which offers several features that enable the user to handle a variety of work tools. This hook is stainless steel with a knurled gripping surface, a robust TD for manual labor. It will be interchangeable with a hand covered by a production cosmetic glove for use outside the work environment. To facilitate easy exchange of the two TDs, a quick disconnect wrist unit will be provided. It is also made of stainless steel to withstand the heavy-duty vocational demands. To preserve as much forearm rotation as possible, flexible hinges are indicated. The hinges will be attached, through a triceps pad, to a figure-of-eight harness. The control cable will be a heavy-duty steel cable.

Following 2 weeks of occupational therapy, the patient is able to return to a limited work schedule as his limb becomes accustomed to use of a prosthesis and he increases proficiency in its use.

Transhumeral Amputation

A 28-year-old man presents with a TH amputation of his right dominant arm. The amputation was the result of a crushing injury sustained 3 weeks earlier while he was working in an ice factory. The amputated limb length is 6 inches from acromion to the bone end. Physical evaluation reveals that healing is progressing satisfactorily, the sutures have been removed, and the limb is cylindrical but edematous. The patient expressed the desire to return to the same factory after his rehabilitation program is completed. The clinic team agreed to initiate prosthetic fitting at this time with a preparatory body-powered TH prosthesis. The preparatory prosthesis will allow for maintenance of bimanual function, which has been demonstrated to positively affect the outcome of upper-limb prosthetic fitting.[25] The prosthesis will have a lightweight aluminum hook interchangeable with a hand with cosmetic glove for better appearance. A quick disconnect wrist will facilitate TD exchange as well as offer the benefit of positively locked wrist rotation. An internal locking elbow with lift assist was prescribed. The lift assist will provide some lift force required for elbow function thereby allowing the cable system to be adjusted to optimize excursion. The socket will be a closed shoulder design to provide good rotational stability and a favorable anchor point for the lateral suspension strap of the harness. The cable system will be a low-friction Spectra cable in a Teflon-lined fair-lead housing.

After 6 weeks of out-patient rehabilitation, the patient was discharged to start a limited work schedule. He is able to don and doff the prosthesis independently, perform activities of daily living, and manipulate basic hand tools using the prosthesis as an assist to the sound hand. A definitive prosthesis will be provided in 4 to 6 months after most of the edema has subsided. The preparatory prosthesis will serve as a prototype for the definitive one, allowing the patient and prosthetic clinic to evaluate the effectiveness of the prosthesis configuration and detect any shortcomings of the component selection.

are more popular than VC designs because VO hooks maintain grip without the need for continued cable tension and are available in a larger array of shapes and sizes. Voluntary-closing hooks offer better feedback regarding prehension forces as well as higher grip strength; however, the user must maintain continuous cable tension or use a locking mechanism to maintain grasp.

Task-specific TDs should be considered for the person with bilateral amputation. Quick-disconnect wrist units facilitate interchange between a utilitarian hook and specific use TDs, such as work tools and kitchen utensils. One innovative approach uses a "hands-free" tool exchanger that allows for automatic release and exchange of one device for another.

A particularly useful arrangement for body-powered system is the Four-Function Forearm Setup originally described by George Robinson and Jim Caywood (Figure 12-6). This system has been used successfully on short TR, TH, and shoulder disarticulation prostheses. The system relies on the single fair-lead control cable to control four components: TD, wrist rotation, wrist flexion, and elbow flexion. The unlocked component is the one that will operate. Positively locking components become a rigid extension of the body that can maintain position under high loads yet when unlocked can be repositioned with ease.

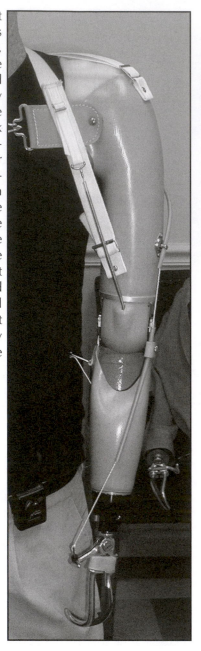

Figure 12-6. The wrist mechanism shown offers integrated wrist rotation, flexion, and a quick release mechanism. Rotation and flexion are controlled by a common control cable that also controls hook opening and elbow flexion; these are the four components actively controlled in a Four-Function Forearm Setup. Note the lever extending from the medial surface near the elbow used to release the rotation lock pin. The wrist flexion lock is released either by pressing a small lever at the wrist level (not visable) or alternately by a cable routed to a more proximal location.

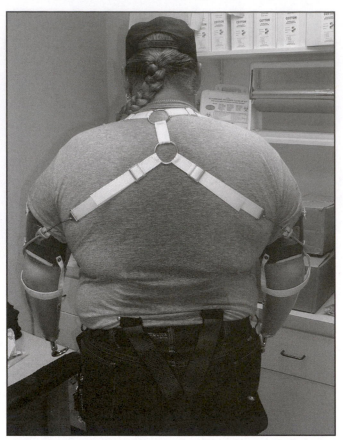

Figure 12-7. The harness for the bilateral transradial simply attaches the two prostheses to each other across the wearer's back. Shown is a double ring design that serves to lower the control straps on the back affording greater excursion.

Harnessing

Compared with the unilateral figure-of-eight harness, the bilateral version eliminates the axilla loop, a frequent area for discomfort, and thus is well tolerated by almost all patients (Figure 12-7). The bilateral TR or TH figure-of-eight harness system, with or without a ring at the cross point, is easy to don and doff independently.

If cable excursion is limited, the harness should not have a ring. If harness straps were allowed to rotate on a ring during functional use, motion would be dissipated. A sewn cross point or a leather pad may be beneficial where the leather is designed to direct the control attachment straps more inferiorly on the scapu-

lae thereby increasing the available excursion. Other options are the addition of a cross-back strap, which keeps the control attachment straps low on the scapulae, and a dual-ring type harness has two rings fixed to each other by a Dacron strap, one below the other.

When the prostheses are harnessed together, each prosthesis serves as the anchor point for the other. When both prostheses use the same harness for control, inadvertent control (sometimes referred to as cross-control) is a risk. One solution to cross-control is to provide a fully body-powered prosthesis on one side and a fully electric prosthesis on the other; the control motions cause no interaction with the operation of any component other than the one intended. Sometimes a socket is fitted for the exclusive purpose of providing an anchor for the contralateral prosthesis. This is often done for people with interscapulothoracic/TH amputations. On the interscapular side, a frame-type socket without distal components will provide a firm anchor for suspension and control of the TH prosthesis and can be shaped to provide shoulder symmetry.[12]

REFERENCES

1. Dillingham T, Pezzin L, Mackenzie E. Limb amputation and limb deficiency: epidemiology and recent trends in the United States. *South Med J.* 2002;95:875-883.

2. Yildirim S, Akan M, Akoz T. Transmetacarpal cross-hand replantation as a salvage procedure in a case of traumatic bilateral upper extremity amputation. *Plast Reconstr Surg.* 2003;112:1350-1354.

3. Wilhelm BJ, Lee WP, Pagensteert GI, May JW Jr. Replantation in the mutilated hand. *Hand Clin.* 2003;19:89-120.

4. Jenkins NJ, Lalikos JF, Wooden WA, et al. Innovative techniques in bony reconstruction to facilitate hand salvage. *Ann Plast Surg.* 2002;48:484-488.

5. Gammal TA, Sayed A, Kotb MM. Resection replantation of the upper limb for aggressive malignant tumors. *Arch Orthop Trauma Surg.* 2002;122:173-176.

6. Bosse MJ, MacKenzie EJ, Kellam JF, et al. An analysis of outcomes of reconstruction or amputation after leg-threatening injuries. *N Engl J Med.* 2002;347:1924-1931.

7. Van Dorsten B. Integrating psychological and medical care: practice recommendations for amputation. In: Meier RH, Atkins DJ, eds. *Functional Restoration of Adults and Children with Upper Extremity Amputation.* New York, NY: Demos Medical Publishing; 2004:73-88.

8. Meier RH, Esquenazi A. Prosthetic prescription. In: Meier RH, Atkins DJ, eds. *Functional Restoration of Adults and Children with Upper Extremity Amputation.* New York, NY: Demos Medical Publishing; 2004:159-164.

9. Atkins D, Heard D, Donovan W. Epidemiologic overview of individuals with upper-limb loss and their reported research priorities. *Journal of Prosthetics and Orthotics.* 1996;8:2-11.

10. Uellendahl JE, Heckathorne C.W. Creative prosthetic solutions for bilateral upper extremity amputations. In: Meier RH, Atkins DJ, eds. *Functional Restoration of Adults and Children with Upper Extremity Amputation.* New York, NY: Demos Medical Publishing; 2004:225-238.

11. Uellendahl JE. Prosthetic socks and liners. In: *First Step: A Guide for Adapting to Limb Loss.* Knoxville, Tenn: Amputee Coalition of America; 2001:56-58.

12. Uellendahl JE. Bilateral upper limb prostheses. In: Smith DG, Michael JW, Bowker JH, eds. *Atlas of Amputations and Limb Deficiencies.* 3rd ed. Rosemont, Ill: American Academy of Orthopaedic Surgeons; 2004:311-326.

13. Carlson L, Veatch B, Frey D. Efficiency of prosthetic cable and housing. *Journal of Prosthetics and Orthotics.* 1995;7:96-99.

14. Ivko JJ. Independence through humeral rotation in the conventional transhumeral prosthetic design. *Journal of Prosthetics and Orthotics.* 1999;11:20-22.

15. McLaurin CA, Sauter WF, Dolan CM, Hartmann GR. Fabrication procedures for the open-shoulder above-elbow socket. *Artificial Limbs.* 1969;13:46-54.

16. Bush G. Powered upper extremity prosthetics programme: above elbow fittings. In: *Rehabilitation Engineering Department Annual Report.* Ontario, Canada: Hugh MacMillan Rehabilitation Centre; 1990:35-37.

17. Anderson MH. Harness and control systems. In: Santschi A, ed. *Manual of Upper Extremity Prosthetics.* 2nd ed. Los Angeles, Calif: University of California; 1958:155-187.

18. Atkins DJ, Heard DCY, Donovan WH. Epidemiologic overview of individuals with upper-limb loss and their reported research priorities. *Journal of Prosthetics and Orthotics.* 1996;8:2-11.

19. Heckathorne CW. Manipulation in unstructured environments: extended physiological proprioception, position control, and arm prostheses. *Proc Int Conference on Rehabilitation Robotics.* 1990;25-40.

20. Childress DS, Weir RS. Control of limb prostheses. In: Smith DG, Michael JW, Bowker JH, eds. *Atlas of Amputations and Limb Deficiencies.* 3rd ed. Rosemont, Ill: American Academy of Orthopaedic Surgeons; 2004:173-197.

21. Simpson DC. The choice of control system for the multi-movement prosthesis: extended physiological proprioception. In: Herberts P, Kadefors R, Magnusson RI, Peterson I, eds. *The Control of Upper Extremity Prostheses and Orthoses.* Springfield, Ill: Charles C. Thomas Publishers; 1974:146-150.

22. Doubler JA, Childress DS. Design and evaluation of a prosthesis control system based on the concept of extended physiological proprioception. *J Rehabil Res Dev.* 1984;21:19-31.

23. Malone JM, Fleming LL, Robertson J, et al. Immediate, early, and late postsurgical management of upper-limb amputation. *J Rehabil Res Dev.* 1984;21:33-41.

Chapter 13

Upper-Limb Externally Powered Prosthetic Designs

Troy Farnsworth, CP and Randall D. Alley, CP

OBJECTIVES

1. Compare externally powered strategies that can be used to control upper-limb prostheses
2. Relate socket designs to various externally controlled strategies
3. Describe the evolution and current types of myoelectric control
4. Discuss microprocessor control used in terminal devices, wrist units, elbow units, and shoulder units
5. Outline the rehabilitation process for patients fitted with externally powered prostheses

---

INTRODUCTION

Over the past decade, the majority of upper-limb prosthetic advancements have related to externally powered systems.[1-3] Although not appropriate for all patients, externally powered components and advanced fitting and training techniques benefit many individuals.

An *externally powered* control strategy is used in an active prosthesis; the strategy is powered by a battery system. Among the input sources are:

- Myoelectric electrodes
- Push switches
- Pull switches
- Touch pads
- Force transducers (servo mechanism)
- Linear potentiometers (servo mechanism)

Other options that may be externally powered are hybrid and adaptive systems. A *hybrid* control strategy uses two or more control strategies. The name "hybrid" is most commonly associated with a transhumeral (TH) prosthesis incorporating an electric terminal device (TD) and a cable-operated (Figure 13-1) or passive elbow unit.[4,5]

An *adaptive* prosthesis can be either an adaptation of an existing prosthesis or a specialized prosthesis designed for a single function (Figure 13-2). Adaptations are commercially produced to facilitate various personal, vocational, and recreational activities; most of the adaptations can be used on any type of externally powered or cable-operated prosthesis equipped with a quick-disconnect wrist mechanism (Figure 13-3).[6]

Most patients are directed to a primary control option based on their physical attributes and intended usage. Often a secondary control option would be desirable to fulfill more functional requirements, thus necessitating multiple prostheses. For example, a plumber might use a cable-driven, heavy-duty prosthesis when working in wet, dirty environment and a more cosmetic myoelectric prosthesis for medium duty and social situations. To further complicate the scenario, assume the user can only tolerate limited use of the cable-operated system because of nerve entrapment, shoulder or back strain, bursitis, or other physical disorder. Alternating wear between two prostheses addresses more of the person's functional requirements. If the same user's physical restriction worsens, the myoelectric may become primary and the cable-controlled prosthesis secondary. When it is impossible to predict the best option, trial fittings can test one or more systems.[7]

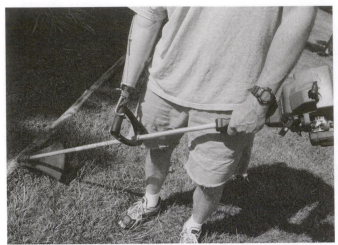

Figure 13-1. Cable-operated prosthesis. (Courtesy of Hanger Orthopedic Group, Inc.)

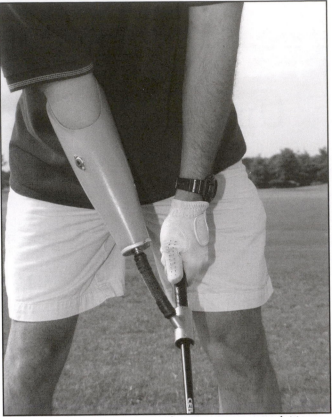

Figure 13-2. Adaptive prosthesis. (Courtesy of Hanger Orthopedic Group, Inc.)

SOCKET DESIGNS

To understand control options, it is necessary to consider the type of socket interface that will incorporate the control mechanism.

Functional performance depends on the attributes of the mechanical components, the control strategy, and the socket. The traditional role of the socket interface is concerned with comfort, appearance, suspension, provision for adequate joint range of motion, and stability.

Recent socket designs also enhance kinesthesia and kinetic transfer. Kinesthesia and proprioception refer to the ability to sense body movement and position, respectively. With regard to prostheses, kinesthesia is a *dynamic* perception concerning the quality and extent of movement, whereas proprioception is a *static* perception of position, posture, and weight. The interface must convey accurate kinesthetic information so the wearer can determine the orientation, movement, and position of the prosthesis precisely. A poorly fitting socket results in inaccurate perceptions of kinesthesia and proprioception and leads to discomfort and deficits in performance.

Whereas kinesthesia involves the gathering and processing of external information, kinetic transfer entails the transfer of human input, whether intrinsically or extrinsically generated, to prosthetic output. An example of intrinsic input is contraction of muscles within the socket to generate electrical signals to facilitate TD operation. Extrinsic human input includes making gross body movements to position a prosthesis or to effect forearm flexion in a cable-driven TH prosthesis.

Newer socket designs offer superior biomechanical advantages over older counterparts. Many patients and practitioners are unaware of innovations because of limited exposure and fear of change. Current design

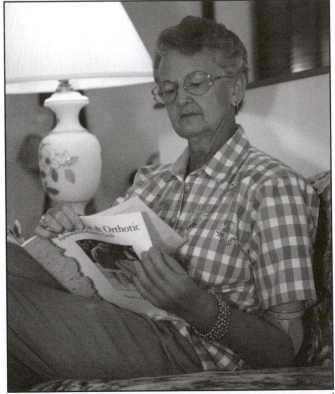

Figure 13-3. Externally powered prosthesis. (Courtesy of Hanger Orthopedic Group, Inc.)

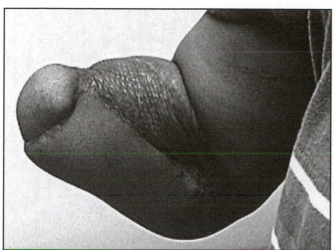

Figure 13-4. Excess antecubital tissue. (Courtesy of Hanger Orthopedic Group, Inc.)

technology often improves the functional outcome without much additional cost.

Advanced Transradial Designs

Incorporating features from several older designs such as the Muenster, Northwestern, and Sauter ¾ sockets, the Anatomically Contoured and Controlled Interface (ACCI) enables better, more comfortable performance.

Its predecessor, the Anatomically Contoured Socket (ACS) developed by NovaCare in the early 1990s was intended for short to mid-length TR limbs or those that had insufficient pronation and supination. It controlled unwanted rotation by extending the medial and lateral trimlines farther on the upper arm than previous sockets. The critical flaw of the ACS was that, although it was designed for shorter limbs, it did not displace loads along the anterior, load-bearing surface of the radius during the initial stages of elbow flexion. A large anterior relief at the antecubital fossa permitted tissue to shift during elbow flexion, causing the main load-bearing area of the socket to rise above the skin without adequate contact until elbow flexion was acute. This was uncomfortable, especially when the user attempted to lift heavy objects. Recognizing this defect in the ACS, radial channels were introduced to increase load-bearing surface. The modified ACS socket contacted the limb in the initial stages of flexion, allowing antecubital tissue room to expand as flexion progressed (Figure 13-4). The channels also helped control axial (longitudinal) rotation of the forearm within the socket by increasing socket pressure and friction.

The most noticeable structural distinctions between the ACCI and earlier designs are the height of the medial and lateral trimlines of the stabilizers and the anteroposterior contour, measured from the antecubital fold to the triceps tendon insertion. These changes in socket contour control axial rotation to enhance stability and protect joints under load, as well as improve suspension throughout the full range of motion.

For longer limbs where active supination and pronation are available, a compromise between rotational control and rotational freedom is achieved by varying the height of the external rigid frame supporting the flexible interface. The individual merely has to overcome the stiffness inherent in the flexible thermoplastic interface to initiate volitional pronation or supination. The relation of the resistance of the thermoplastic socket to the external frame determines the level of rotational control. The flexible interface usually is higher than the outer frame to dissipate shear stress on the skin.

Compared with older designs, the ACCI has a much narrower anteroposterior dimension to increase suspension and to maintain or increase the range of elbow flexion without lowering the anterior trimline.

To achieve suspension through the full range of elbow flexion under a moderate external load, the depth of the ACCI's anteroposterior modification must be great enough to press on the triceps tendon insertion and the antecubital tissues. For adequate elbow flexion, the ACCI has an anterior trimline, which extends into the antecubital fold. Older designs have a lower anterior trimline to allow full flexion and avoid compressing the anterior soft tissue that bulges during elbow flexion. Tissue bulge limits acute flexion as it becomes sandwiched between the anterior brim of the socket and the biceps tendon. Over an extended period of use, the lower trimline tends to exacerbate tissue bulging. Soft tissue increases as it is alternately compressed and stretched during elbow motion. With shorter limbs, the lowered trimline reduces the area of the effective lifting surface, increasing the pressure on this critical region, which is often cited as a zone of discomfort. The ACCI avoids tissue bulging. Its extended anterior trimline has a relief that gives the antecubital tissue a place into which to expand during elbow flexion, yet socket pressure limits tissue expansion at acute flexion.

Other distinctions of the ACCI are: 1) 90 degree angle between the olecranon relief and the raised posterior wall to enhance suspension at full elbow extension and comfort during flexion; 2) medial and lateral supracubital reliefs placed more anteriorly and distally than in the typical supracondylar socket, improving comfort and greatly enhancing suspension during full extension; and 3) slight concavity over the extensor carpi ulnaris to increase stability throughout the full elbow excursion.

Advanced Humeral Interface

The Advanced Humeral Interface (AHI) is a variant of the "Dynamic Andrew Socket" developed by Tom Andrew in the late 1980s. The most distinguishing feature of the AHI is a pair of anterior and posterior stabilizers that extend medially from the proximal portion of the socket just above the level of the axilla. They act as outriggers to control axial rotation and augment stability. The anterior stabilizer compresses the soft tissue overlying the pectoralis major to aid suspension by creating a wedge effect, partially inhibiting distal migration of the socket under load. The AHI compresses a smaller area directed at the center of rotation in the frontal plane as the arm abducts. The compressed area provides partial self-suspension while remaining in the proper location throughout the full range of abduction (Figure 13-5). Similar in concept to the radial channels in the TR ACCI, four small channels in the AHI isolate the distal humerus to improve kinesthesia and kinetic transfer while also helping to control axial rotation.

The lateral trimline is markedly lowered to 1) enhance abduction excursion, 2) increase comfort by eliminating any contact with the bony prominences of the shoulder, and 3) permit more heat dissipation. A slight difference between the "Andrew" socket and AHI is the amount of mediolateral compression. The AHI design has less enlargement of the distal anteroposterior dimension and compresses the mediolateral dimension less, relying on the humeral channels to augment intrinsic stability.

X-Frame for Thoracic Level Fittings

The X-Frame (MicroFrame) was developed to improve performance while reducing the size of the frame commonly used for humeral neck, shoulder disarticulation and interscapulothoracic fittings.

The X-Frame covers much less skin surface. All superfluous material has been removed, including the rigid portion of a traditional socket, which usually covers the superior aspect of the trapezius. The frame resembles an "X," with its four corners rotated inwardly to compress the anteroposterior aspect of the thorax superiorly and inferiorly. The shape uses the outrigger principle seen in other sockets in the superior and inferior regions of contact. The X-Frame provides great stability under a wide range of external forces. Superior compression significantly improves suspension via a wedge effect.

Other structural features of the X-Frame include: 1) scapulospinal suspension, in which the posterior strut of the superior portion of the frame rests on the soft tissue near the medial aspect of the scapular spine; 2) an anteroinferior extension that dissipates both shear and compressive force under load; and 3) a pliable saddle over the trapezius that acts as a suspension strap and

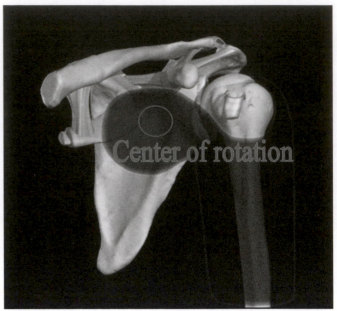

Figure 13-5. Center of rotation. (Courtesy of Hanger Orthopedic Group, Inc.)

an elastic membrane, which maintains electrode contact even when the wearer moves the shoulder through a wide range (Figure 13-6). The X-Frame provides greater stability, suspension, heat dissipation, comfort, and kinesthesia with better appearance than previous socket designs.

In summary, although few controlled studies have been performed on sockets, clinical experience indicates that advanced designs enable greater function, more comfort, and better appearance than traditional counterparts. They can be used with any control strategy and can be easily modified to permit greater joint excursion or more stability depending on the needs of a particular wearer.

POWERED PROSTHETIC CONTROL OPTIONS

Secondary to socket design is the manner in which the powered prosthesis is controlled.[8] Control options determine the extent to which the user integrates the prosthesis into desired activities. Each person's ability depends on strength, range of motion, muscular control, proprioception, amputation limb length, and mechanical aptitude. Choosing a control system is a complicated task that requires understanding of all alternatives.

The purpose of the prosthesis is fundamental in selecting a control system. Terminal device operation and the movements used to position the TD, such as wrist and elbow operation, are "primary controls." Mode selection among operations, system power con-

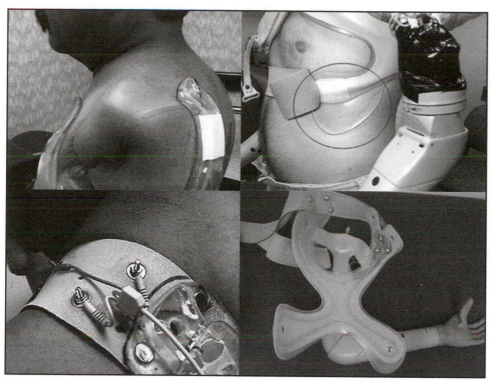

Figure 13-6. Clockwise from upper left: scapulospinal suspension; distal thermoplastic extension; definitive XFrame showing small footprint; soft electrode saddle (Courtesy of Hanger Orthopedic Group, Inc.)

trol, locking, and unlocking of various joints are "secondary controls." Primary controls should be selected first, using methods that produce dependable results easily. Secondary controls are not used as often during normal prosthetic use; they should be chosen so as not to interfere with primary control operations. In most cases, secondary controls are implemented and refined after primary controls are mastered.

Myoelectric Control

Myoelectric control uses electrical signals produced during muscle contraction to control various components. As the user voluntarily contracts the relevant muscle group, a surface electrode embedded in the socket interior detects the microvoltage produced during the contraction. The signal is then filtered, amplified, and sent to a microprocessor, which interprets each signal and compares it to set parameters, then sends the signal to the appropriate components to produce the desired function.

Myoelectric technology is the most commonly used primary externally powered control method. This is probably due to advances in hardware and socket fitting techniques that enhance the user's ability to master the controls. Myoelectric control is relatively easy to use and provides proprioceptive feedback, which enables the patient to relate muscle contractions to prosthetic function. In many cases, a direct relation exists between the extent of muscular contraction and the quality of the prosthetic action. A typical TR myoelectrically controlled prosthesis uses wrist extensor contraction to open the TD and supinate the forearm, while wrist flexors control TD closing and pronation. Myoelectric control can also be used for secondary control options such as mode selection and component locking and unlocking.

Early myoelectric fittings used a threshold of operation level that required the user to contract the given muscle with force above the threshold before the system operated. This produced a fixed speed of operation, known as *digital* control. A limitation of digital control is that the user can not regulate the speed of operation voluntarily, which is potentially hazardous when grasping fragile objects. Currently, digital systems are limited to users who can only produce a very weak electrical signal or those experienced with digital control who are unwilling to change their prosthetic usage.

The next generation of myoelectric control, known as *proportional* control, set parameters to turn the system on and off and allow for variable speed control. Proportional control allows the user to vary the speed of operation depending on the strength of the input electrical signal. Thus a low signal above the threshold produces a slow operation. A strong signal causes faster operation. Proportional control provides the user with enhanced fine prehension ability.[9,10]

In most myoelectric fittings, two muscles (preferably antagonists) control the opposing tasks of a particular component. At the TR level, the wrist extensors open the TD, whether hand, electric hook, or electronic gripper, and supinate the wrist, if applicable, while the wrist flexors control the opposite movements. In the

TH prosthesis, elbow extensors control TD opening, supination, and elbow extension. With shoulder-level fittings, electrode site selection is not as intuitive. The prosthetist chooses among several muscles for control, depending on innervation, size, and the individual's ability to control each muscle. Often the pectoralis major is used to control TD closing, pronation, and elbow flexion, while the infraspinatus or trapezius effects the contrary operations.

Two main types of proportional control systems are used in *dual-site* myoelectric control systems. First, *differential* proportional control evaluates both signals generated by muscle contraction and takes the difference, above the respective thresholds, between two signals. The system is proportional to the relative strength of the difference between the signals. Dual-site systems work well for users who have good voluntary control of both muscle groups and have isolated muscle contractions with little involuntary co-contractions. This type of system does not require the user to relax a contracted muscle group prior to allowing a stronger contraction from the antagonist group to override the system. Consequently, dual-site systems allow responsive opening and closing of the electronic TD.

The second type of proportional control system also evaluates both muscle groups; however, as soon as either signal rises above its threshold, the signal dominates the system so that the signal from the other muscle is ignored. This system works well for individuals who have difficultly isolating independent muscle contractions and who tend to produce high levels of involuntary co-contractions. This system is known as *first come–first served*. It responds proportionally to whichever signal prevails. The major limitation of the first come–first served control method is that both signals are required to relax below their respective thresholds prior to allowing the user to change operation. For example, one cannot change from supination to pronation of an electric wrist without relaxing between the contractions. The need for relaxation slows the operation of the prosthesis.

The most advanced control systems combine *first come–first served* and *differential* control strategies. The first signal over the threshold dominates, but can be overtaken by a second signal that meets specific parameters. This system eliminates the relaxation requirement, thereby speeding the response of the system.

Two main grip control systems exist. With the *time-based grip* system, prehension force is controlled by the duration of muscle contraction above the threshold. In the more advanced *proportional grip* system, grip strength is directly proportional to the muscular signal's strength and speed.

Although most myoelectrically controlled prostheses have two electrodes, sometimes the candidate does not have two suitable sites. A single muscle can be used for control of multiple functions. One signal may be partnered with another control method, such as liner transducers, touch pads, or switches, to create a simulated dual input system. Numerous strategies for *single-site* control allow the user to control the system.

Depending on the hardware, software, and the input signal(s), algorithms with adjustable parameters can be used for configuring a myoelectric system. Hardware systems are manufactured with either predefined or programmable algorithms that can be customized for the individual user.

Critical to fitting a myoelectric system is the ability of the surface electrode to maintain consistent contact at the correct location on the skin. An interruption in electrode contact usually produces a false spike in the input signal, which can cause erratic operation of the prosthetic component. Socket fit and electrode contact are the most common clinical problems.

Many physical factors influence myoelectric control. Skin with scarred or grafted tissue can be fitted; however, due to the varied conductivity of damaged skin, a single electrode should not be placed on both normal and scarred tissue. If the entire surface of the electrode contacts scarred or grafted tissue, myoelectric control can be used without problems.

In most cases, perspiration inside the socket moistens the skin enough to create good signal conduction from the skin to the electrode. Excessive perspiration, however, is detrimental. In very dry climates and in situations where the wearer does not perspire freely, the skin should be moistened with water prior to donning the prosthesis to enable signal conduction.

Other options for controlling powered prosthetic devices include switches, force sensing resistors, and servo mechanisms.[11]

Switch Control

Electronic switches can initiate prosthetic functions. Switches are operated through pushing on a button-like microswitch usually located within the socket or pulling on a transducer in the harness. Switches provide consistent, simple control, but are limited to digital, fixed speed operation. They are most commonly used for secondary operations.

Touch Pads

Touch pads are force-sensing resistors within or external to the socket that serve as momentary switches or can be used for proportional control of primary functions. When the user presses the pad, the output is proportional to the applied pressure. This system is useful for some people with congenital limb deficiency who retain a functional digit. The individual relies on proprioception within the digit and tactile sensation on the skin. Touch pads can also substitute for electrode function in myoelectric systems when the user is unable

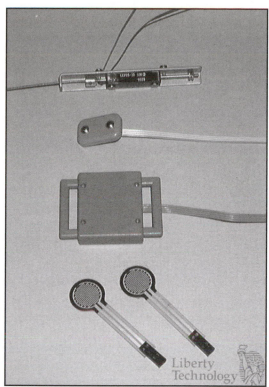

Figure 13-7. Control Input options (Courtesy of Liberty Technology.)

prosthesis needs some method of mode selection, ie, switching among the various components. Mode selection may be accomplished externally by switches or internally by using separate myoelectric signals. For example, a user may have to produce a quick strong contraction to rotate the wrist and a slower signal to operate the TD. Another common method is using voluntary co-contractions to change operational modes. Systems that use the same primary input are *sequential* in operation, with only one device operating at a time.

The other major mode of coordination involves using multiple primary control inputs. Each component may have a *dedicated* control input. An alternative is *simultaneous* operation, involving sharing one input for two components with a different input for additional components. Multiple primary control inputs allow several components to be operated at the same time. A common configuration with simultaneous operation for a TH prosthesis uses myoelectric control to operate the TD and the electronic wrist, while the electronic elbow is controlled by a servo system. Because simultaneous operation imitates physiological functions, it should be used whenever feasible. Attention should be paid to the functional combination and ease of control in simultaneous operations. For example, in TH or proximal level bilateral deficiency, elbow flexion and wrist supination combine to facilitate self-feeding, a task requiring dedicated simultaneous control.[12,13]

Servo Systems

Force and position servo systems can be used for prosthetic control. Typically, the force or position sensors are activated via body motion transmitted through a harness. The servo sensor translates the force or position into proportional operation of a prosthetic component. Servo systems are used primarily when myoelectric control and touch pads are not feasible. For example, a person with TH amputation who has a flail limb because of brachial plexus injury might be a candidate for a servo control system. They are frequently used as a secondary control input for simultaneous control of an electric elbow and TD (Figure 13-7).

Control Coordination

Of equal importance to the control system for each component is the coordination of controls for the entire prosthetic system. If only one component is involved, such as the TD, coordination is simple, with dual-site proportional myoelectric control being popular.

In prostheses with several electronic components, the controls for each component must complement the controls for the other components in the system. One method for controlling multiple components is using the same primary input for all components. The

POWERED PROSTHETIC COMPONENTS

Microprocessors

Powered prosthetic components consist of electronic motors and gearing systems powered by batteries. Individual components are combined to create the desired system. The system's microprocessor coordinates control the components, acting as a kind of "brain."[14]

Microprocessors are of two types. The first type is a central microprocessor that controls all components. The single microprocessor is mounted inside the prosthesis; its function is limited by the generic algorithms specific to the components that it is to control. Alternatively, the prosthesis may have separate microprocessors, each of which controls one component. In this case, the microprocessors are mounted directly on or inside the specific component. Because one microprocessor controls one component, its control algorithms are optimized for the function of that component. Programming and adjustments, however, tend to be more complex with multiple microprocessors.

The algorithms in microprocessors that control the prosthesis can be adjusted through an interface cable system connected to a laptop computer or hand-held personal digital assistant with wireless links.[15] The

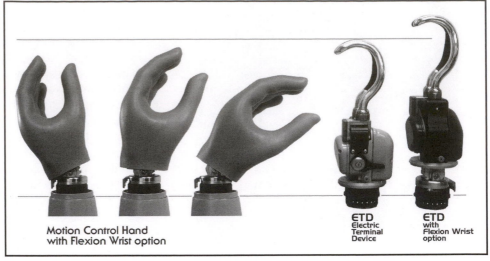

parameters that can be adjusted depend on the hardware and software of the particular system. The most common parameters are:

- Input signal amplification
- Differential gain
- Input signal thresholds (on and off)
- Proportional range of operation
- Mode selection parameters
- Output voltage and currents

Microprocessors regulate the input signals, manage the system power requirements, and regulate the control output to the various components. A rechargeable battery powers the system. Fast-charging high capacity batteries, such as lithium ion or nickel metal hydride cells, do not develop memory problems that could reduce battery function. A battery mounted inside the prosthesis is inconspicuous, whereas a battery set flush on the surface of the prosthesis facilitates installing a fresh battery when necessary.

Terminal Devices

If the microprocessor is the "brain," the TD is the "muscle" of the system. Terminal devices supply most of the function of the prosthesis by providing voluntary prehension. A quick disconnect wrist unit allows the user to change TDs to suit specific activities. Of the various electronic TDs, the most popular is the electric hand (Figure 13-8).

The electric hand moves in the three-jaw-chuck grasping pattern, which gives the user a reasonable blend of function and appearance. Hands are manufactured in sizes to fit people from infants to large adults. Grip strength for the adult size ranges from 0 to 22-29 psi. Specialty hands with thinner attachment plates can be fitted on wrist disarticulation and transcarpal prostheses. The most advanced commercially available electric hand incorporates sensors in the fingers

and hand mechanism to detect if an object is slipping. Slippage causes the hand to compensate automatically by increasing grip force to stabilize the object.[16] Laboratory research and clinical trials have been conducted on electrically powered finger prostheses.[17]

An inner shell covered by a glove protects the electronic system within the hand. Polyvinylchloride (PVC) gloves require frequent replacements because they stain and tear relatively easily, whereas silicone offers a stain-resistant alternative. Production PVC and silicone gloves are manufactured in standard sizes and colors. Custom silicone gloves, although more expensive, offer the best cosmetic restoration.

Electronic hands provide the user with an excellent combination of function and appearance; however, as is true of all prosthetic hands, they obscure part of the object being handled. Because people who wear upper-limb prostheses rely on visual feedback to compensate for loss of hand sensation, blocking the view of the object can interfere with function. Electronic hands allow reasonable observation of a large object, but obscure most of the surface of smaller objects. Another limiting factor of the electronic hand is its fixed prehension geometry. Some tasks are suited for other types of grasp patterns.

The alternative grasping patterns provided by electronic hooks and grippers may be appropriate for some users. Electronic hooks have a lyre or canted hook design with a central axis to produce lateral and tip grasp. Passively, the electronic hook can also be used for hook grasp. One model of electric hook allows the user to operate the system in wet environments without damaging the electronics; however, other usage limitations apply. Similar in function to electronic hooks, electronic grippers have a different shape and movement pattern. Both fingers open and close in a parallel vise-like method, providing cylindrical and spherical grasp. Electronic hooks and grippers are well suited for applications requiring maximum grasp force and durability; however, the wearer must be willing to sacrifice anthropomorphic appearance.[18]

Providing the user with several TDs and a quick change wrist unit enables the person to perform tasks with multiple grasping patterns. Whether an electronic hand, hook, or gripper, each TD has only one grasp pattern. Some people prefer to occasionally interchange an electric TD with a nonelectric one, such as various adaptive accessories. They are ordinarily used with cable-operated systems. If the prosthesis includes other electronic components, such as wrist or elbow units, the user may be able to operate them simultaneously with the adaptive device. For example, electronic wrist rotation may be used while using a feeding utensil.

Wrist Units

Wrist units position the TD either passively or actively. Many electric wrist units allow for quickly disconnecting the TD. In systems without powered wrist rotation, the user must turn the TD, by manually rotating the TD with the contralateral hand or rotating it against a fixed object, or, most conspicuously, rotating the shoulder.

Powered wrist rotation systems can be used on prostheses for long and short TR amputation limbs. They allow the user to orient the TD independently, thus keeping the contralateral extremity free for other tasks.[9] They can be controlled in the same way as TDs. Some electric TDs incorporate fixed passive wrist flexion and extension or ulnar deviation, whereas others have ball-and-socket motion, which allows positioning in any direction. Each user should be evaluated to determine the optimal combination of wrist function, weight, space within the prosthesis, and expense. Giving the user the ability to position the TD can improve function. Overall appearance is better when the wearer can position the TD at the wrist, rather than depending on proximal movements.

Elbow Units

An elbow unit is part of virtually all TH and shoulder level prostheses. The primary function of a prosthetic elbow unit, in combination with the wrist unit, is to orient the TD without gross body movements. The two basic types of elbow units intended for powered prostheses are electrically powered and hybrid cable-operated. Both types are limited by their active ("live") lift capacity. Powered elbow units have lift limited by the power of the motor and drive system, currently 9 pounds maximum.[19] The system performs optimally with minimal loads, such as the weight of the TD and a lightweight article being held. Theoretically, an electric elbow could be designed to provide substantial lifting capacity; however, this is impractical because of the increased weight, size, and noise involved. Electric elbows are most appropriate for users who do not possess sufficient force and excursion to operate hybrid cable-operated elbow units.

Hybrid cable-operated elbow units and their mechanical counterparts are limited in lifting capacity by the user's force and excursion capability. They incorporate an electronic wiring harness and a forearm counterbalance system to offset the weight of the electric TD and wrist unit.[12] An optional electronic lock permits the user to control locking functions without resorting to harnessed body movements and a mechanical lock. A hybrid passive elbow unit is lighter. The user positions it with the opposite hand or by pushing it against a fixed surface.

The maximum lifting capacity of any elbow unit is achieved when the elbow is in its fixed or locked position. Most manufacturers suggest limitations of approximately 50 pounds at the TD.

Shoulder Units

Prosthetic shoulder joints enhance function with prostheses for shoulder disarticulation and thoracic amputations. The joint enables shoulder abduction, flexion, and extension. Prosthetic shoulder joints are sometimes fitted to people with brachial plexus injuries or humeral neck amputations. Such prostheses should have a shoulder-style X-Frame socket.

The most common shoulder joints are friction and locking. Friction joints are manually positioned and support limited weight. Locking joints have a positive lock for the desired flexion angle and use friction for abduction. They have two modes of operation: locked and "free swing" (unlocked). When locked, the joint can withstand substantial force. In the unlocked position, the patient experiences natural arm swing when walking, which dramatically reduces rotational forces within the socket.[20] Unlocking is controlled either by a spring-loaded lever, which unlocks and then automatically relocks, or a two-position lever, which controls locking and unlocking. Recently, an electronic motor activated by any electronic input has become available to lock and unlock the prosthetic shoulder joint.

REHABILITATION

Specific rehabilitation protocols are described in Chapter 14. The most critical factor in successful rehabilitation is teamwork with open communication among clinicians and the patient and family. Other factors influencing success include early management, the prosthetic components and controls, patient-directed training, and regular follow-up.

- Upper-limb prosthetic rehabilitation includes:
  - Preprosthetic management
  - Wound healing
  - Pain management

- ◦ Limb shrinkage and shaping
- ◦ Limb desensitization
- ◦ Hygiene
- ◦ Range of motion exercises
- ◦ Strengthening exercises
- ◦ Training, for myoelectric systems
- Initial prosthetic training
  - ◦ Donning and doffing
  - ◦ Prosthetic wear schedule
  - ◦ Care of the amputated limb and prosthesis
- Prosthetic controls training
  - ◦ Body control motions
  - ◦ Proportional control of muscle contraction
  - ◦ TD training
    - Grasp
    - Release
    - Coordinated movements
  - ◦ Passive and active positioning
- Prosthetic use training
  - ◦ Functional operation training
  - ◦ Activity-based training
    - Daily activities
    - Vocation
    - Recreation
  - ◦ Home and work or school evaluation
  - ◦ Independent home training program
- Follow-up[21]

Follow-Up

Biannual or more frequent re-evaluation is essential to determine the continued adequacy of the system and the individual's function. Re-evaluation should also be performed whenever the user has a major change in body weight or vocation or when a potentially preferable prosthetic design becomes available.

Long-term follow-up and maintenance are as important as the initial care. At the follow-up visit, the prosthetist should assess the fit of the prosthesis, and, together with the rest of the clinic team, determine the patient's perception of the system, usage, any physical, physiological, psychosocial changes, and the person's current and future goals. The visit allows additional prosthetic training and preventative maintenance to avoid unnecessary costs and inconvenience. Follow-up enables outcomes documentation and ongoing patient and staff education.

Funding

Purchasing an externally powered upper-limb prosthesis with essential training can seem an insurmountable burden. The first step to obtain funds, after a thorough evaluation and completion of a rehabilitation plan, is to verify what insurance benefits are available to the patient. Authorization may demand substantiating documentation depending on the funding source. Concise documentation stating medical necessity and all other pertinent information supports the application.

SUMMARY

For many decades externally powered protheses have been used in the rehabilitation of people with all levels of upper-limb deficiencies. The distinct differences between those with upper- and lower-limb amputation affect rehabilitation. Assessment should account for the person's physical, psychological, and psychosocial attributes so that an individualized rehabilitation plan can be implemented. Advanced socket designs are especially critical to provide comfort, stability, control, and performance in externally powered systems that incorporate heavier components and, for myoelectric control, require constant electrode contact. No one system solves all requirements for a given user. Multiple prostheses or components may be required.

Externally powered prostheses can be controlled with various inputs, with myoelectric being the most common. Control strategies depend on input signals and desired control outputs; the parameters can be customized for optimal user performance. Different electronic components can be used to produce the desired function if the user is trained. Success also depends on the quality of long-term follow-up.

REFERENCES

1. Sears H. A new electric system with simultaneous elbow and hand control. Proceedings of the American Academy of Orthotists and Prosthetists; March 2004; New Orleans, La.
2. Hanson W, Mandacina S. Children's prosthetic systems. *O&P Edge.* 2003;2:18-19.
3. Uellendahl J. Upper extremity myoelectric prosthetics. In: Bussell A, ed. *Physical Medicine and Rehabilitation Clinics of North America.* Philadelphia, Pa: Saunders; 2000:639-652.
4. Farnsworth T. Hybrid approach to bilateral upper extremity prosthetic rehabilitation. Proceedings of the American Academy of Orthotists and Prosthetists; March 2003; San Diego, Calif.
5. Alley R. The common humeral hybrid configuration. *O&P Business News.* 2004;13:28-30.
6. Radocy R, Furlong A. Recreation and sports adaptations. In: Meier RH, Atkins DJ, eds. *Functional Restoration of Adults and Children with Upper Extremity Amputation.* New York, NY: Demos Medical Publishing; 2004:251-274.
7. Farnsworth T, Trial fitting of upper-extremity prostheses. *inMotion.* 2001;11.

8. Williams TW. Control of powered upper extremity prostheses. In: Meier RH, Atkins DJ, eds. *Functional Restoration of Adults and Children with Upper Extremity Amputation.* New York, NY: Demos Medical Publishing; 2004:207-224.

9. Sears H, Shaperman J. Electric wrist rotation in proportional-controlled systems. *Journal of Prosthetics and Orthotics.* 1998;4:92-98.

10. Sears H, Shaperman J. Proportional myoelectric hand control: an evaluation. *Am J Phys Med Rehabil.* 1991;70:20-28.

11. Lovely D. Signals and signal processing for myoelectric control. In: Muzumdar A, ed. *Powered Upper Limb Prostheses: Control, Implementation and Clinical Application.* Berlin, Germany: Springer; 2004:35-54.

12. Farnsworth T. A unique application of ballistic motion and linear transducer to control a humeral level hybrid prosthesis. Proceedings of the American Academy of Orthotists and Prosthetists; March 2003; San Diego, Calif.

13. Uellendahl J, Heckathorne C. Creative prosthetic solutions for bilateral upper extremity amputations. In: Meier RH, Atkins DJ, eds. *Functional Restoration of Adults and Children with Upper Extremity Amputation.* New York, NY: Demos Medical Publishing; 2004:225-238.

14. Lake C. Comparative analysis of microprocessors in upper limb prosthetics. *Journal of Prosthetics and Orthotics.* 2003;15:48-65.

15. Limehouse JW, Clinical experiences with animated prosthetics controller and LIMB LINK. Proceedings of the American Academy of Orthotists and Prosthetists; March 2003; San Diego, Calif.

16. Farnsworth T. Clinical application of the "Next Generation—Sensor Hand System." Proceedings of the American Academy of Orthotists and Prosthetists; March 2004; New Orleans, La.

17. Keyberd P, Gow D, Chappell P. Research and the future of myoelectric prosthetics. In: Muzumdar A, ed. *Powered Upper Limb Prostheses; Control, Implementation and Clinical Application.* Berlin, Germany: Springer; 2004:175-188.

18. Sears H. Evaluation studies of new electric terminal devices. Proceedings of the American Academy of Orthotists and Prosthetists; March 2003; San Diego, Calif.

19. Hanson W. Unique capabilities of the Boston Digital Arm System. Trent Prosthetic Symposium; May 2002; Nottingham, England.

20. Anderson C. Adaptations of locking shoulder joints to increase functional range of motion for bilateral upper limb deficiencies. Proceedings of the Myoelectric Controls/Powered Prosthetics Symposium; 1999:146-148.

21. Atkins D. Functional skills training with body-powered and externally powered prostheses. In: Meier RH, Atkins DJ, eds. *Functional Restoration of Adults and Children with Upper Extremity Amputation.* New York, NY: Demos Medical Publishing; 2004:139-158.

Chapter 14

Training Patients With Upper-Limb Amputations

Diane Atkins, OTR, FISPO and Joan E. Edelstein, MA, PT, FISPO

OBJECTIVES

1. Describe early management of patients with upper-limb amputation, including amputation limb care and holistic care
2. Specify the steps in donning and controlling all components of transradial and transhumeral prostheses
3. Suggest means of using the prosthesis as an assistive device in personal care, vocations, and avocations
4. Indicate how the patient should care for the amputation limb and the prosthesis
5. Explain modifications of basic training for children with upper-limb absence and for those with bilateral amputations

INTRODUCTION

Rehabilitation of children and adults who have an amputation at or proximal to the wrist, whether or not the individual has a prosthesis, involves attention to the postsurgical management. If the amputation is acquired, prescription of a suitable prosthesis, and training the individual to achieve maximum function, with and without the prosthesis are indicated. Chapters 3, 4, and 6 on early management, pain, and psychological factors, respectively, are particularly pertinent in understanding comprehensive management of children and adults with upper-limb absence.[1-3]

EARLY MANAGEMENT

Early management includes interventions that emphasize recovery of the amputation limb from surgery and those that enable the patient to resume as many daily activities as possible.[1-3]

Amputation Limb Care

Trauma is the leading cause of upper-limb amputation; consequently, there may be an interval between the accident and amputation. Although the trauma team attempts to save the injured limb, rehabilitation should commence with assessment of joint mobility, skin condition, and motor power in anticipation of amputation surgery. Members of the clinic team should meet with the patient and family to diminish some of the anxiety that accompanies surgery. Introducing them to someone with a similar level of limb loss who has completed rehabilitation is an effective way of helping adopt a realistically optimistic attitude. Amputation limb care is rarely indicated for infants with congenital limb anomaly unless the body segment is surgically revised.

The goal of wound care is a well-healed, nonadherent scar. Wound care commences immediately after amputation. Young adults with traumatic amputation usually heal rapidly. If the trauma that necessitated the amputation was extensive, wound care may involve periodic debridement and other measures to foster nonadherent scarring. Deep burns may require skin grafting with conscientious aftercare.

Unlike patients with leg amputation, volume control procedures are less critical for people with upper-limb amputation. Less soft tissue is transected in the arm

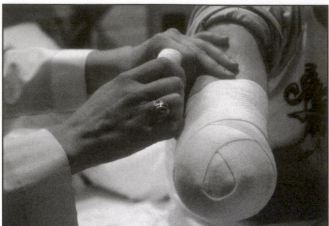

Figure 14-1. Figure-of-eight wrap used to control edema.

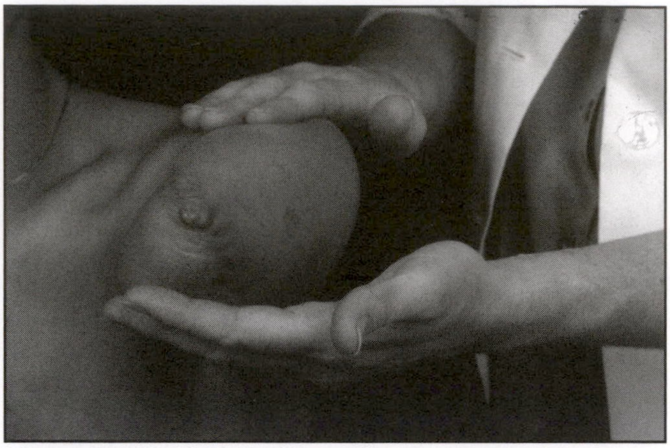

Figure 14-2. Shoulder flexion for transhumeral amputation. This motion is utilized for terminal device operation.

or forearm, and the patient, usually being young and otherwise healthy, is less likely to form much edema. Control of edema, and recording circumferential measurements, is particularly important. Consistent measurements are critical when a myoelectric prosthesis is prescribed as the initial prosthesis. Ongoing fluctuations in edema will cause the socket with electrodes for myoelectric control to loose contact and result in an unsuccessful attempt at utilization. Unna dressings are particularly effective in minimizing postoperative edema and facilitating healing. The gauge bandage permeated with zinc oxide, calamine, glycerin, and gelatin forms an adherent, nonextensible dressing, which can remain on the limb until sutures are removed, approximately 5 days after surgery. A plaster of Paris dressing is an alternative, which will control edema and remains on the limb until suture removal. Plaster, however, is more difficult to apply and remove than Unna dressing. An elastic bandage is another option that assists in reducing edema. It must be applied in a Figure of Eight manner with more pressure applied to the distal end of the residual limb (Figure 14-1). The therapist or someone else must reapply elastic bandage every few hours to maintain limb compression. Elastic shrinker socks are another option, although they tend to roll distally if the arm is fleshy.

Maintaining or increasing joint mobility is an essential part of early management. Adults with transradial (TR) amputations are vulnerable to limitation of pronation and supination, as well as elbow flexion and extension, and shoulder motion. Those with transhumeral (TH) amputations risk losing shoulder mobility (Figure 14-2). These motions are critically important in controlling the prosthesis as well as essential ADL tasks such as dressing, toileting, and functioning in the largest possible workspace.

Because most people with upper-limb amputation do not experience a lengthy period of deconditioning prior to surgery, strengthening exercises play a lesser role in rehabilitation of those with arm amputation as compared with older adults who have leg amputation. Even so, a program of resistance exercises and aerobic conditioning is beneficial to maintain the patient's endurance and functional capacity.

Individuals with proximal amputations are vulnerable to scoliosis. Loss of substantial arm weight alters trunk alignment. Scoliosis is of particular concern in skeletally immature individuals with TH amputations. Not only will appearance and respiration be compromised, but the individual with scoliosis may have more difficulty controlling the prosthesis.

Pain control is a major issue for many people with acquired amputation. Because a large portion of the cerebral cortex is devoted to the hand, interruption of the neurological connection between the brain and the hand can produce marked phantom sensation. The patient perceives the absent hand, which may seem to be in a contorted or painful position. Many interventions reduce the prominence of phantom pain or sensation for most patients; these include ultrasound, percussive or effleurage massage, transcutaneous electrical neural stimulation, acupressure, acupuncture, and bilateral resistive exercise. Edema control is associated with reduction in phantom pain. Local pain may indicate the presence of an irritated neuroma. Although all transected nerves form neuromata, the distal nerve portion can produce pain if it is embedded in scar or fascial tissue. Painful neuromata are a common source of distress in patients with upper-limb amputation. Surgical excision of the neuroma is a common intervention to alleviate symptoms of local pain.

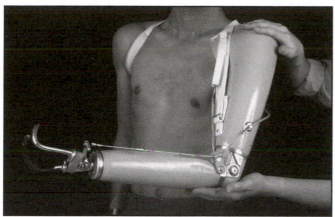

Figure 14-3. Shoulder flexion enables the terminal device to open when a body-powered prosthesis is utilized.

Holistic Care

A principal factor in the rehabilitation of people with arm amputation is attention to psychosocial concerns. The human hand is a visible and important aspect of our ability to communicate in written, verbal and non-verbal ways. Disguising its loss is virtually impossible. Initially, the truncated limb is a constant reminder of the amputation, for the patient and family members. Degree of limb loss does not appear to correlate with the extent of depression, anxiety, or behavioral problems. Parents or the patient may be overwhelmed with guilt for permitting the trauma to have occurred. Birth of an infant with a limb anomaly can be as shocking to the medical staff as to the family. Resulting depression or denial obstructs rehabilitation. Counseling by a psychologist or other mental health caregiver can help the patient and family accept the permanence of the amputation and the reality that the individual with limb loss can learn new ways of accomplishing most tasks.

Change of hand dominance concerns many people with acquired amputation. Whether or not the patient will receive a prosthesis, the device does not have the sensation or dexterity of the anatomic segment. The person should have the opportunity to practice grooming, dressing, toileting, dining, and other activities using the intact limb. The value of tactile and proprioceptive sensation cannot be overstated. Initial attempts are apt to be clumsy, but with practice and encouragement, most people become very facile with unilateral performance. Individuals with unilateral and bilateral amputation also use the teeth, as well as antecubital and axillary fossae, and perform other maneuvers to achieve function. Certain patients receive a temporary prosthesis, which enables bimanual activity; however, the prosthesis lacks the sensory or motor attributes of the sound hand. Some prefer to write with the prosthesis, whereas others change writing dominance as well. Children with congenital limb absence use the intact limb as the dominant side immediately.

Whether or not the dominant hand has been lost, unimanual activities should be part of early management. Clinicians should create a problem-solving environment, which enables the patient to determine the best way to perform daily and recreational activities with the intact hand. The goal of early management is to restore maximum independence and self-reliance to the patient regardless of whether a prosthesis will be fitted and provides active prehension.[4]

PROSTHETIC CONTROLS TRAINING

After the prosthesis is delivered to the patient, it should be evaluated carefully. Ideally, the initial therapy should occur within the first day or two of receiving the prosthesis. Often the occupational therapist or physical therapist performs the detailed evaluation and reports the findings to the clinic team. Training consists of controls training (Figure 14-3), which includes teaching the client to don the prosthesis and control all mechanisms in the prosthesis. Use training involves guiding the patient to incorporate the prosthesis in bimanual activities. Rehabilitation is usually completed when the wearer demonstrates reasonable proficiency in prosthetic control. Additional training focuses on vocational and avocational activities. Training should not proceed until the clinic team is certain that the prosthesis fits and operates properly; otherwise, the wearer is apt to exert unnecessary effort to achieve adequate function.

Transradial Prosthesis

Controls training for the person fitted with a TR prosthesis includes instruction in donning the appliance and operating the terminal device (TD) and wrist unit. The patient must be able to don and doff the prosthesis independently, accurately, and quickly, otherwise it will not be worn on a long-term basis. With a figure-of-eight or figure-of-nine harness, the person first dons a t-shirt to protect the skin from possible irritation by the harness straps. The next step involves encasing the amputation limb in a sock. Cotton, wool, nylon, and silicon are materials commonly used in sock manufacture. Then the individual inserts the amputation limb into the socket. Placing the sound hand through the axillary loop is the final step. A prosthesis with a chest strap requires the patient to place the amputation limb in the socket, then wrap the chest strap around the torso, fastening the strap in the front.

Terminal Device and Wrist Unit Control

The patient needs to control the TD and the wrist unit of the TR prosthesis. A prosthesis with a myoelectric TD has electrodes embedded in the socket. The electrodes are usually placed over the flexor and extensor muscle bellies. Chapter 13 details myoelectric and other forms of external control mechanisms.

A cable-controlled TR prosthesis has a single steel cable that is attached distally to the TD, whether hand or hook, and proximally to the control attachment strap. The cable is encased in a steel tubular housing secured distally to the socket. Proximally the housing is attached to the proximal portion of the socket or to a flexible plastic or leather pad placed over the triceps muscle. The housing prevents the cable from bowstringing when the wearer bends the elbow. The patient flexes the glenohumeral joint or abducts the scapula to apply tension to the cable. The tension is transmitted to the TD to open or close it, depending on its mechanism. Chapter 12 describes body-powered components.

The wrist unit may be manually or myoelectrically controlled. In the former type, the patient rotates the unit with the sound hand or nudges it against a firm surface. In the latter type, microvoltage transmitted from forearm muscles via a skin electrode activates the electric wrist unit mechanism.

The usual method for donning a snugly fitting supracondylar or Muenster socket entails encasing the amputation limb in tubular stockinet, which is approximately twice as long as the limb. The distal end of the stockinet extends beyond the end of the amputation limb. The patient inserts the amputation limb in the socket, taking care to place the end of the stockinet through a hole drilled through the end of the socket. The stockinet continues through another hole in the proximal end of the plastic forearm. The patient tugs on the stockinet to draw the skin and superficial tissue into the socket. If the socket is part of a myoelectrically controlled prosthesis, the patient continues pulling on the stockinet until it is completely pulled from the prosthesis, so that the skin is in direct contact with the socket and its electrodes. If the socket is part of a cable-controlled prosthesis, the patient pulls on the stockinet only until the socket is well positioned, then tucks the end of the stockinet into the forearm cavity.

Cable-controlled TD controls training begins with the prosthesis on the patient. The best position for early training is with the elbow flexed approximately 90 degrees, because the patient can see the TD easily, and the harness and cable are in the most favorable position for ease in TD operation. The therapist resists glenohumeral flexion until the patient observes the TD move. If the device is voluntary opening (VO), it will open; if it is voluntary closing (VC), it will close. The patient practices glenohumeral flexion until the motion can be done without external resistance and the TD operates reliably. The patient should confine the control motion to the amputated side. Tensing the contralateral musculature interferes with performance of bimanual activities in which the contralateral side would be active. The next step in training involves having the

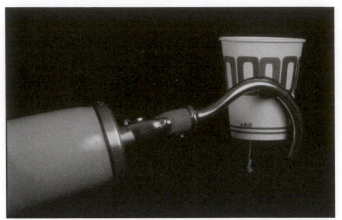

Figure 14-4. Maintaining tension on the cable prevents the paper cup from being crushed by a voluntary-opening terminal device.

patient keep the elbow flexed while attempting to operate the TD by abducting the scapula. When properly executed, the maneuver achieves TD operation close to the body.

With a VC TD, the patient practices closing it gently, then forcefully, and finally at intermediate amounts of force. Control of a VO TD includes drills in opening the hand or hook fully and then at intermediate distances. The patient also practices relaxing cable tension to allow the device to snap closed. The most difficult control procedure requires the wearer to close the device partially by maintaining tension on the control attachment strap (Figure 14-4).

Terminal device operation with a myoelectrically controlled prosthesis begins prior to the construction of the prosthesis.[5-9] The therapist uses a volt meter or a myotester (Figure 14-5) with electrodes to explore the patient's forearm, seeking the site where the patient can register the greatest microvoltage when contracting the flexors forcefully. The procedure is repeated with the extensors. The patient practices isolated contraction of the flexors while maintaining relaxation of the extensors, and vice versa. Once optimal electrode positions are found, the electrodes are embedded in the socket so that they overlie the chosen sites. With the finished prosthesis on, the patient practices opening the TD to various distances, as well as closing the TD with various amounts of force.

After mastering the basic TD opening and closing maneuvers, regardless of design of the TD, the patient then attempts to operate the device with the elbow extended, fully flexed, and at intermediate angles, and with the shoulder in all positions.

Positioning the TD involves using the wrist unit. The therapist teaches the patient to rotate the wrist unit to position the device appropriately. If the wrist unit has a locking mechanism, the individual learns how to unlock it, rotate the unit, and relock it. The person practices

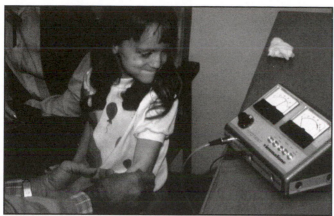

Figure 14-5. A myotester is used to evaluate residual wrist flexors and extensors in the transradial limb.

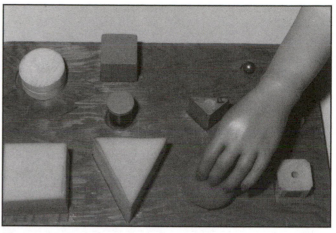

Figure 14-6. A form board is used to practice various grasping patterns with a myoelectric hand or other terminal device.

wrist unit and TD control by grasping objects of various sizes, shapes, and textures on a form board (Figure 14-6). Most objects can be grasped with the TD pronated. However, some items, such as disks, are easier to manage if the TD is placed halfway between pronation and supination. A large, rigid ball is most readily secured in a hook that is turned to the supinated position; with a prosthetic hand, the ball is easier to grasp with the TD pronated. Poor socket fit, improper cable and harness strap position, or component malfunction hamper controlling the prosthesis.

Most adults become proficient in TR prosthetic controls after approximately 5 hours of instruction.

Transhumeral Prosthesis

The easiest way to don a TH prosthesis that has a figure-of-eight harness is with the prosthesis placed on a table with the harness untangled. The patient wears a t-shirt and an amputation limb sock. The individual inserts the sound limb into the axillary loop, then places the amputation limb in the socket. If the prosthesis has a chest strap, the person dons the socket, then encircles the chest with the chest strap, and secures it.

Terminal Device and Elbow Unit Control

Cable control of the TH prosthesis is usually achieved with two cables, each encased in steel housing. One cable extends from the control attachment strap buckled on the back of the harness to the TD. This cable has proximal and distal housing sections. If the elbow unit is unlocked, tension on the cable causes elbow flexion. Controlled relaxation of the cable allows the elbow to extend. If the elbow unit is locked, tension on the same cable activates the TD. The second cable extends from the elbow unit locking mechanism to the anterior support strap of the harness. Alternating tension on this cable locks and unlocks the elbow unit.

Initially, TD operation and positioning it in the wrist unit is taught after the therapist engages the elbow lock.

Terminal device and wrist unit operation are performed in the same way as for a TR prosthesis. The therapist also teaches the patient to rotate the forearm in the horizontal plane by pulling or pushing the forearm so that the elbow unit pivots at the turntable. This enables the individual to work at midline with bilateral activities, such as fastening a belt buckle, snap, or button (Figure 14-7). Additionally, activities such as opening containers and cutting meat are accomplished more easily when the turntable is positioned with the forearm and TD at midline.

Elbow unit control begins with the elbow unlocked. The therapist shows the patient that the same glenohumeral flexion or scapular abduction that operates the TD also flexes the elbow, as the cable connected to the TD passes anterior to the elbow hinge. To extend the elbow, the patient gradually relaxes the shoulder or scapular musculature.

The second step in elbow unit control focuses on elbow locking and unlocking. Training should start with the prosthesis off the patient. The therapist shows the patient that the elbow lock is an alternator mechanism, ie, the first pull on the elbow lock cable locks the unit. The next pull will unlock it. The unit will function only if the elbow lock cable retracts completely. The patient pulls on the elbow lock cable with the sound hand until smooth, reliable action is achieved. With the prosthesis on the patient, the therapist unlocks the elbow and supports the forearm with one hand while using the other hand to resist an oblique movement composed of humeral hyperextension and shoulder girdle depression until the elbow locks. Some degree of humeral abduction may be required initially to exaggerate the motion that is required for elbow lock and unlock control. Abduction helps the learning process. Eventually, the patient should avoid abducting the shoulder for more discrete operation of the

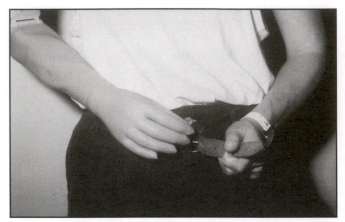

Figure 14-7. Working at midline to close a belt buckle).

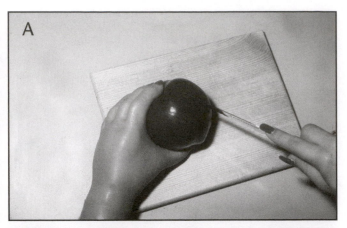

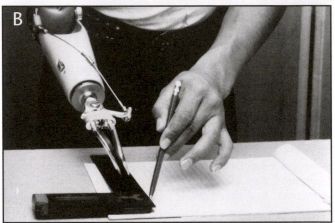

Figure 14-8. (A) A myoelectric hand stabilizes an apple while the sound hand cuts with a knife. (B) The prosthesis and terminal device can stabilize a straight edge in order to draw a line.

prosthesis, because abduction is ungainly and inefficient. Repeating the movement unlocks the unit. Locking and unlocking produce faint sounds, which confirm that the desired movement has occurred. The person then practices rapid elbow locking and unlocking while the therapist continues to support the forearm.

The final step in elbow unit controls training requires coordination of elbow flexion and locking. The patient flexes the elbow to the desired angle, then locks it quickly. If the individual performs slowly, the elbow will extend. Flexion of the elbow hinge requires shoulder flexion, whereas elbow locking needs shoulder hyperextension.

Electrically powered elbow units are activated by switches in the harness or elsewhere in the prosthesis, or by skin electrodes placed over the remnants of the anterior and posterior deltoid muscles. The myoelectric elbow unit may be used in combination with a myoelectrically controlled TD.

Most adults become proficient in TH prosthetic controls after approximately 10 hours of instruction. Elbow operation is often the most difficult and time-consuming aspect of TH prosthetic raining. Positive reinforcement and simple goal-oriented tasks are important to include in functional training.

USE TRAINING

Use training emphasizes employing the prosthesis as an assistive device, complementing maneuvers of the sound hand. Most daily activities, such as drinking from a cup, are naturally performed with one hand.[10,11] The person who wears a prosthesis would do the same, ie, hold the cup in the intact hand. A few tasks, however, are ordinarily done with two hands. These activities form the basis of use training. In general, the TD performs the stabilizing portion of the task (Figure 14-8). The therapist should allow the patient to experi-

ment with various techniques to accomplish endeavors, offering cues only when the individual is stymied. Techniques used by people with hemiplegia often work well for those with an amputation. Some adaptive aids, such as a cutting board with protruding nails, are useful. Use training is beneficial whether the patient has an active or passive TD.

Personal Care

Face washing can be done entirely with one hand. Nevertheless, it is usually easier to stabilize the wash cloth with the prosthesis while soaping it with the soap held in the sound hand. To wash the sound hand, one can hold the bar of soap in the TD while moving the hand over the soap. Individuals with unilateral amputation do not wear a prosthesis when showering or tub bathing. Often those with bilateral amputation also find a way to manage bathing without prostheses.

Grooming may challenge the ingenuity of the patient. Most toiletry appliances, however, can be managed with one hand. A tooth brush, for example is used uni-

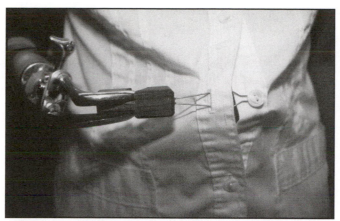

Figure 14-9. A button hook may be used to assist with buttoning.

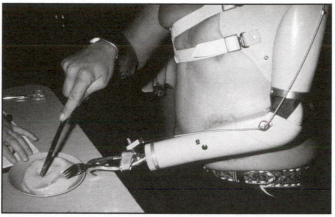

Figure 14-10. The task of cutting meat can be simulated in order to perfect the skill of stabilizing the fork in the terminal device while the sound hand holds a knife.

laterally. Extracting toothpaste from a pump dispenser can be done by pressing on the nozzle control with the forearm on the amputated side while the sound hand holds the brush. With a toothpaste tube, one can also press on the tube with the forearm. An electric or manual shaver suits one-handed use, as do simpler hair styles and makeup.

Practice with buttoning, using a zipper, and managing other garment fasteners is integral to learning to dress. The prosthesis is useful in stabilizing fabric while the sound hand manipulates the closure. Some people use a button hook to facilitate buttoning (Figure 14-9). Shirts, jackets, and coats are most readily donned by slipping the prosthesis into the sleeve, then maneuvering the intact arm in the other sleeve. Pullover shirts and sweaters are most manageable if the garment is laid on a bed or table. The prosthesis enters its sleeve first, following by placing the head through the neck opening and the sound arm into its sleeve.

Trousers and skirts are easy to don if the sound hand holds one side of the waistband and the prosthesis holds the other side. The prosthesis stabilizes the distal end of the zipper while the sound hand pulls the slider.

Meals can be consumed entirely one-handed, depending on the menu. The activity that is most often accomplished with the aid of a prosthesis is cutting meat. The prosthesis holds the fork, while the sound hand grasps the knife (Figure 14-10). After one or more morsels are cut, the wearer switches utensils, to spear food and bring it to the mouth with the fork held in the intact hand.

Writing can be done either with the sound hand or TD. If the nondominant hand was lost, then the person would probably hold the pen in the sound hand. The TD stabilizes the paper, especially when the writing surface is slippery, such as a glass counter at a bank. If the dominant hand was amputated, the patient may have learned to change dominance in the preprosthetic phase of rehabilitation. Alternatively, the individual with TR amputation can hold a pen in the TD, relying on shoulder and elbow motion to shape the letters. A felt marker is a good choice for the beginner because it will work with relatively light pressure and is appropriate for rather large letters. Because they lack natural elbow motion, those with a TH amputation generally find it easier to learn to write with the sound hand.

Vocations

The clerical aspects of most school and professional endeavors are easier to accomplish with the prosthesis serving as a useful tool. Office equipment may be adapted, in most instances with little cost or effort, to suit the capabilities of most people who wear a prosthesis. Keyboard control can be aided with the substitution of a keyboard designed for one-handed use. Alternatively, one can press the key with the tip of the hook or with the eraser end of a pencil held in the prosthetic hand or hook using a one-finger technique. Unlike those with more distal amputations, people with TH amputations will have difficulty reaching overhead with the prosthesis.

Operating an automobile is aided with a spinner knob bolted to the steering wheel. If the patient customarily wears a prosthesis, this change in status should be reported to the licensing agency and automobile insurance company. Instruction with a certified driving instructor is advisable.

Avocations

A wide range of sports is well within the reach of most individuals with amputation, whether or not they wear prostheses.[12] Special TDs can be exchanged for the usual one, to hold a bowling ball or golf club, manage a baseball catcher's mitt, and perform gymnastic stunts (Figure 14-11). Professional football, basketball, and

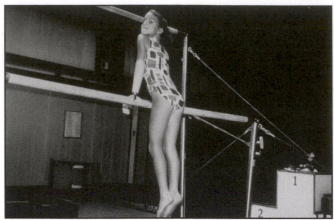

Figure 14-11. A special "mitt like" terminal device can be used in gymnastic activities.

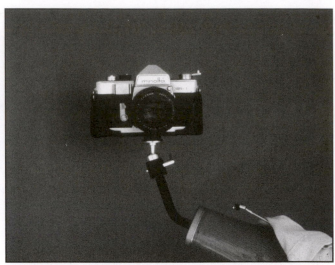

Figure 14-12. Special adaptation to secure a camera.

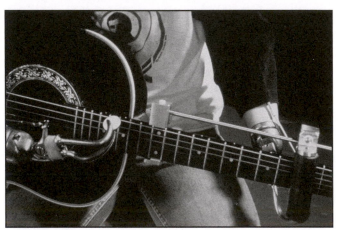

Figure 14-13. A guitar adaptation that enables a bilateral amputee to play with both prostheses.

baseball players with limb deficiencies are role models for their skilled one-handed prowess. Many sports organizations are open to people with disabilities, including those with upper-limb amputations. Participation is a superb way of integrating into the community, as well as garnering the physiological benefits of exercise.

People who wear prostheses can enjoy photography especially if a special TD is worn in place of the customary cable-controlled hook. The device secures the camera, so that the person can use the sound hand to adjust the lens and other controls (Figure 14-12).

Many musical instruments are readily playable by children and adults with amputation.[13] The most accessible are brass winds, because the valves are ordinarily operated with one hand while the prosthesis stabilizes the instrument. One may have to switch hands; for example, a trumpet is designed to be played with the right hand controlling the valves. It can, however, be played with the left hand. Conversely, the French horn, normally played with the left hand, can be operated in reverse. The trombone is well suited to people with amputations because most models have no valves. Strings on guitar and other stringed instruments, ordinarily fingered with the left hand, can have the strings reversed; depending on the instrument, this may also require changing the position of the bridge (Figure 14-13). A pick or bow can be adapted so it is secured in the TD or in an elastic cuff worn on the forearm. Piano compositions for one-handed performance exist in the beginner, intermediate, and advanced repertory. A creative prosthetist can often alter almost any instrument, or adapt the TD, to allow the person with limb loss to have the opportunity to create a unique musical style.

FUNCTIONAL OUTCOME

Factors contributing to ongoing prosthetic use among adults include completion of high school education, employment, emotional acceptance of the amputation, and the perception that the prosthesis is expensive.[14-20] Those with TR amputation are most likely to continue prosthetic use. Early fitting for those with traumatic amputation as well as post-traumatic counseling contribute to continued prosthetic usage. Training increases the patient's efficient and skillful use of the prosthesis. Age, loss of the dominant hand, and marital status do not seem to be determinants of prosthetic use. Because most amputations are unilateral, many individuals eventually opt to discard the prosthesis. Most daily and vocational activities can be accomplished without a prosthesis. Early fitting, good medical management, an experienced prosthetist who provides a well-fitting prosthesis, and a knowledgeable therapist will enhance prosthetic outcome and encourage total independence for all people with unilateral upper-limb amputation. The clinic team is the key to optimal functional outcome.

Caring for the Amputation Limb and the Prosthesis

Instructing the patient and, in the case of children, the family, in the care of the amputation limb and prosthesis is an essential part of rehabilitation.

Amputation Limb

The patient should protect the skin against incipient abrasions, which, if untended, can exacerbate to an extent that prevents wearing the prosthesis comfortably. The patient who has accommodated to daily wear of the prosthesis should check the skin each evening. Reddened or discolored areas should resolve within 10 minutes. If not, the wearer should return to the prosthetist for socket or harness adjustment.

Flexibility and strength should be maintained so that the person can control the prosthesis and perform the full range of activities effectively.

Prosthesis

A cable-controlled hook is the simplest TD to maintain. It should be kept clean and wiped dry if unintentionally immersed. One should check the neoprene lining for deep cracks, which indicate that it needs replacement. Rubber bands on a hook need replacement when they become brittle.

A prosthetic hand, regardless of mechanism, requires care of the glove. This includes avoiding sharp or rough textured objects. The glove can be cleaned with a slightly moistened soapy cloth. One should never place the hand on a varnished surface. The wearer should avoid exposing the glove to solvents, such as gasoline, kerosene, or turpentine, or staining agents such as ballpoint pen ink, newsprint, tobacco, mustard, grape juice, and beet juice. Nail polish can be worn, but must be removed preferably by scraping rather than with acetone. The relatively delicate hand mechanism requires that the patient refrain from immersing the hand in liquid or sand, subjecting it to vibratory stress, or otherwise mishandling it, and must be protected against immersion, debris, and rough usage.

The socket interior should be wiped each evening with a moistened soapy cloth. Unless the prosthesis is myoelectrically controlled, one should wear a fresh sock daily. Most harnesses can be unbuckled from the rest of the prosthesis. The Dacron strap can then be laundered. The housing on the control cable should not become unwound for this would cause it to snag clothing and possibly cause the control cable to break. A clean t-shirt worn under the harness protects the skin and harness.

If the prosthesis has myoelectrically controlled components, the battery must be recharged periodically, preferably nightly. Lithium ion batteries charge faster and provide more power than nickel cadmium ones.

Children With Upper-Limb Absence

Whether the deficit is a congenital anomaly or acquired in childhood, the patient and family are best served by coordinated care provided by an experienced clinic team. Interaction with peer support groups is invaluable, both for family members and for youngsters who will undoubtedly enjoy camping and sports with their peers. The Association of Children's Prosthetic-Orthotic Clinics (6300 North River Road, Suite 727, Rosemont, Ill 60018-4226) is an excellent resource for clinicians. Chapter 15 discusses prosthetic options for children.

Congenital Anomalies

Depending on the functional prognosis, the anomalous limb may or may not be surgically revised to facilitate prosthetic fitting. For example, in most instances of radial absence with or without loss of part of the carpal bones and the thumb, the child retains more function than a prosthesis would provide. Surgery is seldom performed, as the child will learn to use every aspect of the contour and movement of the anomalous limb. Limb sensation provides a major benefit for young children, whereas prostheses eliminate the opportunity to feel objects in the environment. Young children should be encouraged to use their anomalous limb in all encounters with the environment, such as playing in water, sand, and mud. Eventually a prosthesis will be beneficial for performing bilateral tasks in school. Often the school-aged child removes the prosthesis after school for unencumbered play, as well as bathing and sleeping.

If no surgery is performed, the child will not have a scar and will not require wound care or limb volume management. The physical therapist should, however, examine the child carefully to determine whether mobility and strength of the shoulder, elbow, and forearm are compromised.

If the child has had surgery, particularly in the presence of trauma, which results in removal of the distal epiphyseal plate in the humerus or radius and ulna, the clinic team must be alert to the likelihood of overgrowth. The long bones will continue to grow, creating a tender bursa at the end of the amputated limb. The customary treatment, surgical excision of the distal bony tip, may need to be repeated several times during the child's growing years. Preservation of the distal epiphyseal plates avoids the risk of overgrowth. Whether or not the young patient has had surgery, regular visits to the clinic team are important to ascertain when the socket has become outgrown or the length of the prosthesis is inadequate. Ideally, the clinic team should reevaluate the child every 3 months, particularly during ages 1 through 10 years.

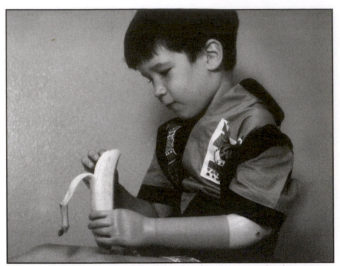

Figure 14-14. A child holds the banana with the myoelectric hand and peels it with the sound hand.

Prosthetic Considerations

Training involves instructing the parent in age-appropriate games, which encourage the young wearer first to hold objects, then to release them, and finally to grasp items in the TD while engaging in bimanual activities.[22,23] Infants respond to stuffed animals, large balls and blocks, and similar toys. Toddlers like bead stringing, sewing cards, rhythm band instruments, construction sets, and card games. Preschool age youngsters can learn basic dressing, eating (Figure 14-14), and drawing skills using the prosthesis as an assist to the sound hand. For those fitted with myoelectric prostheses, adapted electrical toys are especially motivating. For example, a model train can be wired so that flexor muscle contraction causes it to move forward and extensor muscle contraction reverses the direction of the train. This technique is effective in training the child to operate a myoelectric prosthesis. Parental involvement in treatment is associated with ongoing prosthesis use; nevertheless, puberty is a time of higher rejection of the prosthesis. Active prosthetic prehension is common among children older than 6 years of age, whereas relatively few younger patients use prostheses to grasp objects. When school requires bilateral function with stabilization (eg, using scissors, opening packages, and drawing and tracing shapes on paper), prostheses are useful.[24,25]

BILATERAL AMPUTATION

Absence of both hands is comparatively rare, whether by acquired amputation or through congenital anomaly. The loss affects virtually every aspect of daily function and, depending on the length of the amputation limbs, may alter trunk posture and respiration.

Even with a well-fitting prosthesis and a thorough training program, some children conclude that they can manage as well without a prosthesis.[26]

Preprosthetic Care

Wound care for bilateral amputation is similar to that for unilateral loss. Particular attention should be paid to achieving maximum mobility of all upper-limb joints, as well as the trunk and lower limbs. The patient may use the thighs and feet for stabilizing and manipulating objects. Children have great flexibility and can become quite facile using the toes for writing and sewing. For those with acquired amputation, fitting with unilateral or bilateral temporary prostheses is highly desirable. Prostheses and many self-help functional devices enable the patient to regain independence in many aspects of self-care. Children younger than 3 years old with bilateral limb absence are usually fitted with simplified prostheses consisting of a pair of sockets each with a TD and a harness.

Controls and use training proceed in a manner similar to that for patients with unilateral amputation. The dominant side will be that which has the longer amputation limb.

SUMMARY

Preprosthetic care should include maintenance of mobility and strength of all joints proximal to the amputation. Wound care focuses on achieving a well-healed, nonadherent scar. Various modalities alleviate phantom pain for most patients. The clinic team should address the psychological response of the patient and family to the amputation. Early training in one-handed activities is useful and may involve teaching the patient to change hand dominance if the dominant hand was amputated.

Patients don the TR prosthesis by inserting the amputation limb into the socket, then the sound limb into the axillary strap of the harness. Donning the TH prosthesis is usually easier if one begins by donning the axillary strap of the harness. Myoelectric TDs are controlled by contraction of forearm musculature, which transmits an electrical signal to skin electrodes that are wired to a motor in the device. Flexing the shoulder or abducting the scapula operates cable-controlled devices. The elbow unit is flexed by shoulder flexion and is locked by shoulder hyperextension.

The prosthesis assists the sound hand in the performance of bimanual daily, vocational, and avocational activities. The patient needs instruction in the care of the amputation limb and prosthesis. Management of children with limb deficiency should focus on helping the child attain developmental milestones. Patients with bilateral amputation should have an exercise program that emphasizes joint mobility. Their prosthetic rehabilitation and functional training can last a long time, depending on their motivation, coordination, and level of limb loss. Choices of bilateral hook, bilateral electric hand, or one of each, are based on clinic team discussion with the patient. Opportunities to try various types of TDs are invaluable to determine the optimal choice for each person's overall functional independence.

REFERENCES

1. Lipschutz RD. Upper extremity amputations and prosthetic management. In: Lusardi MM, Nielsen CC, eds. *Orthotics and Prosthetics in Rehabilitation.* Boston, Mass: Butterworth-Heinemann; 2000:569-588.

2. Atkins DJ. Postoperative and preprosthetic therapy programs. In: Atkins DJ, Meier RH, eds. *Comprehensive Management of the Upper-Limb Amputee.* New York, NY: Springer; 1989:11-15.

3. Edelstein JE. Preprosthetic management of patients with lower- or upper-limb amputation. *Phys Med Rehabil Clin N Am.* 1991;2:285-297.

4. Fraser CM. An evaluation of the use made of cosmetic and functional prostheses by unilateral upper limb amputees. *Prosthet Orthot Int.* 1999; 22:216-223.

5. Silcox DH, Rooks MD, Vogel RR, Fleming LL. Myoelectric prostheses: a long-term follow-up and a study of the use of alternate prostheses. *J Bone Joint Surg Am.* 1993;75:1781-1789.

6. Edelstein JE, Berger N. Performance comparison among children fitted with myoelectric and body-powered hands. *Arch Phys Med Rehabil.* 1993;74:376-380.

7. Atkins DJ. Adult upper-limb prosthetic training. In: Atkins DJ, Meier RH, eds. *Comprehensive Management of the Upper-Limb Amputee.* New York, NY: Springer; 1989:60-71.

8. Spiegel SR. Adult myoelectric upper-limb prosthetic training. In: Atkins DJ, Meier RH, eds. *Comprehensive Management of the Upper-Limb Amputee,* New York, NY: Springer; 1989:342-345.

9. Edelstein JE. The arm and hand: prosthetic training. In: Murdoch G, Wilson AB, Robinson K, et al, eds. *Amputation: Surgical Practice and Patient Management.* Oxford, United Kingdom: Butterworth Heinemann; 1996.

10. Mayer TK. *One-Handed in a Two-Handed World.* Boston, Mass: Prince-Gallison Press; 1996.

11. Edelstein JE. Special considerations—rehabilitation without prostheses: functional skills training. In: Bowker JH, Michael JW, eds. *Atlas of Limb Prosthetics: Surgical, Prosthetic and Rehabilitation Principles.* 2nd ed. St Louis, Mo: Mosby Year Book; 1992:721-728.

12. Webster JB, Levy CE, Bryant PR, Prusakowski PE. Sports and recreation for persons with limb deficiency. *Arch Phys Med Rehabil.* 2001;82:S38-S44.

13. Edelstein JE. Musical options for upper-limb amputees. In: Pratt R, ed. *The Fourth International Symposium on Music.* New York, NY: University Press of America; 1987:102-107.

14. Burger H, Marincek C. Upper limb prosthetic use in Slovenia. *Prosthet Orthot Int.* 1994;18:25-33.

15. Jones LE, Davidson JH. The long-term outcome of upper limb amputees treated at a rehabilitation centre in Sydney, Australia. *Disabil Rehabil.* 1995;17:437-442.

16. Wright TW, Hagen AD, Wood MB. Prosthetic usage in major upper extremity amputations. *J Hand Surg Am.* 1995;20:619-622.

17. Roeschlein RA, Domholdt E. Factors related to successful upper extremity prosthetic use. *Prosthet Orthot Int.* 1989;13:14-18.

18. Pinzur MS, Angelats J, Light TR, Izuierdo R, Pluth T. Functional outcome following traumatic upper limb amputation and prosthetic limb fitting. *J Hand Surg Am.* 1994;19:836-839.

19. Gaine WJ, Smart C, Bransby-Zachary M. Upper limb traumatic amputees. Review of prosthetic use. *J Hand Surg Am.* 1997; 22:73-76.

20. Lake C. Effects of prosthetic training on upper-extremity prosthesis use. *Journal of Prosthetics and Orthotics.* 1997; 9:3-9.

21. Watts HG, Clark MW. *Who is Amelia? Caring for Children with Limb Deficiencies.* Rosemont, Ill: American Academy of Orthopaedic Surgeons; 1998.

22. Thornby MA, Krebs DE. Bimanual skill development in pediatric below-elbow amputation: a multicenter, cross-sectional study. *Arch Phys Med Rehabil.* 1992;73:697-702.

23. Krebs D, Edelstein J, Thornby M. Prosthetic management of children with limb deficiencies. *Phys Ther.* 1991;71:920-934.

24. Edelstein JE. Rehabilitation for children with amputations. In: Lusardi MM, Nielsen CC, eds. *Orthotics and Prosthetics in Rehabilitation.* Boston, Mass: Butterworth-Heinemann; 2000.

25. Krebs DE. *Prehension Assessment: Prosthetic Therapy for the Upper-Limb Child Amputee.* Thorofare, NJ: SLACK Inc; 1987.

26. Postema K, van der Donk V, van Limbeek J, et al. Prosthesis rejection in children with a unilateral congenital arm defect. *Clin Rehabil.* 1999;13:243-249.

Beyond the Basics

Chapter 15

Special Considerations With Children

Stephen Mandacina, CP, FAAOP; Jack E. Uellendahl, CPO;
Joan E. Edelstein, MA, PT, FISPO

OBJECTIVES

1. Identify the etiologies and incidence of limb deficiencies among children
2. Portray the contributions pertinent to care of children of each member of the rehabilitation team
3. Highlight the unique aspects of surgery and the fitting timetable for children
4. Explore components of upper- and lower-limb prostheses designed for children

PRINCIPLES

Becoming a parent is possibly the most exciting milestone in a person's life. However, when the baby is born without a hand or leg, parents often find themselves confused and depressed. Negative emotions usually subside as they see their infant happy and developing normally. Nevertheless, children with limb deficiencies present distinctive challenges to the family and the rehabilitation team.

ETIOLOGIES AND INCIDENCE

Most limb deficiencies result from either congenital causes or trauma. The term "limb deficiency" designates both congenital and acquired limb absence. Regardless of etiology of the deficiency, most children go on to live very productive lives. Management of patients with congenital absence is termed "habilitation," whereas care of those with acquired amputation is "rehabilitation."

The incidence of congenital limb deficiency has remained relatively constant for the past quarter century, with 25.64 per 100,000 live births in 1996.[1] Upper-limb deficiency predominates, at 58.5%. Approximately 30% of children with congenital anomalies have multiple deficiencies.[2] In most instances, the cause of congenital anomaly in a given case is unknown. Sometimes the loss is due to certain drugs, such as thalidomide or methotrexate, taken during pregnancy, or prenatal exposure to noxious chemicals. Other anomalies result from amniotic band syndrome, in which the amniotic sac ruptures; fibrous tissues adhere to the fetal limb, causing intrauterine amputation.[3]

The International Standards Organization and the International Society for Prosthetics and Orthotics have established a classification system in which congenital deficiencies are termed either transverse or longitudinal.[4] Transverse deficiencies resemble surgical amputation with absence of all structures distally; there is, however, no scar. One names the segment in which the limb terminates, then describes the level within the segment beyond which no skeletal elements exist. In contrast, longitudinal deficiency refers to an anomaly in which skeletal elements are present distal to the abnormal bone(s). The clinician identifies the affected bones, stating whether each bone is totally or partially absent. Common types of longitudinal deficiency are absence of the radius; fibular absence with some or all parts of the foot remaining; and foreshortening of the femur known as longitudinal deficiency femoral partial (LDFP), formerly known as proximal femoral focal deficiency. The most challenging longitudinal deficiency is one in which the hand (or foot) is articulated to the torso. Formerly known as phocomelia, this deficiency is now described as a longitudinal deficiency with total absence of the major long bones of the limb. Whether the deficiency is transverse or longitudinal, it is useful to relate the anomalous limb to a standard amputation level, such as long transradial or standard transhumeral.

Acquired amputation in children is most often the result of trauma, particularly caused by farm machinery, lawn mowers, and vehicular and railroad accidents. Malignant tumors, such as osteosarcoma, may lead to amputation, especially among adolescents. Limb salvage procedures have reduced the incidence of amputation for this cause,[1] although the long-term functional results of amputation and limb salvage are similar. Few children experience infections and vascular malformations that lead to amputation.

REHABILITATION TEAM

As with other specialties in prosthetics, treatment of children is best managed by those well versed in their particular issues. The team approach, described in Chapter 1, helps ensure that all needs of the child and family are addressed.[5-8] A useful resource for

identifying teams treating children with limb deficiency is the Association of Children's Prosthetic Orthotic Clinics (ACPOC) (6300 North River Rd, Suite 727, Rosemont, IL 60018-4226).

Finding a prosthetist with considerable experience in fitting children is helped by considering several questions:

- Is the prosthetist certified with the American Board for Certification in Orthotics and Prosthetics?
- How much pediatric experience does the prosthetist have?
- Does the prosthetist belong to the American Academy of Orthotists and Prosthetists, Amputee Coalition of America, and ACPOC?
- Can the prosthetist provide funding resource information?
- Does the prosthetist have access to limb banking, which refers to recycling used components, especially myoelectric units?
- Is the prosthetist experienced with traditional and recent components from the leading manufacturers?

The physical therapist and occupational therapist should be adept at training children. Most therapy takes place at school or home; therefore, having therapy homework assignments and educating the parents regarding appropriate activities are essential.

The family of an infant with limb deficiency should be referred to a center specializing in limb deficiencies as soon after birth as possible. In fact, if prenatal sonograms reveal limb deficiency, consultation with the parents can begin prior to the baby's birth.

In most instances, the evaluation process starts when the infant is 3 months old, although fitting will not occur for another few months when the child and family are ready for the prosthesis. The first evaluation focuses on answering parents' questions and developing a treatment plan based on the scope of the disability. It is most helpful to introduce new parents to the family of a child with a similar absence who is succeeding with habilitation. Successful care depends on continuous re-evaluation by experienced practitioners, appropriate components, timely fittings, and ongoing therapy.[7]

Prosthetic management of children differs somewhat from that of adults. Children are not simply smaller versions of adults. Physically, children's posture, gait, manual dexterity, coordination, and activities differ from those of mature individuals. Children grow in stature and girth. Although it is impossible to predict exactly how much growth will occur over a specific period of time, one thing is certain—growth will occur. The prosthesis needs to be designed to prolong its usable life by incorporating designs and materials that will allow for easy enlargement.

Vigorous activity tests the limits of prosthetic durability in ways that most adult wearers can only dream of, as children care little about damaging their prostheses—in short, they behave like children!

Intellectually, children have few or no preconceptions about the appearance of prostheses, or experience with the consequences of intemperate play. Emotionally, the very young child with a congenital deficiency may have no sense of loss. Eventually, however, even babies sense the reactions of family and meddlesome strangers. A child old enough to interact with peers in the playground and nursery school will eventually notice anatomic differences. In contrast, an older child who loses a limb because of trauma or disease is apt to experience a profound sense of loss and undergo a period of readjustment.[5] In addition, children are legally and financially dependent on their parents or guardians and thus must yield to the family's preferences regarding rehabilitation. Thus, parents should work with clinicians to develop a routine that causes the child to expect that the prosthesis will be put on consistently. It is important that children like their prostheses and want to wear it, not because mom and dad make them wear it.[9]

SURGERY AND POSTOPERATIVE CARE

Whenever suitable, surgical amputation in children should be performed as a disarticulation rather than a mid shaft ablation. Disarticulation preserves the distal epiphyseal growth plate, allowing for the longest possible lever for prosthetic control, and prevents bony overgrowth. Overgrowth generally presents as a spike-like prominence, which can be palpated at the end of the tibia, fibula, humerus, and less commonly, the femur. The end may be tender and inflamed; a bursa may form or the bone may protrude through the skin.[10] The prosthesis should be designed to accommodate the early stages of bony overgrowth by incorporating distal padding that can be removed as the overgrowth occurs. Eventually, surgical revision will be required.

Following surgery, wound healing, edema control, and range of motion and strengthening exercises are implemented.[11] Volume management can be addressed with an elastic soft dressing, Unna semirigid dressing, or a removable rigid plaster or fiberglass dressing. Sometimes an immediate postoperative prosthesis is prescribed. Otherwise, the prosthesis should be provided as soon as sutures are removed. When residual limb volume fluctuates, as when a child is undergoing chemotherapy, an adjustable socket is advantageous.

PROSTHETIC PRINCIPLES

Prosthetic management should complement the child's development. Although the rate of development varies widely, most children with limb deficiency reach developmental milestones in the same sequence and at the same time as able-bodied peers. Limb absence, however, may affect how the child performs tasks, such as crawling and bimanual prehension. Fitting a prosthesis should not take place until the child and family are psychologically ready and the young patient is developmentally and physically able to benefit from the device.

Optimally, evaluations should take place approximately every 3 months until the young person reaches adolescence. Growth spurts may necessitate more frequent clinic visits and socket adjustments. The family and teacher should evaluate the skin regularly to identify potential areas of skin breakdown. Although the socket is continuously modified for growth, after approximately 12 to 18 months of wear, a new socket or a completely new prosthesis may be necessary. If the child has a backup prosthesis, it should also be adjusted. The fitting process is repetitive and predictable, an important consideration for insurance and therapy planning.

During habilitation or rehabilitation, parents should write instructions for teachers and other adults who interact with the child so that the child receives consistent responses regarding prosthetic wear and use. The more the child wears the prosthesis, the more it will be incorporated in daily life. Acceptance among peers will increase if the child wears the prosthesis frequently

MANAGING CHILDREN WITH UPPER-LIMB DEFICIENCIES

Fitting Timetable

At 6 months, many children exhibit functional reaching, orienting the hand and moving the arm toward an interesting object. The baby discovers bimanual grasp at about the same age. By 8 months, most youngsters can sit without support and are starting to pull to the standing position. Ten-month-old infants usually can pull up to stand, crawl, and support themselves with their hands on sturdy furniture.

Evaluation anticipating prosthetic fitting should commence by 8 or 9 months of age to ensure adequate time for discussion by the rehabilitation team and family of fitting procedures and insurance authorizations. A simple prosthesis aids the infant in attaining basic skills. Most children with unilateral deficiency will perform virtually all of the activities of their able-bodied peers. The prosthesis also accustoms the family to incorporating it in the daily routine. The child is seen as having a "helper-hand," rather than no hand at all. Because the prosthesis discourages the child from relying on tactile sensation on the abnormal limb to explore objects, it should be removed periodically so that the young person can explore with the amputation limb. Fitting may be postponed without adverse consequences to bimanual function if the clinical team deems the delay appropriate. Insurance complications and component problems should be resolved promptly to avoid delaying the learning process.

As the child develops, the prosthesis becomes a useful tool, especially for bimanual tasks, such as donning socks or stringing beads. Wearing the prosthesis in nursery school is important because the child performs many supervised bimanual activities there. Teachers and parents should encourage the child to hold objects with the prosthesis, not in the antecubital fossa or under the arm.

Prosthetic Components

Children are fitted with a wide variety of components, depending on the level of amputation and other physical considerations, anticipated activities, and financial issues.

Transradial Prostheses

Most of the prosthetic options designed for adults are also manufactured in smaller sizes. Hooks are made to suit infants younger than 1 year of age. Small hands compatible with the physique of a 12- to 15-month-old child are also available, although the hand's mechanism differs from that of the adult size.[12] Basic options

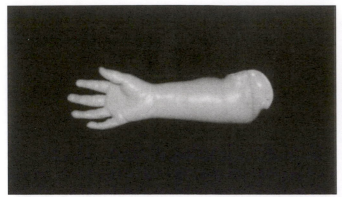

Figure 15-1. Foam-filled hand.

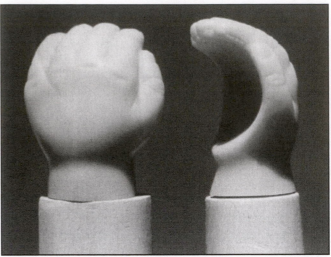

Figure 15-2. Hand used for opposition (eg, holding a bottle).

include passive oppositional, cable-operated, and electrical prostheses. In addition to the basic prosthesis, many children benefit from one or more recreational devices.

Passive Oppositional Prostheses

Although called "passive," this type of prosthesis enables the child to engage in bimanual activities, such as holding a large teddy bear (Figure 15-1). A passive prosthesis can be fitted when the infant is 8 months old. At this age, the baby no longer needs the hands for trunk support, and thus can reach and hold objects. The child becomes aware of a prosthetic "helper-hand" to be incorporated in bimanual activities. Typically, the passive oppositional prosthesis is made of plastic foam or rubber. Some terminal devices (TDs) for youngsters are suitable for holding a bottle (Figure 15-2) or crawling (Figure 15-3). Some parents insist on fitting their child with the infant passive mitt. Although it does not provide palmar opposition, the mitt disguises the amputation with a stylized version of a hand. Even when the child is fitted with a prosthesis offering active prehension, a passive prosthesis is a good backup device for use when the rambunctious youngster engages in vigorous play, such as running down the soccer field.

Cable-Operated Prostheses

Cable-operated prostheses (Figure 15-4), also known as body-powered prostheses, have a harness and cabling system, enabling the youngster to control and operate either a voluntary-opening (VO) or a voluntary-closing (VC) TD via body movements. Often a self-suspending socket eliminates the suspension strap of the harness; such sockets allow a looser fitting, more comfortable harness. A flexible socket in a rigid frame is particularly comfortable and facilitates alteration of socket size to accommodate growth.

Terminal devices are typically VC hands (Figure 15-5). Parents often request a hand rather than a hook for cosmetic reasons. This preference often changes after a

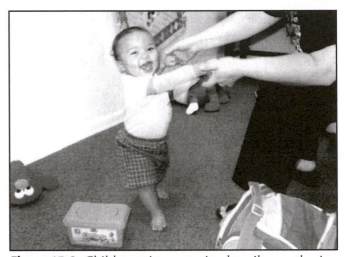

Figure 15-3. Child wearing a semiprehensile prosthesis.

few years when many parents accept either a hook or a hand. The VC style is usually easier for the beginner to operate. When the shoulder muscles are more developed, a VO hook or hand may be provided. The smallest VO and VC hooks are covered with pink or brown plastic to mask the metallic look. The VO CAPP (Child Amputee Prosthetics Project, University of California at Los Angeles) TD is an option that does not have as mechanistic an appearance as a hook.[12] Another VO variation is the wafer hook, which has thicker fingers and thus may be cosmetically more acceptable to the family. Ideally, the child, rehabilitation team, and parents can try different styles.

Because the cable-operated prosthesis for the infant is not fitted with a cable, it may be considered a passive prosthesis. Nevertheless, the infant uses the TD to hold rattles and similar objects placed there by the parent or

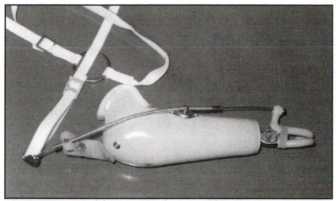

Figure 15-4. Cable-operated arm with voluntary-opening hook.

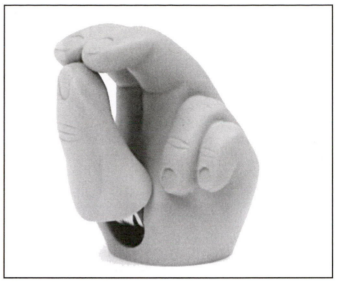

Figure 15-5. Cable-operated voluntary-closing hand.

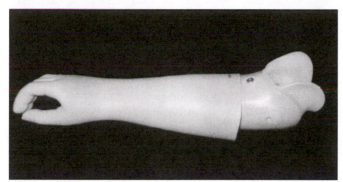

Figure 15-6. Myoelectric hand.

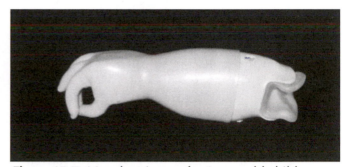

Figure 15-7. Myoelectric arm for 1-year-old child.

therapist. At 12 to 18 months, depending on the child's maturity, the cable is added. Most patients learn release prior to the grasping maneuver.[13]

Electrical Prostheses

The third main option is the externally powered prosthesis, usually with a hand TD (Figure 15-6).[14] Similar to the adult version, TD control is achieved via a battery-powered motor and an input device, either skin electrodes or a switch. An electrical prosthesis can be fitted to a child as young as 1 year of age.[15-18] The prosthesis needs to be simple, lightweight, and comfortable and should provide prehension with operational ease (Figure 15-7).[19] Myoelectrical prostheses are attractive because they offer simple control without being appreciably heavier than the cable-operated or passive prosthesis because of contemporary microprocessors and batteries. With a self-suspending socket, no harness straps are needed for suspension or control of a myoelectric prosthesis. Switch-controlled prostheses, however, are rarely fitted to patients with transradial deficiency; they are typically fitted to children with high longitudinal anomalies.

The input device is typically one or two electrodes. Testing to determine electrode site is difficult with children. Newer myotesters, operating on the principle of a volt meter, can be used with a computer that has

a digital image of a hand. The child controls the computer image through electromyographic (EMG) signals, enabling understanding of the relation of muscle contraction to prosthetic hand action. Initial training involves having the child extend the wrist on the sound side. The youngster soon realizes that the same motions that move the sound wrist and hand will control the prosthetic hand. Infants younger than 1 year of age are usually unable to cooperate with testing. Palpating the amputation limb enables finding the apex of the muscle belly, which will be a good starting point for the electrode.[19]

Rather than nickel-cadmium batteries, new smaller lithium-ion ones increase use time to nearly 3 days on one charge, have a quick charge time, and offer the ability to add to a partial charge. Batteries can often be installed inside the forearm shell to improve the appearance of the prosthesis while protecting the batteries, with less corrosion of the contacting elements.

The myoelectric prosthesis for a young child often has single-site control. One electrode receives a myoelectrical signal above a threshold, causing the TD to open. Relaxing the muscle contraction closes the TD.[20] A site can control the hand with an electrical signal as low as 5 µV. A small override switch may be placed on the socket exterior to allow an adult to open the hand if the child cannot do this. Single-site electrode control provides the child with a more physiological control of the hand as compared to a body-powered system. Additionally, the isometric contractions used to signal the electrode will probably increase muscular development.

The electrode is placed on the wrist extensor muscle group. The extensor muscles usually open the TD in the adult prosthesis. Thus, to plan for the time when the patient will graduate to a prosthesis with dual-site control, it is less confusing if the same muscle group continues to be used to open the TD. The socket must allow complete, continuous contact between the electrode and the skin. Otherwise, the child may produce an inadvertent or erratic signal causing unpredictable hand operation.

Periodic re-evaluation of the child wearing a single-site system should focus on how well the youngster controls the TD as well as maintaining good fit of the prosthesis. When the child can understand controlling the TD with two EMG signals, often at age 2½ years, it is timely to change to a dual-site system. The dual-site prosthesis is generally fitted when a new, larger prosthesis is needed. The second electrode is placed on the wrist flexor muscle belly to control TD closing. Closing of the device is no longer automatic; with a dual-site system, closing is voluntary. Most microprocessor controls permit changing the control strategy by changing a coding plug, located inside the forearm of the prosthesis, by connecting to a computer or by a wireless link to a hand-held personal digital assistant. Any of these changes can be done with a single visit to the prosthetist.

The child may use increasingly larger versions of the cable-operated or electrical prosthesis through adolescence and on to adulthood. A 2½- to 3-year-old child is beginning to be much rougher on the prosthesis. The toddler is starting to dress independently, climb stairs and furniture, and kick and throw a ball. Parents should encourage the child to use the prosthesis in these activities (Figure 15-8).[21] Active, undisciplined youngsters can hurt themselves, another person, or a pet if they use the prosthesis to poke or pinch. Although VO TDs only pinch with approximately 2 pounds of force, the pressure can still be uncomfortable. Grasp force of a VC TD and a myoelectric hand is even greater.

Recreational Prostheses

Outdoor activities, such as climbing and running, may cause children to fall and injure themselves and the prosthesis. Consequently, the family might consider having the child wear a passive prosthesis with or without a sport-specific TD on the playground. It becomes a backup or dirty arm and is a lightweight option for

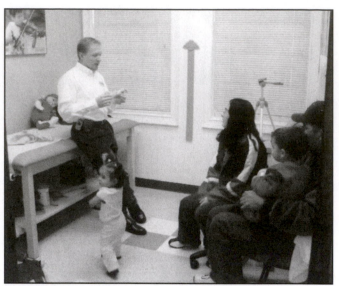

Figure 15-8. Educating and involving parents.

gymnastics and beach sports. Most importantly, parents should allow the child to be a child, without limiting age-appropriate activities; otherwise, the youngster will feel different from his or her friends (Figure 15-9). The recreational (activity-specific) prosthesis allows the child to perform functions beyond the usual grasp-release. A quick-disconnect wrist unit enables rapid interchange of TDs on the basic prosthesis, thereby avoiding the need to obtain a separate device for a particular activity. Playing the violin and riding a tricycle or bicycle (Figures 15-10 and 15-11) are easier with a recreational prosthesis. Viewing the prosthesis as a "tool-box" enables the child to pursue a wide range of activities. Many prosthetic components and gadgets are available for different activities. Although it is important to provide children with these tools, it is more important to pace their introduction to complement their ability to use them.

Socket Designs

As with adult prostheses, socket design is the most critical factor influencing the functional success of the child with limb deficiency. Of course, therapy, components, and parental involvement are important; however, if the socket does not fit well, is uncomfortable, or restricts joint range of motion, the child will not want to wear the prosthesis. Therefore, special attention must be directed at designing a socket that will suspend the weight of the components, allow for growth, and, in the case of a myoelectric prosthesis, maintain electrode contact.

Newer plastics enable achievement of these goals. Flexible thermoplastics can be shaped to provide a comfortable fit and modified easily to accommodate growth. Sockets made of these plastics can be fitted

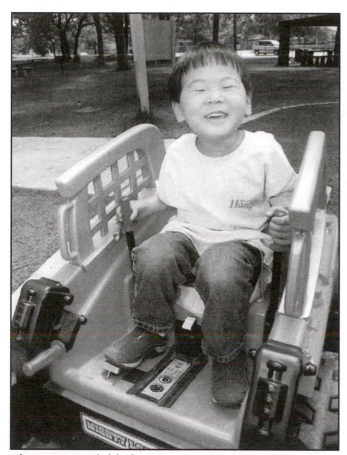

Figure 15-9. Child playing.

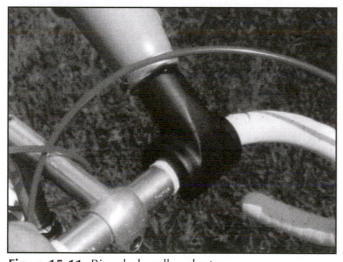

Figure 15-11. Bicycle handle adaptor.

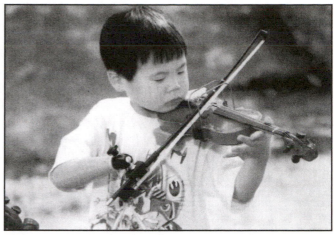

Figure 15-10. Recreational violin bow adaptor.

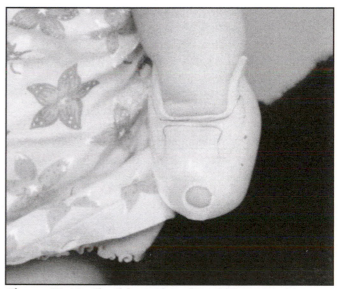

Figure 15-12. Flexible socket showing aggressive suspension and dots for electrode placement.

snugly to achieve optimum suspension and control (Figure 15-12). By age 1 year, the muscles and skeleton have developed sufficiently to tolerate the weight of a prosthesis with a self-suspending socket. Younger children may either receive self-suspending sockets or a looser socket with a suspension sleeve.

Transhumeral Prostheses

The initial prosthesis for the 1 year old with transhumeral amputation will probably have a harness, socket, friction elbow unit, forearm shell, and a cable-controlled or myoelectric TD. Initially, the TD will be used to hold objects passively without reliance on a cable or electrode. Eventually, the child can be fitted with a hybrid prosthesis, which typically includes a myoelectrically controlled TD with electrodes on the triceps and biceps bellies. Cable control of the TD is another popular option. The friction elbow unit does not have a locking mechanism, making it simpler to control than a unit with a cable or electrical lock.

The key factor in evaluating children with higher level deficiencies is judging whether the patient can tolerate the weight of the prosthesis. Once the child can control the weight of the prosthesis, a locking elbow unit can be installed with harnessing for control. The child may need 1 year or more of wearing a passive elbow before being ready to change to a locking elbow. The 3 year old should be evaluated for harnessing the elbow. A cable-operated elbow should be used for 2 to 3 years before an electric elbow is considered. Some children benefit from an electric elbow unit if they can cope with its weight and control complexity. All children should have the opportunity to try recreational TDs.

The child with longitudinal deficiency who has functional digits may be able to use them to control electric switches or a modified cable system. Tactile feedback enhances the control of the prosthesis.

Bilateral Prostheses

Children with bilateral transradial deficiencies can be fitted with a pair of prostheses initially. Those with high level limb absence are likely to accommodate better to being fitted one side at a time, typically first on the longer, more dominant side. Within 3 months, the opposite side should be fitted so that the patient can balance the weight of the first prosthesis and learn bimanual activities as soon as possible. Keeping the prostheses lightweight and simple is likely to improve functional success and therefore the psychological response of the child and family.

The more complicated the system, the more difficult it will be to operate. Additionally, until the muscular and skeletal systems are strong, the child cannot tolerate the weight and extensive skin coverage of high level, bilateral prostheses.

Well before, as well as throughout, prosthetic fitting, the child should be taught foot skills. By pinching the great toe and second toe together, patients can accomplish many tasks, such as writing and sewing. Loosely fitting shoes and specially sewn socks facilitate foot use. Some activities are easier to perform with the mouth and teeth. Holding items is much easier, because the prehension force of the jaw is strong and is controlled through proprioceptive and tactile feedback. Regular dental care is imperative. When circumstances permit, it is preferable to stabilize objects with prostheses, the feet, and the chin, rather than the mouth.

MANAGING CHILDREN WITH LOWER-LIMB DEFICIENCIES

The focus of habilitation of children with lower-limb deficiencies is standing, walking, and other ambulatory activities, in contrast to the emphasis on prehension in upper-limb management.

Surgical Revision

Children with longitudinal lower-limb deficiency are more apt to have surgical revision than are those with upper-limb anomalies because the lower limbs are essential for weight bearing and walking. For example, a person with a severe fibular deficiency would have to wear a very high shoe lift or have the foot removed with a Syme's or Boyd's amputation.[22] Absence of the fibula results in a less bulbous distal end than a standard Syme's and therefore the prosthesis may need to have auxiliary suspension.[23] The juvenile Syme's limb is short enough to accommodate a sophisticated prosthetic foot-ankle assembly either initially or as the patient grows and the length discrepancy increases. The child functions in a manner comparable to a person with transtibial (TT) amputation.

For unilateral LDFP, ablation of the foot enables fitting with a socket, knee unit, shank, and foot-ankle assembly. The end of the thigh on the amputated side approximates the level of the sound knee. If the end of the amputation limb is longer than the sound thigh, external knee hinges are needed. As the child grows and the length discrepancy between amputated and sound sides becomes relatively greater, a standard endoskeletal knee unit is suitable. Function is similar to that of an individual with transfemoral (TF) amputation.

A less common surgical alternative for longitudinal deficiency, particularly LDFP, is the Van Nes rotationplasty. The procedure rotates the leg 180 degrees so that the foot points posteriorly. The ankle must have adequate range of motion to function as a knee and be at approximately the same level as the contralateral knee. A socket encases the foot for weight bearing. A pair of single-axis hinges attached to a thigh corset provides suspension. Although individuals with rotationplasty look well in their prostheses and function in a manner comparable to TT amputation, some people object to the unusual appearance of the bare limb.[11]

If surgical conversion of longitudinal deficiency is not performed, the foot may be placed in plantar flexion inside an equinus prosthesis to accommodate leg-length discrepancy.

Regardless of prosthetic design and surgical treatment, the unstable hip associated with LDFP causes the patient to walk with lateral trunk bending.

Fitting Timetable

The first lower-limb prosthesis should be fitted when the child begins to pull to stand at 6 to 8 months. Independent walking occurs at about 1 year[19]; the child starts walking by contacting the floor with the entire plantar surface and keeps the knees extended. By 18 months of age, most children have matured to achieve heel contact. By 2 years of age, the child can jump, run, kick a ball, and hop.[19]

Prosthetic Components

Lower-limb prostheses for children include smaller versions of many of the components available for adults.

Transtibial Prostheses

Prosthetic feet sized for children are available in most of the designs intended for adults. Most commonly, infants are fitted with a Solid Ankle Cushion Heel (SACH) foot. It offers a simple, robust, and cost-effective solution for the youngest of prosthesis users. The immature gait pattern of a 1-year-old child precludes benefiting from a more sophisticated foot-ankle assembly. As the child grows, however, feet with dynamic response and compliance at loading response become more suitable. For the young woman, an ankle with height adjustability may be a welcome component.

Normally, during most of stance phase, the leg rotates externally.[20] This kinesiological mechanism is lost with TT or more proximal amputations. Therefore, it is beneficial to install a torque absorber to minimize the rotational shear forces that would otherwise be experienced between the skin and socket.

Transfemoral Prostheses

Pediatric prosthetic knee units have improved considerably in recent years. The first TF prosthesis may have an articulating knee unit, which provides the youngster with reasonable symmetry in walking.[24] Sometimes, however, the initial prosthesis has a locked knee or no knee unit. A polycentric unit enables more natural function than a locked knee. If the thigh is too long to accommodate a knee unit having internal mechanism placed distal to the socket, then outside hinges are indicated. Whenever possible, however, it is preferable to fit a knee unit that offers friction control and an extension assist because the gait is more natural than with hinges. As the child grows, space beneath the distal end of the socket will become available to accommodate a fluid-controlled mechanism providing cadence response. School-aged children can be fitted with dynamic stance-flexion control, whereas adolescents can benefit from a hydraulic unit with microprocessor control. Their prostheses should have a shock-absorbing mechanism to facilitate playing basketball and other active sports.

Suspension Options

Suspension of the prosthesis is critical to overall success. For the very young child, suspension needs to be secure enough to resist displacement during crawling. Silicone suction sockets (3S) have proven successful on both TT and TF prostheses. Suspension is attained with a roll-on silicone interface. Additional gel caps in the 3S system offer a convenient method for managing bony overgrowth. For TT prostheses, suspension sleeves provide good suspension and can be used with a variety of interface materials, such as textile socks and gel materials. At the TF level, elastic suspension belts are frequently used as an alternative to the 3S socket.

Whenever the distal aspect of the limb is bulbous, it may be used for suspension with a socket design that surrounds the broad contour snugly.

Socks and liner materials facilitate accommodating growth. Thicker materials can be used initially and then as growth occurs, thinner ones can replace the original layer or be removed altogether. If a flexible thermoplastic material is used within a frame, the thermoplastic can be heated and stretched into the windowed area. To keep up with growth of the contralateral limb, the child should be seen by the prosthetist three or four times a year for prosthetic adjustment. The average replacement frequency during childhood is 18 months.[5]

Bilateral Prostheses

Functional goals for the child with bilateral lower-limb amputations usually include ambulation. Children with bilateral TT deficiency develop considerable walking proficiency. Those with bilateral TF absence who have arms with which to balance should also be expected to walk independently.[6] For the infant with bilateral TF deficiency, stubbies (short, nonarticulated prostheses) lower the center of gravity giving the child more stability, thus making it much easier for the toddler who is beginning to cruise, then walk in the erect position with less fear of falling.[25,26] As the individual grows and matures, articulated prostheses are indicated. The prostheses will probably be somewhat shorter than the child's predicted height. A common concern of children with bilateral amputation is maintaining height comparable to peers; consequently, in addition to enlarging the socket, the prosthetist will also have to lengthen the prostheses periodically. Gait is slower than that of non-disabled peers, with lateral trunk bending to both sides. Maintaining good physical strength and avoiding obesity are key factors in the long-term success of the child with bilateral lower-limb prostheses. The child should also have a wheelchair for long distance travel.

CONCLUSION

Prosthetic components for children with upper- or lower-limb deficiency generally mirror those available for adults. Prescription should balance function, durability, ease of growth accommodation, and cost with the size and maturity of the child.

REFERENCES

1. Dillingham TR, Pezzin LE, Mackenzie EJ. Limb amputation and limb deficiency: epidemiology and recent trends in the United States. *South Med J.* 2002;95:875-883.
2. Watts H. Multiple limb deficiencies. In: Smith DG, Michaels JW, Bowker JH, eds. *Atlas of Amputations and Limb Deficiencies.* 3rd ed. Rosemont, Ill: American Academy of Orthopaedic Surgeons; 2004:923-929.

3. Walter JH, Goss LR, Lazzara AT. Amniotic band syndrome. *J Foot Ankle Surg.* 1998;37:325-333.

4. International Organization for Standardization: ISO 8548-1. Prosthetics and orthotics—limb deficiencies, Part 1: method of describing limb deficiencies present at birth. Geneva, Switzerland: International Organization for Standardization; 1989:1-6.

5. Fisk JR, Smith DG. The limb-deficient child. In: Smith DG, Michaels JW, Bowker JH, eds. *Atlas of Amputations and Limb Deficiencies.* 3rd ed. Rosemont, Ill: American Academy of Orthopaedic Surgeons; 2004:773-777.

6. Gaebler-Spira D, Uellendahl J. Pediatric limb deficiencies. In: Molnar G, ed. *Pediatric Rehabilitation.* 3rd ed. Philadelphia, Pa: Hanley & Belfus; 1999:331-350.

7. Novotny M, Swagman A. Caring for children with orthotic/prosthetic needs. *Journal of Prosthetics and Orthotics.* 1992;14:191-195.

8. Area Child Amputee Center. *Children With Limb Loss Series: Birth to Five, Six to Twelve, and Adolescents and Children with Hand Differences.* Grand Rapids, Mich: Area Child Amputee Center; 1990.

9. Rubenfeld L, Varni J, Talbot D, et al. Variables influencing self-esteem in children with congenital or acquired limb deficiencies. *J Assoc Child Prosthet Orthot Clin.* 1988;23:85.

10. Watts HG. Surgical modification of residual limbs. In: Smith DG, Michaels JW, Bowker JH, eds. *Atlas of Amputations and Limb Deficiencies.* 3rd ed. Rosemont, Ill: American Academy of Orthopaedic Surgeons; 2004:931-943.

11. Coulter-O'Berry C. Physical therapy. In: Smith DG, Michaels JW, Bowker JH, eds. *Atlas of Amputations and Limb Deficiencies.* 3rd ed. Rosemont, Ill: American Academy of Orthopaedic Surgeons; 2004:831-840.

12. Uellendahl JE, Riggo-Heelan J. Prosthetic management of the upper limb deficient child. *Phys Med Rehabil Clin N Am.* 2000;11:221-235.

13. Shaperman J, Landsberger S, Setoguchi Y. Early upper limb prosthetic fitting: when and what do we fit. *Journal of Prosthetics and Orthotics.* 2003;15:11-19.

14. Patton JG. Training the child with a unilateral upper-extremity prosthesis. In: Meier RH, Atkins DG, eds. *Functional Restoration of Adults and Children With Upper Extremity Amputation.* New York, NY: Demos Medical Publishing; 2004:297-316.

15. Herring JA, Birch JG, eds. *The Child With a Limb Deficiency.* Rosemont, Ill: American Academy of Orthopaedic Surgeons; 1998.

16. Berke G, Nielsen C. Establishing parameters affecting the use of myoelectric prostheses in children: a preliminary investigation. *Journal of Prosthetics and Orthotics.* 1991;3:162-168.

17. Datta D, Ibbotson V. Powered prosthetic hands in very young children. *Prosthet Orthot Int.* 1998;22:150-154.

18. Brenner C. Electric limbs for infants and preschool children. *J Prosthet Orthot.* 1992;4:184-190.

19. Hubbard S, Koheil R, Heger H, et al. Development of upper extremity myoelectric training methods for preschool congenital amputees. *J Assoc Child Prosthet Orthot Clin.* 1984;19:9.

20. Meredith JM, Uellendahl JE, Keagy RD. Successful voluntary grasp and release using the cookie crusher myoelectric hand in 2-year-olds. *Am J Occup Ther.* 1993;47:825-829.

21. Edelstein JE. Developmental kinesiology. In: Smith DG, Michaels JW, Bowker JH, eds. *Atlas of Amputations and Limb Deficiencies.* 3rd ed. Rosemont, Ill: American Academy of Orthopaedic Surgeons; 2004:783-788.

22. Inman VT, Ralston HJ, Todd F. Human locomotion. In: Rose J, Gamble JG, eds. *Human Locomotion.* 2nd ed. Baltimore, Md: Williams & Wilkins; 1994:1-22.

23. Glancy GL. Fibular deficiencies. In: Smith DG, Michaels JW, Bowker JH, eds. *Atlas of Amputation and Limb Deficiencies.* 3rd ed. Rosemont, Ill: American Academy Orthopaedic Surgeons; 2004:889-896.

24. Giavedoni BJ. The use of prosthetic knees in infants and toddlers. Alignment. *Can Assoc Prosthet Orthot.* 2000:25-26.

25. Kruger LM. Stubby prostheses in the rehabilitation of infants and small children with bilateral lower limb deficiencies. *Rehabilitation.* 1990;29:12-15.

26. Uellendahl JE. Bilateral lower limb prostheses. In: Smith DG, Michaels JW, Bowker JH, eds. *Atlas of Amputations and Limb Deficiencies.* 3rd ed. Rosemont, Ill: American Academy of Orthopaedic Surgeons; 2004:621-632.

Chapter 16

Rehabilitation Outcomes

Joan E. Edelstein, MA, PT, FISPO

OBJECTIVES

1. Compare the characteristics and results of subjective and objective studies related to prosthetic rehabilitation
2. Differentiate among subjective instruments of function, including the Stanmore Harold Wood Mobility Scale, Prosthetic Evaluation Questionnaire, Locomotor Capabilities Index, and Amputee Mobility Predictor, as well as quality of life scales
3. Relate amputation level and various prosthetic components to objective assessments of rehabilitation outcome, including energy consumption and walking speed
4. Comment on rehabilitation outcome of people with upper-limb amputation

INTRODUCTION

Long-range planning is an integral part of medical care. The responsible clinician must make a rational forecast of the likely function of each patient based on clinical experience with other individuals who share similar physical attributes and are fitted with comparable prostheses. Over- or underestimating a given person's function is a cruel deception, on the one hand establishing frustratingly unattainable goals and on the other hand shortchanging the patient. Research provides broad guidelines that can help the clinic team form plausible predictions. The problem is complicated because so many factors influence rehabilitation outcome, and so few well-designed studies have been published.

OUTCOME STUDIES

Two major types of outcome studies pertaining to people with amputations are those that use subjective instruments, typically questionnaires, and objective evaluations of oxygen consumption, gait kinematics, and kinetics. Studies may concern particular populations, especially adult men with traumatic amputation,

or specific components, such as energy-storing feet. Regrettably, both types of research suffer from such small sample sizes that the results can be generalized only with great caution.

Subjective Instruments

Subjective instruments are intended to evaluate the overall function of individuals with lower-limb amputations.[1] No published questionnaire measures all aspects of mobility. Meta-analysis of studies published between 1978 and 1998 demonstrated that the Stanmore Harold Wood Mobility Scale[2] was most frequently cited.[1] Follow-up of all patients with unilateral amputation revealed that 1 year after discharge from the rehabilitation center almost all those aged younger than 50 years were walking in the community. Among the older adults, half of those with transtibial (TT) amputation and less than a quarter of people with transfemoral (TF) amputation were functional ambulators.[3] The Prosthetic Evaluation Questionnaire has a four-item functional scale, two mobility scales, and four psychosocial questions[4]; scores are inversely correlated with walking distance among adults with unilateral TT amputation.[5] Balance confidence accounted for most of the mobility performance as measured by the Prosthetic

Evaluation Questionnaire and the Houghton Scale.[6] This scale is also responsive to functional change in adults with amputations caused by trauma or vascular disease.[7] The Locomotor Capabilities Index,[8] a 14-item self-report with demonstrated internal consistency and test-retest reliability, confirmed that those with TT amputation were more independent than individuals with TF amputation. Another confirmation that amputation level affects rehabilitation outcome is the Amputee Mobility Predictor[9]; its scores are correlated with the Medicare 5-level coding scale.[10]

Amputation level is not the only determinant of rehabilitation outcome. Quality of life appears to be more affected by body image, as indicated on the Amputee Image Body Scale, than by age, level of amputation, or number of comorbidities.[11] The Sickness Impact Profile-68 predicted functional outcome in 69% of 46 patients older than 60 years with unilateral amputation caused by vascular disease.[12] The Trinity Amputation and Prosthesis Experience Scales[13] has been used to assess consumer satisfaction; troublesome areas include delay in fitting the first prosthesis and negative perceptions regarding prosthetists' interpersonal manner.[14,15] The Orthotics and Prosthetics Users' Survey[16] is a self-report of functional status, general health, employment, and satisfaction with clinic services, which demonstrates internal consistency and construct validity. Interviews of 32 adults who averaged 1 year between amputation and return to work indicated that reintegration into the workforce was delayed by problems with the amputation limb, particularly wound healing; many individuals were employed in less physically demanding jobs after rehabilitation.[17]

Objective Instruments

Among the objective assessments of rehabilitation outcome are physiological measures. Electrocardiography and peak heart rate have shown that the average physical and cardiac condition is poor in adults with vascular amputation, most of whom having succeeded in prosthetic training with or without a walker.[18]

Energy Consumption

The most common type of outcome assessment involves measurement of oxygen consumption, an indication of the energy cost of activity. The demand of walking with a prosthesis is similar to that of those who do not have amputations when the amount of oxygen is measured on the amount consumed per minute. When, however, oxygen consumption is related to the distance walked, many studies confirm that prosthesis users consume more energy and walk slower than age-mated, able-bodied adults.[19-25]

Amputation level influences energy demand. Adults with Syme's amputation caused by vascular disease walked 33% slower and consumed 30% more energy per unit distance than nondisabled subjects.[20] Healthy young men with nonvascular TT amputation walked 12% slower than normal with 12% higher energy cost per unit distance. Subjects with longer amputation limb lengths had less energy overuse than those with shorter limbs while walking at a comparable pace.[21] In a study comparing adults with TT amputation caused by vascular disease to those of similar age who had traumatic amputations at comparable levels, the dysvascular group was found to walk 44% slower. Adults with traumatic amputation walked 11% slower than able-bodied subjects. The rate of oxygen consumption per unit distance was increased by 58% for the dysvascular group and by 33% for those who had trauma.[22]

Transfemoral amputation exacts a much steeper energy cost per unit distance, as much as 116% more than nondisabled adults.[20] Comfortable walking speed is slower after amputation, most likely because of the increased energy demand.[23] Eight adults with hip disarticulation walked 41% slower than normal, whereas 10 subjects with transpelvic amputation walked 51% slower. The energy cost per unit distance was 43% and 75% greater than normal for these groups, respectively.[24]

Walking Speed

Several small-sample studies of individuals with bilateral amputations were in agreement that walking speed was decreased from 15% for those with bilateral TT amputation to 48% for those with bilateral TF amputation, with as much as a 200% rise in energy cost per unit distance.[24] Six elderly adults with bilateral TT amputation selected a walking speed half that of nondisabled peers with a 123% increase in energy cost per unit distance. Two adults with TT/TF amputations walked 56% slower than normal, with a 118% increase in net cost of walking. Those with bilateral TF amputation chose a walking speed 71% slower, and at this speed their energy cost per unit distance was 260% higher than normal. Five young adults with bilateral TF amputation spent 91% more energy per unit distance while walking 40% slower than normal.[19]

For individuals with bilateral TT or more proximal amputations, wheelchair use may be a more functional mode of mobility than ambulation with a pair of prostheses. Two investigations have demonstrated that those with bilateral TT amputations[26] and those with bilateral TF amputations[27] were more efficient when propelling a wheelchair. Six adults with bilateral TT amputations caused by peripheral vascular disease (PVD) averaged a 12% reduction in velocity at a 157% greater energy cost when walking as compared with wheeling. A 41-year-old woman with traumatic TF amputations walked at a velocity 31% of her wheelchair propulsion velocity at an oxygen cost seven times that needed for wheelchair use.

Adults with unilateral TT amputation due to PVD had resting heart rates similar to able-bodied age mates, although those with amputation were much less active as measured by an electronic activity monitor.[28] Heart rate does not account for the lower activity found with patients having amputation. Prospective study of 46 elderly adults with unilateral amputation due to PVD confirmed a low functional level 1 year after amputation; poor one-leg balance on the sound leg and cognitive impairment were most predictive of diminished future function.[12]

It is apparent that physiological response is strongly affected by amputated limb level and etiology of amputation, whether or not the broader issue of quality of life is directly affected by such factors.

Comparison of Components

Data are inconclusive with regard to the effect of various prosthetic components. Published research consists largely of studies on small, heterogeneous samples, with subjects not blinded to the component being evaluated, and components seldom applied in a random manner.[29]

Many studies involve comparison of various types of prosthetic feet. Some investigators comparing the energy cost between the SACH and various dynamic elastic response feet have failed to show a significant difference.[30,31] Other research suggests the greater efficiency of dynamic response feet, particularly the Flex-Foot. Seven young adults with traumatic TT amputation who used the SACH foot and the Flex-Foot (Ossur North America, Aliso, Calif) showed a minimal difference in oxygen consumption per unit distance at slower walking speeds; at more rapid velocity, however, those wearing the Flex-Foot demonstrated a 10% decrease in oxygen consumption while walking at an average 9% higher self-selected walking velocity.[32] Physically active young men used slightly less energy with a foot having a shock-absorbing spring, as compared with walking and running with a SACH or Flex-Foot.[33] Six young adults fitted with shock-absorbing pylons consumed 5% to 9% less oxygen when walking 130% to 160% of normal velocity.[34]

Although the kinematics of TF gait with a locked knee unit differ markedly from those with a freely swinging knee, no statistically significant difference in energy consumption has been reported; however, a significant energy increase occurred when subjects walked with the knee setting to which they were unaccustomed. The older group walked faster with the locked knee, whereas the younger group fared better with the unlocked knee.[35] As compared with other knee units, young adults fitted with TF prostheses having computerized knee units walked more rapidly with less energy expenditure.[36-38] Lower energy cost and faster speed was exhibited by subjects wearing an ischial containment TF socket as compared with the quadrilateral design.[39]

Other components also affect function. Thirteen subjects with unilateral traumatic TT amputation averaged 83% more steps per day when wearing a polyethylene foam liner as compared with an elastomeric gel liner.[40] Ten adults with TF amputation caused by vascular disease walked at similar velocity regardless of the weight of the prosthesis, with as much as 1625 g added to the basic prosthesis.[41]

Upper-Limb Prosthetic Studies

Few studies have investigated the rehabilitation outcome of individuals with upper-limb amputation. Early fitting for those with traumatic amputation, as well as post-traumatic counseling, contribute to continued prosthetic usage.[42] Because most upper-limb amputations involve only one hand, many individuals eventually opt to discard the prosthesis.[43] Most daily and vocational activities can be accomplished without a prosthesis. Factors contributing to ongoing prosthetic use among adults include completion of high school education, employment, emotional acceptance of the amputation, and the perception that the prosthesis is expensive. Those with TR amputation are more likely to persist with prosthetic use, as compared with people having other levels of amputation.

CONCLUSION

Many factors affect the rehabilitation outcome, especially amputation level and etiology, and to a lesser extent, prosthetic components. Larger, better controlled studies are needed to enable more accurate prediction of the long-term status of people with lower- or upper-limb amputation.

REFERENCES

1. Rommers GM, Vos LD, Groothoff JW, Eisma WH. Mobility of people with lower limb amputations: scales and questionnaires. *Clin Rehabil*. 2001;15:92-102.

2. Hanspal RS, Fisher K. Prediction of achieved mobility in prosthetic rehabilitation of the elderly using cognitive and psychomotor assessment. *Int J Rehabil Res*. 1997;20:315-318.

3. Davies B, Datta D. Mobility outcome following unilateral lower limb amputation. *Prosthet Orthot Int*. 2003;27:186-190.

4. Legro M, Reiber GD, Smith DG, et al. Prosthesis Evaluation Questionnaire for persons with lower limb amputations: assessing prosthesis-related quality of life. *Arch Phys Med Rehabil*. 1998;79:931-938.

5. Trantowski-Farrell R, Pinzur MS. A preliminary comparison of function and outcome in patients with diabetic dysvascular disease. *Journal of Prosthetics and Orthotics*. 2003;15:127-132.

6. Miller WC, Deathe AB, Speechley M. Psychometric properties of the Activities-specific Balance Confidence Scale among individuals with a lower-limb amputation. *Arch Phys Med Rehabil.* 2003;84:656-661.

7. Devlin M, Pauley T, Head K, Garfinkel S. Houghton Scale of prosthetic use in people with lower-extremity amputations: reliability, validity, and responsiveness to change. *Arch Phys Med Rehabil.* 2004;85:1339-1344.

8. Franchignoni F, Orlandini D, Ferriero G, Moscato TA. Reliability, validity, and responsiveness of the Locomotor Capabilities Index in adults with lower-limb amputation undergoing prosthetic training. *Arch Phys Med Rehabil.* 2004;85:743-748.

9. Gailey RS, Roach KE, Applegate EB, et al. The Amputee Mobility Predictor: an instrument to assess determinants of the lower-limb amputee's ability to ambulate. *Arch Phys Med Rehabil.* 2002;83:613-627.

10. Levin AZ. Functional outcome following amputation. *Topics Geriatr Rehabil.* 2004;4:253-261.

11. Miller CA. Factors related to quality of life in elderly persons following lower limb amputation. *J Geriatr Phys Ther.* 2004;27:115.

12. Schoppen T, Boonstra A, Groothoff JW, et al. Physical, mental, and social predictors of functional outcome in unilateral lower-limb amputees. *Arch Phys Med Rehabil.* 2003;84:803-811.

13. Dillingham TR, Pezzin LE, Mackenzie EJ, Burgess AR. Use and satisfaction with prosthetic devices among persons with trauma-related amputations: a long-term outcome study. *Am J Phys Med Rehabil.* 2001;80:563-571.

14. Gallagher P, MacLachlan M. The Trinity Amputation and Prosthesis Experience Scales and quality of life in people with lower-limb amputation. *Arch Phys Med Rehabil.* 2004;85:730-736.

15. Pezzin LE, Dillingham TR, MacKenzie EJ, et al. Use and satisfaction with prosthetic limb devices and related services. *Arch Phys Med Rehabil.* 2004; 85:723-729.

16. Heinemann AW, Bode RK, O'Reilly C. Development and measurement properties of the Orthotics and Prosthetics Users' Survey (OPUS): a comprehensive set of clinical outcome instruments. *Prosthet Orthot Int.* 2003;27:191-206.

17. Bruins M, Geertzen JH, Groothoff JW, Schoppen T. Vocational reintegration after a lower limb amputation: a qualitative study. *Prosthet Orthot Int.* 2003;27:4-10.

18. Cruts HE, de Vries J, Zilvold G, et al. Lower extremity amputees with peripheral vascular disease: graded exercise testing and results of prosthetic training. *Arch Phys Med Rehabil.* 1987;68:14-19.

19. Gonzalez EG, Edelstein JE. Energy expenditure during ambulation. In: Gonzalez EG, Myers SJ, Edelstein JE, et al, eds. *Downey & Darling's Physiological Basis of Rehabilitation Medicine.* 3rd ed. Boston, Mass: Butterworth Heinemann; 2001:417-447.

20. Waters RL, Perry J, Antonelli D, Hislop H. Energy cost of walking of amputees: the influence of level of amputation. *J Bone Joint Surg Am.* 1976;58:42-46.

21. Gailey RS, Wenger MA, Raya M, Kirk N. Energy expenditure of trans-tibial amputees during ambulation at self-selected pace. *Prosthet Orthot Int.* 1994;18:84-91.

22. Pagliarulo MA, Waters R, Hislop HJ. Energy cost of walking of below-knee amputees having no vascular disease. *Phys Ther.* 1979;59:538-543.

23. Jaegers SM, Vos LD, Rispens P, Hof AL. The relationship between comfortable and most metabolically efficient walking speed in persons with unilateral above-knee amputation. *Arch Phys Med Rehabil.* 1993;74:521-525.

24. Nowroozi F, Salvanelli ML, Gerber LH. Energy expenditure in hip disarticulation and hemipelvectomy. *Arch Phys Med Rehabil.* 1983;64:300-303.

25. Waters RL, Mulroy SJ. Energy expenditure of walking in individuals with lower limb amputations. In: Smith DG, Michael JW, Bowker JH, eds. *Atlas of Amputations and Limb Deficiencies.* 3rd ed. Rosemont Ill: American Academy of Orthopaedic Surgeons; 2004:395-407.

26. DuBow LL, Witt PL, Kadaba MP, Reyes R, Cochran V. Oxygen consumption of elderly persons with bilateral below knee amputations: ambulation vs. wheelchair propulsion. *Arch Phys Med Rehabil.* 1983;64:255-259.

27. Wu Y-J, Chen S-Y, Lin M-C, Lan C, Lai JS, Lien IN. Energy expenditure of wheeling and walking during prosthetic rehabilitation in a woman with bilateral transfemoral amputations. *Arch Phys Med Rehabil.* 2001;82:265-269.

28. Bussmann JB, Grootscholten EA, Stam HJ. Daily physical activity and heart rate response in people with a unilateral transtibial amputation for vascular disease. *Arch Phys Med Rehabil.* 2004;85:240-244.

29. van der Linde H, Hofstad CJ, Geurts ACH, et al. A systematic literature review of the effect of different prosthetic components on human functioning with a lower-limb prosthesis. *J Rehabil Res Dev.* 2004;41:555-570.

30. Torburn L, Powers CM, Guiterrez R, Perry J. Energy expenditure during ambulation in dysvascular and traumatic below-knee amputees: a comparison of five prosthetic feet. *J Rehabil Res Dev.* 1995;32:111-119.

31. Casillas JM, Dulieu V, Cohen M, et al. Bioenergetic comparison of a new energy-storing foot and SACH foot in traumatic and below-knee vascular amputations. *Arch Phys Med Rehabil.* 1995;76:39-44.

32. Nielsen PH, Schurr DG, Golden JC, et al. Comparison of energy cost and gait efficiency during ambulation in below-knee amputees using different prosthetic feet. *Journal of Prosthetics and Orthotics.* 1989;1:24-31.

33. Hsu MJ, Nielsen DH, Yack HJ, Shurr DG. Physiological measurements of walking and running in people with transtibial amputations with 3 different prostheses. *J Orthop Sports Phys Ther.* 1999;29:526-533.

34. Buckley JG, Jones SF, Birch KM. Oxygen consumption during ambulation: comparison of using a prosthesis fitted with and without a tele-torsion device. *Arch Phys Med Rehabil.* 2002;83:576-581.

35. Isakov E, Susak Z, Becker E. Energy expenditure and cardiac response in above-knee amputees while using prostheses with open and locked knee mechanisms. *Scand J Rehab Med Suppl.* 1985;12:108-111.

36. Schmalz T, Blumentritt S, Jarasch R. Energy expenditure and biomechanical characteristics of lower limb amputee gait: the influence of prosthetic alignment and different prosthetic components. *Gait Posture.* 2002;16:255-263.

37. Chin T, Sawamura S, Shiba R, et al. Effect of an Intelligent Prosthesis (IP) on the walking ability of young transfemoral amputees: comparison of IP users with able-bodied people. *Am J Phys Med Rehabil.* 2003;82:447-451.

38. Perry J, Burnfield JM, Newsam CJ, Conley P. Energy expenditure and gait characteristics of a bilateral amputee walking with C-leg prostheses compared with stubby and conventional articulating prostheses. *Arch Phys Med Rehabil.* 2004;85:1711-1717.

39. Gailey RS, Lawrence D, Burditt C, et al. The CAT-CAM socket and quadrilateral socket: a comparison of energy cost during ambulation. *Prosthet Orthot Int.* 1993;17:95-100.

40. Coleman KL, Boone DA, Laing LS, et al. Quantification of prosthetic outcomes: elastomeric gel liner with locking pin suspension versus polyethylene foam liner with neoprene sleeve suspension. *J Rehabil Res Dev.* 2004;41:591-602.

41. Meikle B, Boulias C, Pauley T, Devlin M. Does increased prosthetic weight affect gait speed and patient preference in dysvascular transfemoral amputees? *Arch Phys Med Rehabil.* 2003;84:1657-1661.

42. Weed R, Atkins DJ. Return to work issues for the upper extremity amputee. In: Meier RH, Atkins DJ, eds. *Functional Restoration of Adults and Children with Upper Extremity Amputation.* New York, NY: Demos Medical Publishing; 2004:337-351.

43. Datta D, Selvarajah K, Davey N. Functional outcome of patients with proximal upper limb deficiency—acquired and congenital. *Clin Rehabil.* 2004;18:172-177.

Chapter 17

Adaptive Prostheses for Recreation

Kevin Carroll, MS, CP, FAAOP; Randy Richardson, RPA; Katherine Binder, CP

OBJECTIVES

1. Introduce the concept of adaptive prostheses for sports and other recreation
2. Relate a physical fitness program to prosthetic use
3. Describe lower- and upper-extremity adaptive prostheses
4. Link activities of varying levels of intensity with specific prosthetic demands and options
   a. Lower intensity activities: gardening, fishing, walking, golfing
   b. Intermediate intensity activities: cycling, skating, swimming, football
   c. High intensity activities: mountaineering, running, skiing, skydiving
5. Explore the prosthetic options available for participation in professional sports

INTRODUCTION

Prosthesis users of every amputation level share a universal desire: they want to be able to do more. They want to walk, run, carry, dance, work, and play. These wishes have fueled the development of an array of adaptive prosthetic components by large companies and small specialty manufacturers. Hundreds of innovative designs are enabling prosthesis wearers to participate in various recreational sports activities. This trend is a positive move from the widely held misconception that people who use prostheses should not expect to reach high levels of activity or be able to participate in activities they enjoyed before amputation. A survey of lower-limb prosthesis users indicated participation in activities including basketball, bicycling, bowling, camping, dancing, fishing, hunting, gardening, golfing and walking.[1] Although every person is unique and must be evaluated individually, no one should be discouraged from pursuing favorite activities.[2]

The term "adaptive prostheses" has multiple meanings depending on the person and the activity. Sometimes an adaptive prosthesis is a separate device used for a specific activity. In other situations, a person may wear the everyday prosthetic arm or leg but change a single component. Occasionally, simple modifications to the basic prosthesis can enhance performance. Often, prosthetists work closely with their patients to modify the prosthesis or to fashion unique components so the client can engage in a particular activity.

Snow skiing outriggers are an example of adaptations. Advances in the primary prosthesis including improved socket technology, gel liners, and computerized upper- and lower-limb components provide users with more comfort and greater performance capability.

People who seek an adaptive prosthesis cross the spectrum from the older adult who wants to garden to the competitive athlete who wants to win the triathlon. Through the expanding world of adaptive prosthetics, people are able to enjoy the self-confidence and personal growth that spring from sports and other recreational involvement. The person who combines intense personal motivation with cutting-edge prosthetic technology may pursue virtually any activity (Figure 17-1).

PHYSICAL FITNESS

In general, people who participate in sports are committed to a regular program of physical fitness and conditioning. The US Department of Health and Human Services *Healthy People 2010* lists physical activity among the top 10 leading health indicators. The highest risk of death and disability is found among those who do not engage in regular physical activity.[3] Therefore, it is essential for everyone who has sustained amputation—and may have spent time being sedentary—to follow a program of gradually increasing exercise. Physical therapists and occupational therapists can outline a strengthening and flexibility exercise program for both upper- and lower-limb prosthesis users. Beginning with simple stretching exercises and moving to intensive athletic activities, physical conditioning is the foundation for a healthy, active lifestyle. The largest group of prosthesis users—adults over the age of 50—must make a special effort to remain active to help control other age-related disorders such as weight gain, cardiovascular disease, diabetes, osteoporosis, and depression.[4]

Consider that:

- Regular exercise plays a key role in preventing many health problems
- Excess weight is a major contributing factor in cardiovascular disease, the onset of diabetes, and the progression of existing diabetes
- Excess weight negatively affects prosthetic fit and performance
- Cardiovascular disease is the leading cause of death in the United States
- About 60% of men older than 60 and women aged 80 and older will experience major narrowing of the arteries
- Vascular problems and diabetes are the primary causes of amputation in older adults
- After age 50, osteoporosis will cause most women to lose approximately 30% of their bone tissue, whereas men will average a 17% loss
- More than 1.5 million American women sustain fractures annually
- Walking, running, skating, aerobic exercise, weight lifting, dancing, tennis, and basketball are bone-strengthening activities
- Emotions play a vital role in physical health
- Exercise can help counter feelings of sadness and fear
- Regular exercise stimulates the release of chemical endorphins that help counteract depression

Clearly, staying active is an essential part of health and wellness that should be encouraged for prosthesis users of all ages.

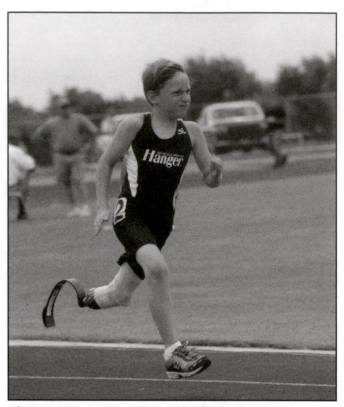

Figure 17-1. Motivation embodied. The person who combines intense personal motivation with cutting-edge prosthetic technology may pursue virtually any recreational activity he or she desires.

LOWER-LIMB ADAPTIVE PROSTHESES

Adaptive prostheses can be as sophisticated as a sleek sprinting leg for an elite athlete, or as simple as a rubber pod that serves as a stable, waterproof foot for use at the beach. Some users have an adaptive prosthesis designed for a specific activity such as running, snow skiing, or scuba diving. This allows them to wear a regular prosthesis for everyday activities and switch to the adaptive prosthesis as needed. More likely, however, the average person applies adaptive components or accessories to the regular prosthesis to use it for recreation. For example, a shock absorber can be added for playing tennis, a torque absorber is helpful when golfing, and poles fitted with outriggers enable skiing. Some people wear the same socket all the time and use a small adaptive device known as a quick disconnect coupler (Ferrier Coupler, North Branch, Mich; www.ferrier.coupler.com) to change the lower portion of the prosthesis. For transfemoral (TF) users, the coupler can be mounted on the distal end of the socket or below the knee unit; transtibial (TT) prostheses have the coupler on the distal end of the socket. A threaded pin locks the coupler securely in place. This allows the user to

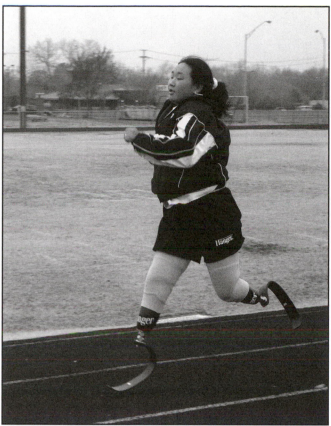

Figure 17-2. Bilateral TT user has returned to running and cycling since being fitted with dynamic sockets.

quickly and easily disconnect the bottom portion of the prosthesis and attach a different ankle, foot, or knee to the regular socket. The coupler also preserves the alignment of the prosthesis in the presence of adaptive components.

Some prosthetic feet are adapted for specific activities. Nevertheless, in most cases, multi-axis and dynamic response feet are optimal for active users. Multiaxis feet allow rotation, inversion/eversion, and dorsiflexion and plantar flexion of the foot-ankle assembly. Such feet increase stability and comfort for those who walk on uneven surfaces such as golf courses or hiking trails. Dynamic response feet enable a more natural gait, permitting users to be more active for longer periods by providing good energy return.[5] Some of the energy the person expends during mid and late stance is stored within the foot and then released to advance the wearer through swing phase. Patients with Medicare functional levels of K3 or K4—especially children, young adults, and athletes—may benefit from using dynamic response feet that absorb and release energy.[6] Most dynamic response feet incorporate carbon fiber to increase the energy storing characteristics and reduce the overall weight (see Figure 8-8).

For TF prostheses, computerized knee units increase stability. Some of these offer the additional advantage

of two separate modes. Typically, the first mode is programmed for walking; the second mode is programmed to accommodate recreational activities. To switch to the second mode, the person simply taps the toe of the prosthesis on the ground.[7] Sophisticated units can be severely damaged if water, sand, or dirt penetrates the electronic components. Therefore, they are not suited for some activities. For a detailed discussion of computerized knees, refer to Chapter 9.

Advanced components are irrelevant if the socket causes discomfort. Chapters 8 and 9 describe dynamic sockets. Thermoplastic sockets can be adjusted easily. For example, as exercising muscle increases in volume, the socket can be enlarged (Figure 17-2).

Lower-limb prosthesis users may prefer not to wear a prosthesis when participating in some activities, such as swimming or water-skiing. A limb protector should be considered to protect the limb from injury. Even so, the ability to perform most activities, on average, is much higher when wearing a prosthesis.[1]

Finally, one should not overlook the recreational capabilities of hip disarticulation and transpelvic (HD/TP) prosthesis users. Historically, they have often been labeled permanently disabled, strongly discouraged from believing they can be active. Recent improvements in prosthetic components and socket designs have promoted increased mobility. An excellent source, HD/DP Help (www.hphdhelp.org) lists 24 recreational activities in which they can participate, from archery through wheelchair racing. Some HD/TP prosthesis users even enjoy extreme activities such as mountaineering and ice climbing.

UPPER-LIMB ADAPTIVE PROSTHESES

Many individuals with upper-limb deficiency choose not to wear a prosthesis. Approximately 5000 people are fitted with their first upper-limb prosthesis annually; at the end of 1 year, only 50% of them were still using it.[8] Some clinicians are discouraged by this low rate of usage and are working to educate potential users about prosthetic advances. A patient who is not fitted within one month of amputation usually begins to function unimanually. Others have had a negative fitting experience that involved pain or poor function. Some people become adept at specific activities without using a prosthesis.[2] Others use a prosthesis in daily life but engage in recreation without it. Therefore, upper-limb prosthesis users who pursue sports with an adaptive prosthesis are special individuals who display a lot of motivation. Some of the most popular adaptive designs have been developed by people with amputations who wanted to find a better way to participate in their favorite activities.

An early consideration is whether an adaptive prosthetic arm should be body-powered or externally pow-

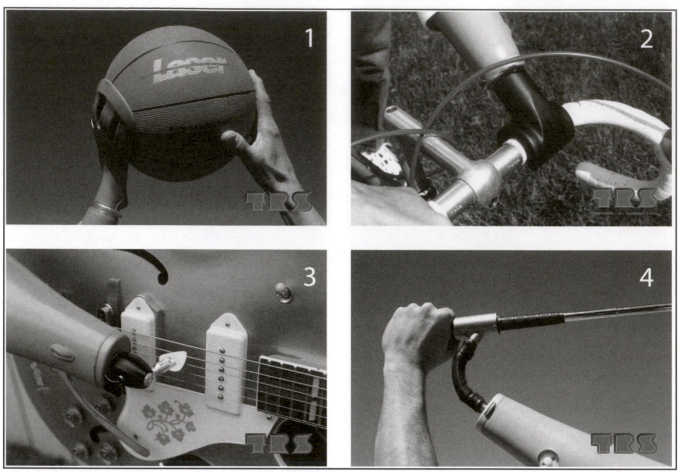

Figure 17-3. Terminal devices: (1) Supersport; (2) bicycle TD; (3) guitar pick holder; (4) golf TD.

ered. Although myoelectric technology has refined the appearance and some of the function of prosthetic elbows and hands, the body-powered prosthesis remains the more common choice.[9] Externally powered prostheses are heavier, tend to respond more slowly, are more fragile, and have greater sensitivity to moisture and temperature extremes. The cosmetic glove can be easily stained, punctured, or torn. A high percentage of users who wear externally powered prostheses are children who are likely to subject the prosthesis to many potentially damaging activities. Many users of body-powered prostheses state they can move both the elbow and hand quickly, a factor often important in recreational pursuits. These prostheses are substantially less expensive, increasing the likelihood that an active user could own two prostheses, namely a cosmetically pleasing functional prosthesis for day-to-day use and a rugged one for recreation

The terminal device (TD) is the part of the prosthesis that substitutes for the anatomic hand. Many TDs are manufactured. When combined with a rapid disconnect wrist unit, the TD can be easily removed, so that the client can replace one TD with another. Someone with

a myoelectric prosthesis can interchange the hand with the more durable, clamp-like device called a greifer. Recreational prostheses almost always incorporate a rapid disconnect wrist. By placing a rubber washer or O-ring on the threaded screw at the base of the TD, the user has better control over incremental rotation of the hand.[10] Specific TDs have been developed for archery, baseball, basketball, bicycling, canoeing, fishing, football, golf, gymnastics, hockey, musical instruments, photography, pool, snow skiing, swimming, weight lifting, and windsurfing (Figure 17-3).

As is the case with those who have lower-limb amputation, people with upper-limb amputation who may prefer not to wear a prosthesis when participating in some activities should wear a limb protector.

LOW STRESS ACTIVITIES

Showering

Slippery surfaces, such as wet tile, require a cautious approach from those who have lower-limb amputation. Balancing on one leg while showering increases the risk

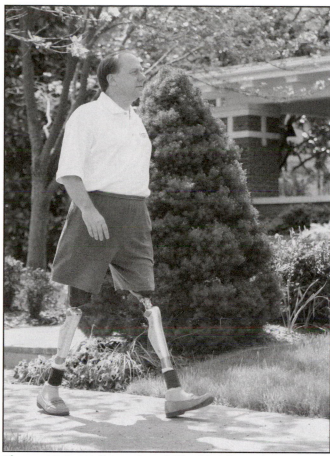

Figure 17-4. Walking downhill with bilateral computerized knee units.

ing to the open road. Computerized knee systems are helpful because they have a second mode that can be programmed to limit knee flexion while driving, yet still allow for extension to move safely between the accelerator and the brake pedals. This feature is helpful to some bilateral TF users, allowing them to drive without hand controls.

Upper-limb prosthesis users typically rely on the sound hand to turn the steering wheel, although many TDs can help with two-handed steering. Those who wear hooks must exercise care to not catch them on the steering wheel. The Hosmer Driving Ring (www.hosmer.com) is a fixture that attaches easily to the steering wheel. People who wear bilateral upper-limb prostheses may prefer to have a vertical handle placed on the wheel to facilitate steering. Some people with transradial (TR) amputation, whether bilateral or unilateral, prefer to drive without any prosthesis.

All clients should check with their insurance company and the state drivers' licensing agency for any special requirements that pertain to driving with or without a prosthesis.

Walking

People take walking for granted until they experience the loss of a lower limb. Following amputation, many people rely on crutches or a wheelchair until they are fitted with a prosthesis. They quickly realize how difficult it is to carry objects while using crutches and that wheelchair ramps are not always conveniently located. Therefore, most are eager to pursue prosthetic fitting so they can resume a level of mobility similar to what they had before amputation.

Most individuals want a smooth, natural gait. This accomplishment is considerably easier for patients with TT and Syme's amputation. Transfemoral and HD/TP patients require more extensive gait training. Walking is the basic form of mobility for most prosthetic users and is also an excellent form of exercise. By adding distance and speed, walking can become the foundation of a physical fitness program that is simple, economical, and effective.

A lightweight energy-storing foot is often beneficial, although initially it may take more effort to learn to control.

Computerized knees facilitate walking for active TF users. The unit adjusts its stability when the sensors detect uneven terrain. For example, when walking down a hill with a traditional knee unit, the user may find it safer to descend sideways; if the person were to attempt to go straight down the hill, the knee may collapse, causing a serious fall. In contrast, the computerized knee instantly adjusts to the new angle, drastically reducing the likelihood of excessive knee flexion. With practice, users learn to trust the knee and master walking downhill facing forward (Figure 17-4).

of falling. Thus using a shower chair is a simple solution, particularly for older adults. Another option is a basic "shower leg" that enables users to stand while showering; this is particularly practical when a person is traveling and does not have access to a shower chair. Prosthetists can fabricate a shower leg that incorporates a rubber distal pod instead of a foot. The Aqualimb by Endolite (www.endolite.com) is a simple TT shower leg with an anti-slip tread pattern on the sole of the foot. Waterproof covers by XeroSox (www.xerosox.com) are available in both upper- and lower-limb models. They are made of thick surgical latex, providing an airtight vacuum seal. The lower-limb version features a nonskid sole.

Driving

Driving is one of the first activities people are eager to try, often before they receive a prosthesis. Most people with a unilateral prosthesis find they can drive with their sound limb after a period of acclimation. Driving is more challenging for those who wear a right lower-limb prosthesis. Transfemoral users will find driving more difficult than clients with TT prostheses, and both will need many hours of practice before tak-

Gardening

Sometimes the most functional adaptive prostheses are the least sophisticated. One example is an all-terrain foot that looks like a rubber pod on a short pylon. This foot can be obtained from a prosthetist. These feet are often used on a temporary prosthesis. Some people continue to wear them for tasks such as yard work or gardening. The simple design provides a stable base, especially on uneven ground. Because rubber is flexible, the user can bend, twist, and turn readily. When this foot gets muddy or wet, it can be washed.

Upper-limb prosthesis users who want to garden will probably prefer a voluntary-closing (VC) hook. Myoelectric hands are not appropriate become they are not waterproof, and the cosmetic gloves are easily punctured and stained. Another option is the Electronic Terminal Device (ETD) from Motion Control (www.motioncontrol.com), which integrates water-resistant housings with a hook. Using a quick disconnect wrist unit, the user can remove the myoelectric hand and switch to the ETD for any activity that requires a more rugged device.

Fishing

People who wear a unilateral upper-limb prosthesis can use the prosthesis either to hold the rod or turn the reel handle for line retrieval. Reels can be purchased as either right- or left-handed models. The controlled grasp of VC TDs and electrically powered hands enable them to work well for fishing, whereas voluntary-opening (VO) hooks tend to slip off the reel handle. The unique "One Armed Fishing Bandit" is a combination of a rod attached to a waist belt, designed specifically for fishing with one hand. A line of electric reel systems for one-handed control are available through Electric Fishing Reel Systems (www.elec-tra-mate.com).

Lower-limb prosthesis users can wear a waterproof prosthesis or a waterproof cover when they go fishing. The rubber pod foot increases stability on wet surfaces (eg, docks, rocks, and boat decks). The everyday prosthesis can also be worn if the knee component is protected from water and dirt. Most feet can be cleaned if they get wet or dirty.

Because fishing can disturb balance, clients who are fishing from a boat or near rushing or deep water should also wear a life jacket.

Flying

People who are or want to become pilots usually will be able to use their everyday prosthesis without special modifications. Most unilateral TT and TF users can perform every task necessary for safe flight. Those with bilateral lower-limb prostheses may find it necessary to install a hand brake in private planes. Several people, some with multiple amputations, are pilots. The late

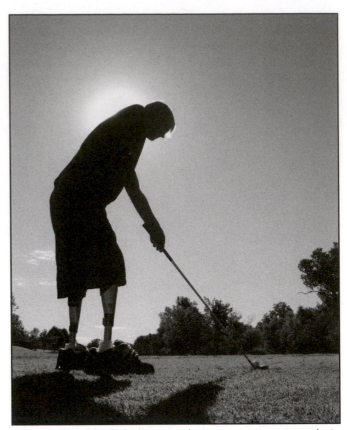

Figure 17-5. Golf helps prosthetic users increase their coordination, flexibility and confidence, while also providing a social dimension.

Ed Hommer, who wore bilateral lower-limb prostheses, was a pilot for American Airlines. He died while mountain climbing. Transfemoral prosthesis user Bill Dunham is a private pilot and an active member of the Civil Air Patrol. Dana Bowman is a helicopter pilot and instructor who wears bilateral lower-limb prostheses.

Upper-limb prosthesis users need no modifications to pilot a small plane. Some find that a myoelectric prosthesis provides better control than a body-powered one. Mike Penwich wears a pair of upper-limb prostheses when piloting stunt planes.

Golf

Golf is a sport that people with limb loss can enjoy. Golf helps clients increase their coordination, flexibility and confidence in a social environment. The National Amputee Golf Association (NAGA), incorporated in 1954, has more than 4000 members. The NAGA offers the First Swing Program, which teaches golf techniques to those with physical disabilities at more than 30 clinics across the country each year (Figure 17-5).[11]

Most TT users wear their everyday prosthesis. Shock absorbers and torsion adapters help create a more natural pivot when swinging the golf club. These compo-

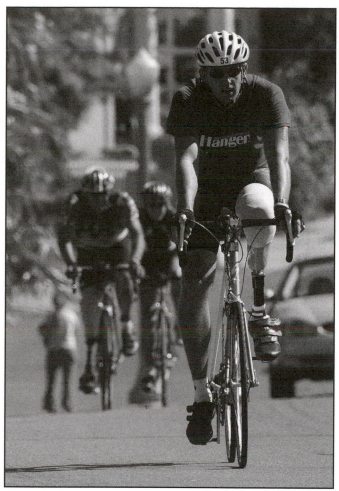

Figure 17-6. Bicycling. (Courtesy of Hanger Prosthetics and Orthotics.)

Individuals who wear an upper-limb prosthesis may use a TD that holds a golf club and has a flexible wrist for smooth transition during the golf swing. A cable-operated hook or an electric hand are other options; however, without a flexible wrist, the game is essentially played with the sound arm only. Some golfers hold the club and swing using the sound hand and arm. People with bilateral TR prostheses can try using a TD and a flexible wrist on both prostheses. Golfing is much more difficult for those with bilateral TH prostheses.

INTERMEDIATE STRESS ACTIVITIES

Cycling

Most people learn to ride a bicycle when they are children, relishing the sensations of wind, speed, and motion. Fortunately, the simple pleasures of cycling are still available to many upper- and lower-limb prosthesis users, usually on a standard bicycle with inexpensive modifications. Most children can ride a standard tricycle or child's bicycle. Hand-pedaled tricycles are an option for people with lower-limb amputation.

Juan de la Roca Perez, a TF user, has a high activity prosthesis that allows him to enjoy bicycling, running, and swimming—the same sports in which he participated prior to amputation. His socket features a lower trim line, allowing greater range of motion and more comfort during cycling.

Safety is always a factor in cycling, but especially when relearning how to ride. The ability to balance is key. Because people who wear prostheses do not have equal weight on both sides of their body, maintaining balance can be a challenge that takes time to master. Beginners should learn to ride on mowed grass, making a much softer landing than concrete. Protective gear, including a helmet, fingerless gloves with padded hands, knee and elbow pads, sunglasses, and appropriate clothing are important. Children who are learning to ride should have a one-speed bicycle that is size-appropriate; adults who wish to ride should obtain a sturdy bicycle with multiple speeds.

Among children with limb differences, bicycle riding is as natural as for other children. Children with amputations stated they were equal to their friends when cycling. Nearly all preferred to wear a prosthesis when cycling. Wearing foot straps or stirrups on both pedals is helpful, as is the assistance of another person when learning to ride.[13]

Several specialized bicycle designs are appropriate for prosthesis users. Two popular styles are hand-pedaled bicycles and recumbent bicycles. Both position the rider much lower than on a standard bicycle and provide comfortable seats with good back support. Hand bicycles usually have three wheels—two in the

nents also absorb the shear forces that occur with lower body rotation, reducing stress on the residual limb. Adding shock or torsion adapters increases the weight of the prosthesis. Some people prefer not to wear golf shoes with spikes because this decreases the ability to rotate on the prosthetic side.[12] The Swivel Golf Shoe, developed by the War Amputations of Canada, is a rotational device installed in a regular golf shoe.

People with TF prostheses benefit from standard or computerized hydraulic knee systems that incorporate stance control. These units provide hydraulic resistance as the prosthetic knee bends when the wearer prepares to hit the ball, allowing the person to develop a golf swing similar to that of an able-bodied player. A few people opt not to wear a prosthesis when golfing, balancing on one leg to swing and using crutches to walk.

Clients with bilateral amputation enjoy golf. For those with a TF prosthesis on one or both sides, a computerized knee system dramatically improves function. With some modifications, golf can also be played in a seated position from a wheelchair or electric cart.

rear and one in the front—with the pedals located in front of the chest for easy hand turning. Recumbent bicycles have two or three wheels with a short or long wheelbase. Most riders, especially people with bilateral TF and HD/TP amputations, describe hand bicycles and recumbent bicycles as feeling more stable and more comfortable than standard bicycles.

Lower-limb prosthesis wearers can ride with their everyday prosthesis; however, they may want to add a toe clip on the pedal or wear special bicycle shoes. Competitive cyclists often prefer a pedal clip in place of the prosthetic foot. Transfemoral users benefit from computerized knees with the second mode programmed to allow free swing during cycling. A hydraulic knee should be set in the free swing mode, bypassing stance phase resistance and making it much easier to pedal. Some people cycle without a prosthesis. A simple toe clip installed on the pedal on the sound side enables them to push and pull the pedal. The unused pedal can be removed. Another option for TF users who are competitive cyclists is to have a custom-made socket attached to the saddle of the bicycle. The amputation limb slips into the socket when riding and slips out when the cyclist leaves the bicycle.

The coauthor (K.C.) has fitted several HD/TP patients who ride standard bicycles wearing their prostheses. They have the anatomically correct HD/TP socket design outlined in Chapter 10.

People who wear upper-limb prostheses are frequently able to use standard bicycles. Usually the TD is used for steering, balance, and stability while the sound hand controls the levers for gears and brakes. The shift and rear brake lever on the handlebars needs to be positioned on the side the user prefers—usually the sound side. Any bicycle shop can move the levers. Bicycles should be equipped with a dual brake control that activates the front and rear brakes simultaneously (see Figure 17-3). For body-powered prostheses, a VC TD can grip the handlebars securely. An externally powered hand would be damaged in a fall. Some individuals with bilateral upper-limb amputation like the stability of a recumbent bicycle.

Rollerblading/Skating/Ice Skating

Transtibial and TF users will find it easier to skate if the prosthesis is aligned to tilt slightly forward. A simple way to tilt the prosthesis is by inserting a soft plastic or foam wedge under the heel of the foot.[14] When selecting the foot, the heel height of the skate must be considered. An adjustable ankle makes it much easier to obtain the proper ankle/foot alignment, especially if the skate has a Cuban heel style. For TF users, the flexion of the prosthetic knee needs to be adjusted to enable the knee to swing the lower leg forward quickly for the next stride.

Those who wear an upper-limb prosthesis will have better balance if they wear the prosthesis while skating. People who prefer not to wear the prosthesis should consider wearing a limb protector on the amputation limb.

Aerobic Exercises

Aerobic exercises provide good cardiovascular conditioning without much specialized equipment. Because of the repeated impact of jumping and bouncing, lower-limb prosthesis users may prefer to use a shock- and torque-absorbing pylon on the prosthesis. A flexible, energy storing foot is also helpful. For TF users, a computerized knee can have the second mode of the knee set specifically for the demands of the exercise. Whether the person wears an upper-limb prosthesis while exercising is a matter of personal preference.

Tennis

Unilateral upper-limb wearers can rely on their sound hand to hold the racquet and use a specially adapted socket or TD, such as the custom-made ring device from Therapeutic Recreations Systems Inc (www.oandp.com/products/trs), to hold the tennis ball so it can be tossed in the air for serving. Terminal devices are specifically designed to hold a tennis racquet.

A lower-limb prosthesis with the addition of a shock absorber and torsion adapter works well. Because tennis requires bending of the knee and rapid movement of the feet, TT users will fare better than those with TF prostheses. A multi-axis, dynamic foot is desirable. Transfemoral wearers benefit from a hydraulic knee unit, preferably computerized. Tennis shoes usually have a flat sole, necessitating insertion of a soft plastic or foam wedge under the prosthetic heel (Figure 17-7).

Water Sports

Consumer demand has led to the creation of numerous waterproof prosthetic components and accessories for swimming, snorkeling, scuba, boating, and water-skiing. Transtibial users can wear the waterproof leg described in the section on showering for walking at the beach and around the swimming pool, and while boating/fishing and gardening. Some waterproof prostheses have holes in the outer shell to allow the limb to fill with water to reduce buoyancy; water drains through the hole.[14]

Instead of purchasing a waterproof prosthesis, some people opt for inexpensive covers that protect the prosthesis from getting wet, such as XeroSox. The cover should be used for 30 to 45 minutes, and then opened to allow air to circulate inside for a few minutes before resealing the vacuum seal. Although these covers work fairly well, a waterproof prosthesis is a better option.

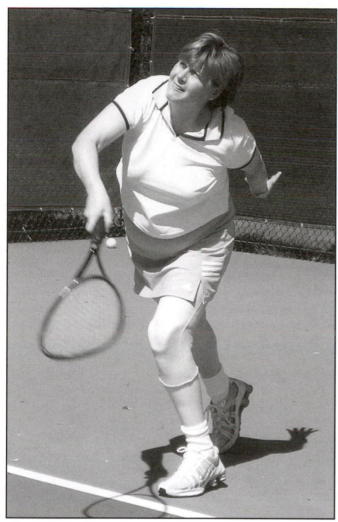

Figure 17-7. Tennis.

Swimming

Swimming is an excellent exercise that conditions the body, especially the cardiovascular system. Swimming can be enjoyed either with or without a prosthesis. Depending on the level of amputation, some people find that a specially designed swimming prosthesis increases their ability. Swimming with a prosthesis strengthens the muscles of the amputation limb. For lower-limb users, Rampro (Leucadia, Calif, www.rampro.net) has two options, the Swimankle and the Activankle. Both are constructed from non-corroding Delrin and stainless steel and have two locking positions, one for walking and one with 70 degree plantar flexion for swimming. They can be worn with or without fins, making them particularly useful for snorkeling or scuba diving. The Activankle has a protective covering to keep sand out of the mechanism. When unlocked, the Activankle allows for unlimited dorsiflexion, making it suitable for jet skiing, wind surfing, and snow skiing. Those who

wear bilateral TF prostheses may find that attaching a Swimankle to the distal end of each socket will allow them to wear swim fins for increased mobility in the water. Additionally, by keeping the attachment close to the distal end of the socket, less effort is required. People with TT amputation may want to wear a knee orthosis to increase knee stability and protect it from water resistance.

Upper-limb prosthesis wearers may find that a custom-designed swimming prosthesis improves stroke resistance. The Freestyle Therapeutic Swim Device (Therapeutic Recreation Systems) can be used with a custom swimming prosthesis. The device flares open during the power stroke, for resistance and propulsion, and collapses during the backstroke to conserve energy. A custom-molded flexible socket minimizes socket pistoning during swimming. Some people with TR amputation strap a plastic swimmer's training paddle to the amputation limb to improve their stroke resistance.

Many individuals engage in water activities while wearing an everyday prosthesis that is not waterproof. Prostheses with electronic components should never come in contact with water. Any prosthesis exposed to salt water should be cleaned with dish washing liquid soap and fresh water, thoroughly dried, and sprayed with WD40 to prevent corrosion (Figure 17-8).

Team Sports

Athletes who wear upper- or lower-limb prostheses compete in football, basketball, volleyball, baseball, and soccer. Organized sports hold great attraction for numerous children and adults. Those who wear a lower-limb prosthesis need a socket with a cushioning gel liner, a pylon with shock and torque absorbers, and a dynamic response foot with an adjustable ankle. The TF prosthesis should have a pneumatic, hydraulic, or computerized knee unit. Several college football players wear a reinforced lower-limb prosthesis built for high impact.[15] Most individuals play sports wearing their ordinary, unmodified prosthesis. Commonly, people with lower-limb amputation play soccer with crutches without a prosthesis.

Those with upper-limb amputation often prefer not to wear a prosthesis when participating in football, basketball, or baseball. If the person chooses to wear a prosthesis during sports it should have a flexible socket and TD manufactured specifically for the particular sport. Therapeutic Recreation Systems offers a diverse selection of TDs, including the Grand Slam Baseball, the Hi-Fly Fielder, and the Power Swing Ring, for baseball; the Mills' Re-Bound Pro Basketball Terminal Device; and the Super Sport Hand and Free Flex Hand, both with wrist flexion and extension, for football, basketball, and volleyball.[14]

HIGH STRESS ACTIVITIES

Bodybuilding/Weight Lifting

Individuals wearing lower-limb prostheses can generally lift weights without any prosthetic adaptations. Whether standing, sitting, or lying, wearing a prosthesis while lifting significantly improves stability and balance.

Upper-limb prosthesis users who wish to engage in weight lifting can use a VC Grip Prehensor (Therapeutic Recreation Systems). By modifying the prehensor with a locking pin accessory, the person can manage dumbbells, barbells, and cable-controlled weights. Mike McElheny, who wears a TR prosthesis, is an accomplished weight lifter and bodybuilder. Professional weight lifters can use a steel clasp, designed to grasp and lock onto handles and bars, for extreme weight bench pressing, dumbbell flies, dead lifts, and squatting.

Mountaineering

Rock and technical climbing is an elite sport even for the able-bodied. These intense activities require a great deal of stamina, strength, and perseverance. Climbing requires specialized instruction and equipment and is hazardous even for highly experienced experts. Stringent safety measures require climbers always to work in pairs or teams, never alone, and to be belayed with a top rope for protection from falls.

The challenge and accomplishment of climbing Mounts McKinley, Everest, and El Capitan have been experienced by several people who wear lower-limb prostheses, including Warren McDonald, Tom Whittaker, and Ed Homer. Kyle Underwood has an HD amputation yet is also an ice climber. These men have developed unique adaptations to their prostheses that enable them to pursue their passion for mountaineering. A mountaineering prosthesis should be rugged enough to be banged into rocks and exposed to moisture. Many times, when being fitted with a new prosthesis, these athletes will keep and modify the older prosthesis, using it exclusively for outdoor adventuring.

Warren Macdonald sustained bilateral TF amputation when his legs were crushed in a rock climbing accident in 1997. After his amputations, he was not willing to give up his active lifestyle, which included hiking, camping, rock climbing, and ice climbing. He worked closely with the co-author (K.C.), helping design a series of adaptive prosthetic devices that enabled him to continue with his activities. For mountain climbing, he prefers to wear prostheses with very short pylons and all-terrain feet. This combination gives him a lower center of gravity, plenty of stability, and the ability to make quick, agile movements for getting over rocks and up and down steep mountain inclines. He has three adap-

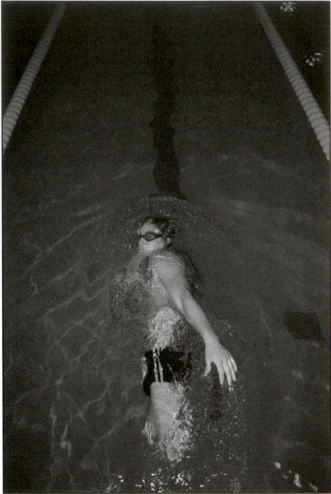

Figure 17-8. Swimming is an excellent, low-stress exercise that conditions the body and the cardiovascular system. Swimming can be enjoyed with or without a prosthesis.

tive feet: all-terrain feet for ascending; all-terrain feet with shock and torque absorbing pylons for descending; and spiked, crampon-style feet for rock climbing, ice climbing, and hiking. All of these feet attach to a flexible socket that can be adjusted to accommodate the increased muscle volume in the amputation limbs, which develops during intense exercise[16] (Figure 17-9).

People who have upper-limb amputation can engage in rock and technical climbing if they have a reliable prosthesis with a heavy-duty TD that can be wedged between rocks and can grip rough surfaces. Stainless steel VC TDs are useful for climbers. Aron Ralston, a rock climber who was forced to amputate his own arm after spending 5 days trapped beneath a boulder, now wears a rugged TR prosthesis. Incredibly, just 4 months after his accident, Ralston competed in the Adventure Duluth race, which included 11.5 miles of sea kayaking, 4 miles of whitewater canoeing, and a 12-mile trail run.[15]

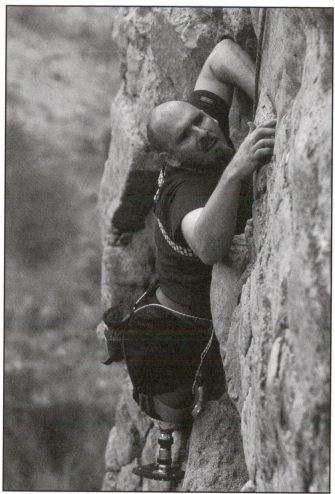

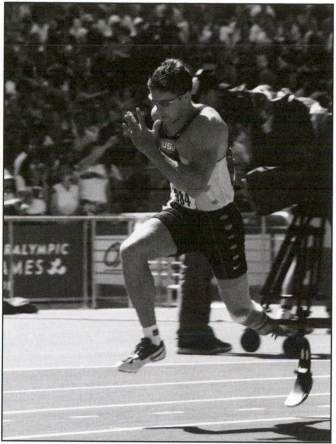

Figure 17-10. Running. (Courtesy of Hanger Prosthetics and Orthotics.)

Figure 17-9. Mountain climbing. These climbers have developed unique adaptations to their prostheses that enable them to pursue their passion for mountaineering. This person prefers to wear legs with very short pylons and all-terrain feet. This combination gives him a lower center of gravity, plenty of stability, and quick, agile movements for getting over rocks and up steep mountain inclines.

Running

Running was once considered almost impossible for people who had lower-limb amputation. Now it is an activity that many pursue. It is much easier for those who wear TT prostheses to run, as compared with those who need TF prostheses, who expend substantially more energy, and face a higher risk of falls. People who wear HD/TP prostheses have the most difficult challenge when attempting to run but the very determined person who is in great physical condition can run. Most prosthesis wearers will not have a symmetrical running gait. Successful runners are usually not overweight, are in good physical condition, usually have relatively long amputation limbs, and have healthy skin on the amputation limb. Often, they were runners before they

sustained amputation. People with unilateral or bilateral TT amputations can probably run on their current prostheses if they are equipped with energy-storing feet. For optimum results, serious runners have a second prosthesis with a specially designed foot that is aligned for running (Figure 17-10). Knee disarticulation and TF users find it takes a lot of trust in the prosthesis to achieve running.

Some components, such as nonenergy storing feet, rigid sockets, and computerized knee units, are not suitable for running. A conventional hydraulic knee unit must be set differently for running than for walking. If the unit has stance phase control, this must be bypassed for running. A hydraulic knee unit with swing control is preferred. The flexion resistance must be set to a high level to limit the amount of knee flexion, and extension resistance must be set to a low level to allow the knee to extend freely. It may be necessary to externally rotate the knee to get the proper alignment for running. Alternatively, the client can learn to externally rotate the amputation limb when running. With a sprinting foot, most runners find that a significant amount of plantar flexion of the foot is necessary to achieve optimal running motion. Extra socket flexion improves the running

Figure 17-11. Skydiving.

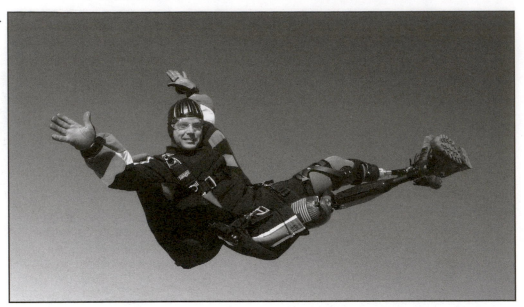

gait. Some people with bilateral TF prostheses, such as Laurens Molina, have had success with running. An internationally competitive wheelchair marathoner, Molina spent 8 years in a wheelchair before being fitted with lightweight, adaptive prostheses that feature sprinting feet and hydraulic knees.

Skydiving

Skydiving is an extreme activity that attracts a small number of people. Most prefer to wear their prosthesis to restore symmetry to the body and make the freefall portion of the experience more stable. Most divers land favoring the sound leg for added control. Dana Bowman sustained TF amputation of one leg and TT amputation of the other leg in a skydiving accident. He now jumps with two adaptive prostheses. They feature heavy-duty shock-absorbing feet and pylons that compresses up to 1 inch on ground contact for maximum shock absorption (Figure 17-11).

Snow Skiing and Snowboarding

Snow skiing is an exhilarating sport, made accessible to prosthetic users through an array of adaptive equipment and programs. Historically, snow skiing has been the leader among organized sports in appealing to people with physical challenges.

Many unilateral lower-limb prosthesis users prefer to ski without a prosthesis. Transtibial wearers, however, are more likely than TF users to wear a prosthesis. People who ski with a prosthesis need to talk to their prosthetist about modifying prosthetic alignment to obtain additional flexion. Adjustable ankles are useful when skiing; Rampro's Activankle can be unlocked for snow skiing, flexing freely without rotation or lateral movement.

Regular ski poles may be used; however, poles with outriggers are a popular option. Outriggers look like forearm crutches with a miniature ski attached to the bottom of the pole. The aluminum poles are available in various lengths. The ski attachment can be flipped vertically from a control lever located near the handle. Two popular brands are the LaCome FlipSki (Taos, NM) and the Superlite line of adaptive poles from Enabling Technologies Inc (Washington DC, www.abledata.com) (Figure 17-12).

People who wear bilateral prostheses, as well as some unilateral users, may prefer a sit-ski or mono-ski. The person is strapped into the seat of the ski and uses outriggers to guide it. Sleds and mono-skis are often equipped with shock absorption and evacuation harnesses. Yetti, Enabling Technologies Inc, and Mountain Man are three American manufacturers (www.abledata.com). High level bilateral users should consider the option of snowboarding; a bucket-like socket in which the user sits can be attached to the snowboard.[14]

Adaptive TDs for upper-limb prostheses make snow skiing easier. The All Terrain Ski Terminal Device by Therapeutic Recreation Systems Inc features a quick disconnect pole. The Hosmer Ski Hand is a molded silicone hand with an opening that holds a ski pole. People with upper-limb amputation can ski without a prosthesis although using poles or outriggers on both sides improves balance (see Figure 17-3).

Water-Skiing

Water-skiing is an exciting sport that helps balance and trunk strength. Skiers and boat passengers should always wear life jackets. Beginning skiers are encouraged to slowly work their way to longer times and greater speeds. Some people prefer to water-ski with-

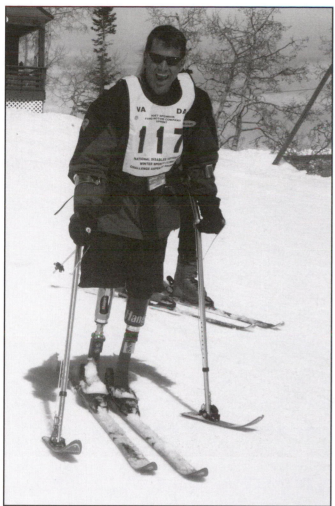

Figure 17-12. Snow skiing. (Courtesy of Hanger Prosthetics and Orthotics.)

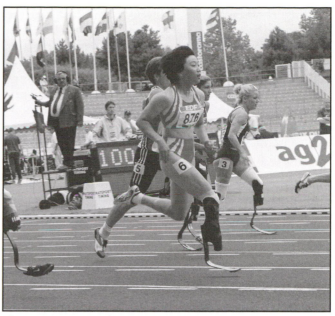

Figure 17-13. Paralympic Games.

out using a prosthesis. Slalom skiing, with or without a prosthesis, is a popular option. When slalom skiing with a lower-limb prosthesis, it is generally easier to position the sound leg in front of the prosthesis. The prosthesis can be made slightly shorter to place weight farther back on the ski. The knee should be outset and externally rotated to allow for clearance of the sound knee. If using two skis, the ski on the prosthetic side should be kept 3 to 6 inches ahead of the other one. If the skier starts with the prosthesis trailing, the force of the water is likely to wrench the prosthesis off.[12] Other options, particularly for people wearing bilateral prostheses, include the mono-ski and sit-ski for water-skiing. Both devices look more like a surfboard than a ski and allow the skier to be seated, either directly on the board or in a specially designed seat. Dana Bowman, who wears bilateral prostheses, has designed a hybrid slalom water-ski that uses the bindings from snow skis. His waterproof feet snap into the binding, and when he falls, the feet release just as in snow skiing.

People with upper-limb amputation can water-ski without a prosthesis, using the sound hand to hold the rope. Some adaptations are available for those who want to ski with their prostheses include a water-skiing system with a single ski rope handle works with a simple shallow hook TD. A self-suspending supracondylar socket usually provides adequate suspension yet will release when pulled or twisted if the hook fails to twist off during a fall.[10] Prostheses should always be covered with a neoprene sleeve to allow them to float.

The boat should have a quick disconnect system to allows a skier to release the rope instantly in the event of a fall. For this approach to be safe, the passenger must be attentive to the skier, releasing the rope immediately upon a fall. Skiers should never lock onto a ski rope handle with any type of TD, nor should they wear a prosthesis that requires a harness and cable, or wear an externally powered prosthesis in the water.

PROFESSIONAL SPORTS

High performance sports legs for the professional athlete are at the top end of the spectrum of adaptive prosthetics. How great is the need for this type of prosthesis? Almost 4000 athletes from 136 countries competed in the 2004 Paralympic Games in Athens, Greece. Sprinting, track and field, swimming, tennis, and triathlon are some of the events where Paralympians vie to win medals. The adaptive prostheses that propel them across the finish line are lightweight, sleek, and engineered for maximum impact and energy return (Figure 17-13).

Many running and sprinting feet consist of a curved strip of carbon fiber composite with no heel; the toe has gripping studs attached to the plantar surface to prevent slippage. For other events, athletes choose high performance feet that have toe and heel springs, which are customized for the individual's weight and activity. Some feet have cushioning bumpers at forefoot, heel, and midstance, and an ankle bushing. These soft components are used to customize the foot to suit the user. Bumpers and bushings dampen and absorb shock. Heavy-duty vertical shock-absorbing pylons are commonly used; many athletes also have added torque absorbers (Figure 17-14). The flexible socket has pressure relief in areas of the amputation limb, sustaining high impact or friction. The socket is adjustable to accommodate the changes in muscle volume that occur during intense physical activity. Usually, the athlete will wear a cushioning liner between the amputation limb and the socket to absorb shock. Gel liners are particularly effective. As a further safeguard against skin abrasion, many athletes use liquid silicone to reduce friction and carry special protective fabric that can be layered over sensitive areas. Ensuring the suspension of the prosthesis during competition is critical, thus many athletes rely on an auxiliary suspension system. For example, pin lock suspension can be supplemented with a suction sleeve or a securing strap.

The speed gap between Paralympic and able-bodied runners is quickly closing with the development of high performance prosthetic components. Paralympic sprinters are setting world records that are scarcely more than one second off the world records set by able-bodied Olympic sprinters.[17]

Lightweight carbon composite feet designed specifically for sprinting are the first choice for most runners. Several manufacturers offer feet specifically for running. Some designs are more suited to sprinting, providing a solid, quick release of energy return for short distance running. Other models are more appropriate for longer distance running. Transtibial athletes may choose a different type of foot than TF athletes due to the control provided by the anatomic knee. The socket must fit well, especially when the athlete participates in high-impact activities.

Closing Thoughts

Adaptive prostheses are leveling barriers to activity that once seemed firmly in place. Rather than discouraging people who wear prostheses from pursuing recreational activities, clinicians should encourage them to try adaptive prostheses and accessories. The achievements of outstanding athletes can inspire people who possess the health and the motivation to be active.

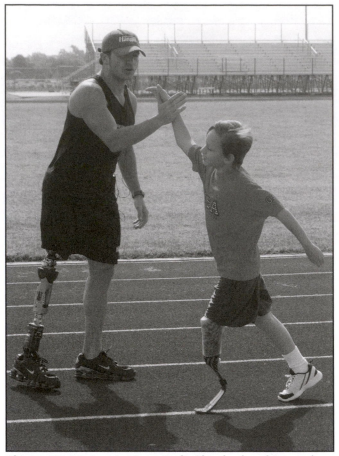

Figure 17-14. Inspiration. (Left) Shock absorbing pylon. (Right) Prosport foot.

References

1. Legro MW, Reiber GE, Czerniecki JM, Sangeorzan BJ. Recreational activities of lower-limb amputees with prostheses. *J Rehabil Res Dev*. 2001;38:319-325.

2. Bowers R. Encouraging the dream. *inMotion*. 2003;13:48-49.

3. US Department of Health and Human Services. *Healthy People 2010*. Available at: http://www.healthypeople.gov. Accessed January 2005.

4. Carroll K. Prosthetics and aging: mobility for the long run. *First Step: A Guide for Adapting to Limb Loss*. 2001;2:43-45.

5. Lehmann JF, Price R, Boswell-Bessette S, et al. Comprehensive analysis of energy storing prosthetic feet: Flex Foot and Seattle Foot versus standard SACH foot. *Arch Phys Med Rehabil*. 1993;74:1225-1231.

6. Trost F. Energy storing feet. *J Assoc Child Prosthet Orthot Clin*. 1989;24:82-85.

7. Dupes B. What you need to know about knees. *inMotion*. 2004;13:24-26.

8. Wiley G. Upper limb replacement. *Orthopaedic Technical Review*. 1999;1(3).

9. Atkins DJ, Heard D, Donovan W. Epidemiologic overview of individuals with upper-limb loss and their reported research priorities. *Journal of Prosthetics and Orthotics*. 1996;8:2-11.

10. Radocy B. Prosthetic adaptations in competitive sports and recreation. In: Smith DG, Michaels JW, Bowker JH. *Atlas of Amputations and Limb Deficiencies*. 3rd ed. Rosemont, Ill: American Academy of Orthopaedic Surgeons; 2004:327-338.

11. National Amputee Golf Association. History of NAGA. Available at: http://www.nagagolf.org. Accessed June 2004.

12. Kegel B. Adaptations for sports and recreation. In: Bowker JH, Michael JW, eds. *Atlas of Limb Prosthetics*. 2nd ed. St Louis, Mo: Mosby Year Book; 1992:623-654.

13. Vander Hoek M. Bike riding: Does limb difference make a difference? *inMotion*. 1999;9:12-14.

14. *The War Amputations*. Available at: http://www.waramps.ca. Accessed January 2005.

15. Bieze J. These athletes redefine "normal." *BioMechanics*. November 2003. Available at: http://www.biomech.com. Accessed January 2005.

16. Carroll K. Adaptive prosthetics for lower extremity amputees. *Foot Ankle Clin*. 2001;6:371-386.

17. Edwards A. Amputee spring records fall twice in June. BioMechanics. August 2003. Available at: http://www.biomech.com. Accessed January 2005.

Resources

ActiveAmp.org
PO Box 9315
Wilmington, DE 19809
1-302-683-0997
www.acitveamp.org

Adaptive Adventures
PO Box 2245
Evergreen, CO 80437
1-877-679-2770
www.adaptiveadventures.org

American Academy of Orthotists and Prosthetists
526 King Street, Suite 201
Alexandria, VA 22314
1-703-836-0788
www.oandp.org

American Amputee Hockey Association
www.amputeehockey.org

American Amputee Soccer Association
www.ampsoccer.org

American Orthotic and Prosthetic Association
330 John Carlyle Street, Suite 200
Alexandria, VA 22314
1-571-431-0876
www.aopanet.com

American Physical Therapy Association
1111 North Fairfax Street
Alexandria, VA 22314-1488
1-800-999-2782
www.apta.org

Amped Riders (skateboarding)
1-610-404-0824
www.ampedriders.com

Amputee Coalition of America
900 East Hill Avenue
Knoxville, TN 37915-2568
1-888-267-5669
www.amputee-coalition.org
Amputee Web Site
www.amputee-online.com

Canadian Amputee Hockey Association
www.canadianamputeehockey.ca

Canadian Association for Disabled Skiing
27 Beechwood Ave, Suite 310
Ottawa, ON K1M 1M2
1-613-842-5223
www.disabledskiing.ca

Challenged Athletes Foundation
2148-B Jimmy Durante Boulevard
Del Mar, CA 92014
1-858-793-9293
www.challengedathletes.org

Disabled Sports USA
451 Hungerford Drive, Suite 100
Rockville, MD 20850
1-301-217-0960
www.dsusa.org

Fishing Has No Boundaries Inc.
PO Box 175
Hayward, WI 54843
1-800-243-3462
www.fhnbinc.org

HP/HD HELP
Box 25033
Santa Anna, CA 92799
www.hphdhelp.org

International Paralympic Committee
Adenauerallee 212-214
53113 Bonn
Germany
+49-228-2097-0
www.paralympic.org

National Ability Center
PO Box 682799
Park City, UT 84068
1-435-649-3991
www.nac1985.org

National Amputee Golf Association
11 Walnut Hill Road
Amherst, NH 03031
www.nagagolf.org

National Sports Center for the Disabled
PO Box 1290
Winter Park, CO 80482
1-970-726-1540
www.nscd.org

One Arm Bandits Inc. (softball)
Victor Rosario: 1-305-266-4256
Patricia Bewsey: 1-561-791-1544
www.onearmbandits.com
O & P Edge (on-line magazine)
Western Media LLC
12910 Zuni Street, Suite 500
Westminster, CO 80234
1-866-613-0257
www.oandp.com

Spokes 'n Motion
2226 South Jason Street
Denver, CO 80223
1-303-922-0605
www.spokesnmotion.com

Todd Albaugh's Handicapped Hunting Resource Guide
4008 West Michigan Avenue
Jackson, MI 49202
1-517-343-4868
www.disabledhunting.net

USA Water Ski
1251 Holy Cow Road
Park City, FL 33868-8200
1-863-324-4341
www.usawaterski.org

US Adaptive Recreation Center
PO Box 2897
43101 Goldmine Drive
Big Bear Lake, CA 92315
1-909-584-0269
www.usarc.org/html/equipment.html

US Hand Cycling Federation
PO Box 3538
Evergreen, CO 80437
1-303-679-2770
www.ushf.org

US Paralympic – US Olympic Committee
One Olympic Plaza
Colorado Springs, CO 80909
1-719-866-2030
www.usparalympics.org

US Sled Hockey Association
2236 East 46th
Davenport, IA 52807
1-563-344-9064
www.usahockey.com

USA Swimming – Adapted Swimming Committee
1 Olympic Plaza
Colorado Springs, CO 80909
1-719-866-4578
www.usaswimming.org

War Amputations of Canada
1 Maybrook Drive
Scarborough, ON M1V 5K9
www.waramps.ca

MANUFACTURERS

Achievable Concepts
ABN. 66 093 173 552
PO Box 361
Moonee Ponds, 3039
Victoria, Australia
+(61) 3 9370 0217
www.achievableconcepts.us

Electric Fishing Reel Systems
PO Box 20411
Greensboro, NC 27420
1-336-273-9101
www.elec-tra-mate.com

Enabling Technologies Inc.
2225 South Platte River Drive
Denver, CO 80223-4017
1-303-936-0232

Endolite
105 West Park Road
Centerville, OH 45459
1-800-548-3534
www.endolite.com

Ferrier Coupler Inc.
3461 Burnside Road
North Branch, MI 48461
1-800-437-8597
www.ferrier.coupler.com

Hosmer Dorrance Corporation
561 Division Street
Campbell, CA 95008
1-408-379-5151
www.hosmer.com

Howell's Tackle Company
PO Box 5323
Emerald Isle, NC 28594
1-252-393-2311
www.howellstackle.com

Lacome Inc.
PO Box 77
Taos, NM 87571
1-505-758-5816
(snow skiing outriggers)

Motion Control. Inc.
2401 South 1070 West, Suite B
Salt Lake City, UT 84119
1-888-696-2767
www.utaharm.com

Mountain Man
720 Front Street
Bozeman, MT 59715
1-406-587-0310
(adaptive snow skiing)

Quickie Designs (formerly Magic in Motion)
20604 86th Avenue South
Kent, WA 98032-1224
1-800-342-1579
(Shadow mono ski)

Rampro
2021 Sheridan Road
Leucadia, CA 92024
1-800-4941404
www.rampro.net

Therapeutic Recreation Systems
3090 Sterling Circle, Studio A
Boulder, CO 80301
1-800-279-1865
www.oandp.com/products/trs/

XeroSox Products
6702 Netherlands Drive
Wilmington, NC 28405
1-888-XEROSOX
www.xerosox.com

Chapter 18

In the Future:
Prosthetic Advances and Challenges

Matthew A. Parente, PT, CPO; Mark Geil, PhD; Brian Monroe, CPO

OBJECTIVES

1. Introduce current and historical computer-aided design/computer-aided manufacture theories and designs
2. Relate developments in materials science to prosthetics
3. Examine the future role of external power sources, including battery and artificial muscle technology
4. Describe microprocessor controlled knee systems and research for future systems
5. Trace the development of modern concepts related to upper-limb prosthetics

INTRODUCTION

Prosthetics is a dynamic, continually evolving field. What research is on the horizon? How will insurance companies and other payment sources affect the field?

Prosthetics demonstrates amoeboid characteristics, in that it is ever changing. Although the fundamental principles of the field remain relatively invariate, some aspects use concepts from outside worlds. Once a new and potentially beneficial idea is identified, it may be integrated into the field. One example is the striking similarity between the cable used in bicycles and in upper-limb body-powered systems. Another illustration is the microprocessor, which was part of computers long before it was used to control a prosthetic knee unit. When concepts are "borrowed," they usually create possibilities far beyond their original use.

The central nervous system displays two possibilities for the future of prosthetics. The first is the principle of convergence, demonstrated by the motor pathways. Convergence enables diverse information from many sources to be organized and delivered to a single target.[1] Does the possibility exist where the fields of prosthetics, orthotics, physical therapy, and other disciplines bond to form a single entity? A more likely scenario would be a transition away from specialization within the field, evolving into an "off-the-shelf" environment, allowing practitioners to simplify the prosthetic experience.[2]

The opposite of convergence is divergence, observed primarily by sensory pathways. A single bit of information can be distributed simultaneously to many targets.[1] The analogy with prosthetics is clear—continued specialization within segments of the field. The potential benefits of having individuals and companies specialize in a single aspect of prosthetic treatment should ensure a high level of expertise regarding that component. A potential drawback would be that a patient might require several experts to create a suitable prosthesis.

The goal of prosthetic design is to mimic some aspect of a functional limb. The prosthesis has the daunting task of enabling movement with efficiency similar to that of the human body.

Prostheses combine plastics, alloys, carbon, and a wide variety of other materials. These materials can improve the way prosthesis wearers function. Likewise, better ways of fabricating prostheses and innovations in components of upper- and lower-limb prostheses can also help some people achieve a more satisfying life style. The motivation for improving prostheses is asking ourselves, "How do I make this device _____?" Fill in the blank for yourself, but potential answers include smaller, lighter, stronger, faster, easier, and better.

CAD/CAM

Computer-aided design (CAD) and computer-aided manufacture (CAM) are technologies used in many applications to, quite simply, make things. In its most basic application, a designer can use a computer to draw the shape of an object. Let's say it's a cell-phone housing. Once the shape is satisfactory, the computer communicates the shape directly to a machine that builds a prototype of the cell phone housing. The process is quick and efficient, and is used to make everything from tiny stents to airplanes.

The simple example understates the power of CAD/CAM. Modern CAD also enables analysis, so the designer can make sure the parts of the housing fit one another, view samples of the final outcome to determine the best surface colors and patterns, and even evaluate the potential for mechanical failure of the part using various materials, all before a single prototype has been made. CAM software checks the designer's work before the first cut, saving costly prototype failures, and can convert the shape to be manufactured in a wide variety of formats recognized by multiple machines.

CAD often starts with capturing an existing shape and importing that shape into the computer.[3] This process, called *digital shape capture*, is common in prosthetic applications. Once the shape is in the computer, modification can take place using CAD software. Several CAD programs have been customized for use in prosthetics and orthotics. The modification tools mirror those used in fabrication laboratories. Such tools include carving, filling, and adding or subtracting volume of the socket. The modified shape is then exported into a file format that can be used by the machine that will manufacture it (the CAM part).

In prosthetics, the shape that is captured is usually a patient's amputation limb. The prosthetics-tailored CAD software then displays a three-dimensional model of the limb so that the prosthetist can modify the shape to produce a well-fitting socket.

Certain socket designs, such as a transtibial patellar-tendon-bearing socket, require specific modifications that change the shape substantially in certain areas (eg, the patellar bar). The final modifications cause the shape to look more like a socket than an amputation limb. Trim lines and flares are added, an appropriate distal end is added from a library of shapes, and the entire shape is angled appropriately for manufacture. The part that is manufactured is usually not the socket, but a positive model of the modified amputation limb, which is in turn used to fabricate a socket by traditional methods.[4] In essence, the CAM-produced positive, usually made out of plastic foam, takes the place of the plaster positive model made from the traditional plaster cast method.

CAD/CAM function depends on mathematics. The quality of the resulting prototype socket depends markedly on the appropriate choice of CAD modeling.

Instructions sent for manufacturing to a computer numerical control (CNC) milling machine or a rapid prototyping machine also vary. Some file formats are long strings of numbers, with each line providing specific coordinates for a milling machine cut. The size of the file depends on the number and complexity of the cuts required.

One aspect of CAD/CAM has had a significant impact on the practice of prosthetics. Because the file produced by the CAD software is a simple digital computer file, and because it essentially contains all of the modifications that will be manufactured into the socket, the CAM step can occur in another geographic location and can be directed by someone other than the prosthetist. Consequently, central fabrication has become an effective means for prosthetists to produce sockets without the large overhead expense associated with CAM milling machines or a complete prosthetic fabrication laboratory. The process can be as simple as an e-mail sent to a central fabrication site with a CAD file attached. Of course, prosthetists must determine the method of capturing the shape and must develop relationships with central fabrication personnel to understand their file formats and manufacturing practices. Several companies have marketed their methods of digital shape capture. Although each method is distinctive, all accomplish a similar result.

The first system commercially available for prosthetic and orthotic use was produced by the VORUM Research Corporation (Vancouver, British Columbia). The creator, Carl Saunders, developed a comprehensive suite of CAD/CAM software and hardware called the CANFIT-PLUS Systems. This product line includes shape-scanning technology, design modification software, and CNC milling machines. The CANFIT scan-Gogh scanning and imaging system incorporates a hand-held, noncontact optical scanner, which can capture an image of almost any part of the body. The image is modified with the use of CANFIT Visual CAM software and design programs. Then the image is sent to a 4-axis CANFIT tabletop carver for milling. The system is completely proprietary, and therefore has great compatibility with its own devices.

The Ossur (Aliso Viejo, Calif) CAD/CAM system, previously CAPOD (Computer Aided Prosthetic and Orthotic Design), features similar components and objectives to the VORUM system. CAPOD was a recent acquisition of Ossur. This backing could provide the system with the support for continued research and design. The system itself consists of a portable Digital Free Scan, prosthetic workstation for transtibial and transfemoral scanning, and milling machines. Ossur CAD/CAM software is designed solely for the collection of Ossur products. This system also offers the ability for orthotic design applications, such as knee and spinal bracing.

Ohio Willow Wood (Mt Sterling, Ohio), a prosthetic supplier, also has designed a means of digital shape capture. The Omega system is used for digital shape capture, image modification, component selection, and online ordering. The Omega T-Ring captures limb shapes with the push of a button. The patient dons a mapping liner, and the prosthetist identifies landmarks for proper image acquisition. The T-ring is then placed around the limb for the "snapshot." The ring is centered with the use of a positional assist that is in contact with the distal end of the amputation limb. The system also offers the ability to capture an image with the use of the Omega Tracing Pen. The handheld pen is used to sweep over the patient's body part that is being imaged. The pen offers clinicians the ability to have contact with the patient, similar to the casting process. The system also incorporates a personal digital assistant (PDA) and computer software that allows for navigation throughout the system to modify the image and document the patient's information.

Hanger Orthopedic Group (Bethesda, Md) has also developed a hand-held digital capture system, called Insignia This unique undertaking is an attempt to develop a product solely for its certified practitioners. The Insignia system consists of a hand-held laser scanner, processing unit, modification software, and milling machines. Each component of the Insignia system was developed by Hanger, and is proprietary. The image capture is performed by the FastSCAN Cobra system. A wand creates a three-dimensional image when it is swept over the scanning surface. It automatically eliminates overlapping sweeps that would create redundant data.

Laser imaging and data acquisition systems are being used by the US Armed Services. The Insignia scanner uses two embedded motion sensors that allow the patient to move during the scanning process. This is a tremendous advantage for the practitioner who can now work with all types of patients, especially children. Once the image is obtained, it may be modified on a computer with the use of Hanger's Zander CAD. Zander enables the clinician to modify the image in a unique file format, OP3. This file allows the practitioner to modify the image across any axis. The overall benefits of the system include portability, speed, movement tracking, and a nationwide clinical support network. The Insignia system is supported by an extensive initial educational requirement and then supplemented by regional continuing education seminars.

Other methods of digital image capture and image modification programs are available. An advantage of using software for the modification process is the continuing ability to update information. New versions of the software deliver the most recent technology to the clinician. Research and development does not end with the initial launch of the product. Software updates indicate a company that understands the changing environment of technology.

HISTORY OF CAD/CAM

The C's in CAD and CAM imply that the technologies have their origins in the advent of computing. Computer-aided design was invented in 1963 by Ivan Sutherland, who designed a computer drawing program that used a light pen and an 8-inch monitor for his PhD dissertation at the Massachusetts Institute of Technology.[5] The first CAD programs were two-dimensional (2-D) drafting tools. Although the programs did essentially what a draftsman could do, CAD did guarantee a neat drawing. The power of CAD came from the leap beyond the flat pane of the computer monitor screen to three-dimensional (3-D). The 3-D CAD programs used in the early 1980s ran on workstations served by enormous mainframe computers. Manufacturing machines have been capable of running from pre-coded sets of instructions for decades, but the power to manufacture a 3-D object was dramatically improved when the object could be designed on a computer.

Because prosthetics and orthotics involve the design and manufacture of 3-D objects, often with customized modifications, the field is a natural application of CAD/CAM. A 1985 special issue of the *Prosthetics and Orthotics International* dealt with the then-emerging technologies. Authors compared the potential efficiency of digital techniques with traditional methods, proposing extraordinarily improved socket manufacturing rates.[6] Despite the early recognition of CAD's potential, most sockets fabricated today are created through manual casting and measurement methods. Nevertheless, an increasing number of prosthetics facilities throughout the United States use some type of CAD/CAM system.[7] At one point in the evolution of CAD/CAM, cast digitization was suggested as a hybrid of digital and manual techniques; however, this approach saved little time and most practitioners viewed the additional cost of CAD/CAM as unjustifiable.

Today, digital methods incorporating additional applications are used for socket fabrication. Digital systems can include prosthetic liners into a socket shape and can match cosmetic covers to the patient's skin tone. In orthotics, CAD/CAM has been used for design and production of insoles, shoe lasts, ankle-foot and knee-ankle-foot orthoses, spinal orthoses, the cervical orthoses, custom seating, and helmets for reduction of positional plagiocephaly. Applications involving the foot have taken longer to perfect due to the difficulty in digitally modeling complex anatomical shapes. Carl Saunders has stated that, "CAD/CAM for orthotics has evolved to the point where 'plaster-free,' efficient, high quality design and manufacture of most custom orthotic devices is a reality."[8]

An alternative technique avoids the digital shape capture step entirely. Instead, anthropometric measurements are taken from the amputation limb and a digital shape is produced by the software based in the library of standard limb shapes.[4] Modification and manufacture then continue as usual. This "by the numbers" approach is particularly appealing when digital shape capture is challenging or impossible (eg, short transfemoral amputation).

Shape-Capture Technologies

Two primary technologies represent the most commonly used systems for digital shape capture:
1. Electromagnetic-field based digitization
2. Optical-based measurement

Electromagnetic-field based digitization is a contact scanning system, in which the scanning device comes into direct contact with the patient's limb. Because a magnetic field has known spatial characteristics, a magnetic field emitter can produce a small grid of recognized coordinates. When a magnetic field sensor is positioned in that field, both its position within that grid and its 3-D orientation are constantly known.

Consequently, if the sensor is used to trace the surface of an amputation limb, the limb's 3-D shape can be captured and visualized in real time on a computer. Some practitioners like having direct patient contact, with the ability to introduce the same sorts of socket shape manipulations they would use if they were applying a plaster cast by applying varying amounts of pressure to the magnetic field sensor. The system requires the patient to remain relatively still for a few minutes while the limb is mapped,. Also, the technology requires a nonmetallic environment near the magnetic field emitter.

Optical-based measurement is a noncontact approach. Several systems exist. Light amplification by stimulated emission of radiation (LASER) scanning is widely used in general engineering industries for shape capture. In prosthetics, the shape of the limb is captured as a visible but harmless laser beam passes over the entire limb. Systems include fixed boxes into which a limb is placed and hand-held scanners. Other optical techniques involve camera/pattern systems and digital photo reconstruction. At least two images of an object are required to reconstruct the 3-D shape of that object. These systems use images from multiple viewpoints to capture the shape. Optical systems do not allow manual manipulation of the shape, but often do allow digitiza-

tion of landmarks if small marks are placed on the limb surface.

Increasingly, digital shape capture techniques are being complemented by large libraries of typical limb shapes and, for the proximal region of limbs, prosthetic socket brims. Some software manufacturers are allowing hybrid approaches to capture the shape of the residual limb. Hybrid approaches use digital shape capture of certain areas of the socket, such as the distal portion, where an accurate custom fit is important, and "by-the-numbers" scaling of reference shapes to form the proximal part of the socket.[9]

Outlook

CAD/CAM technology continues to advance. Yet, its clinical acceptance is less easy to quantify. It is instructive to compare the state of clinical opinion on CAD/CAM from over a decade ago to today. In 1993, Kristinsson wrote, "It is not considered that CAD has anything to offer yet besides documentation and ease of fabrication. This hopefully will change in the near future as the systems evolve."[10] In 2001, Smith and Burgess noted that, "The fabrication techniques that are currently being used with CAD/CAM systems are still rather traditional techniques. Most devices are still laminated or formed over computer-carved models."[4] Both statements suggested untapped potential of CAD/CAM technology. In its current state, CAD/CAM benefits the prosthetics and orthotics industry. It improves efficiency and has enabled the practice of central fabrication. Various CAD systems can make precise, reliable volume measurements of both simple geometric shapes and residual limb models[11,12] CAD/CAM is taking modern prosthetics throughout the world, representing a method for manufacturing cheap, reliable sockets in developing countries, as has been demonstrated in the Prosthetics Outreach Foundation's clinic in Hanoi, Vietnam.[13]

Research should explore underutilized qualities of CAD/CAM. Structural data obtained from digitization can be stored and used for more sophisticated structural analyses. Limb geometry data could be used as part of computational models to further the understanding of biomechanical forces translated from amputation limb via the socket to other prosthetic components during physical activity. It may be possible to use data from a digitized amputation limb to calculate an "ideal" socket design in real time.

An additional untapped advantage of CAD/CAM comes from the fact that the socket to be manufactured will eventually be coupled with prosthetic adapters and other components to form a complete prosthesis. Because the CAD-designed socket is already on the computer, this coupling can be planned on the computer with the appropriate software. Otto Bock has developed design software that allows the practitioner to plan component selection, heel height, and adapters. The software confirms that the chosen components will work together and suit the specific patient.

Finally, it seems inefficient to use CAD/CAM to design a socket and manufacture a positive model instead of a finished socket. With rapid prototyping technology, it should be possible to use CAM to produce a finished socket directly, avoiding the traditional step of forming a socket over a positive model. Researchers in Australia have produced sockets using Fused Deposition Modeling.[14] Lokhande and Crawford[15] have demonstrated a similar technique using Selective Laser Sintering. At Northwestern University the extrusion technique called "Squirt Shape" enables a socket to be directly manufactured by adding a continuous bead of molten plastic, layer upon layer in a spiral, until the entire socket is fabricated. Wall thickness is uniform, and favorable material properties have been documented.[16] Questions remain regarding the strength of sockets manufactured through rapid prototyping.[17] If these sockets prove to be durable and well-fitting, then rapid prototyping technologies could further improve the efficiency and long-term cost savings of CAD/CAM.

BATTERIES

In addition to a comfortable socket, an increasing number of upper- and lower-limb prostheses include externally powered components, as noted in Chapters 9 and 13. Power depends on battery technology. New batteries are smaller, lighter, and more powerful than older ones. The prosthetics industry has outgrown the household alkaline battery. Rechargeable batteries are a necessity for prostheses. The patient needs a battery that enables making the prosthesis operate through a whole day without recharging or replacing it.

Many types of batteries are on the market. Each has unique qualities. Deep Cycle Lead Acid batteries are inexpensive, reliable, and provide a relatively long life cycle, but also have a low energy density and pose several hazards.[18] Other fuel cell options, such as lithium ion, nickel-cadmium, and nickel metal hydrides, have been explored as replacements to the lead acid-based batteries.

Within the battery, the chemical reactions that produce energy involve many factors. Theoretically, one of the best cathode materials is hydrogen, but it is problematic as a material for batteries. At normal temperatures and pressures, hydrogen is difficult to manufacture into a battery cell due to its low atomic weight. In the late 1960s, scientists discovered that some metal alloys could store atomic hydrogen 1000 times their volume. These alloys, termed hydrides, are usually based on compounds such as $LiNi_5$ or $ZrNi_2$. In properly designed systems, hydrides can provide a storage sink of hydrogen that can reversibly react in battery cell chemistry.

The most common cells that use hydride cathodes use the nickel anodes from nickel-cadmium (NiCad) cell designs. They typically have an electrolyte of a diluted alkaline solution of potassium hydroxide. Substituting hydrides for cadmium in battery cells has several advantages, the most obvious being that such cells eliminate a major toxic material, cadmium. Without cadmium, cells should be free from the memory effect that plagues NiCad cells. Hydrogen, as a metal hydride, presents a 50% increase in storage density as compared with NiCad cells.

The primary drawback of cells based on nickel and metal hydrides, Ni-MH cells, is that most such cells have a substantially higher self-discharge rate than do NiCad cells. In many ways, NiMH cells are interchangeable with NiCads. They have a similar ability to supply high currents, although not quite as much as NiCads. NiMH cells also endure many charge/discharge cycles, typically up to 500 full cycles, but are not a match for NiCads.

Another battery for prostheses is the lithium ion. Lithium, the most chemically reactive metal, provides the basis for compact energy storage. Nearly all high-density storage systems use lithium because it has an inherent chemical advantage. Lithium is very reactive, and depending on the anode, cells with lithium cathodes can produce from 1.5 volts to 3.6 volts per cell, higher voltage than any other material. Lithium batteries offer a 50% higher storage density than nickel-metal hydride. Lithium-ion cells also lack the memory effect that plagued early NiCad cells. In general, current lithium cells also have a higher internal resistance than NiCad cells and consequently cannot deliver high currents. The life of lithium cells is more limited than that of nickel-based designs, although lithium-ion cells do withstand hundreds of charge/recharge cycles.

The major difficulty with lithium is that it is too reactive. It reacts violently with water and can ignite into flame. Batteries based on lithium metal were manufactured in the 1970s and in the 1980s, some companies introduced commercial rechargeable cells based on metallic lithium, quickly raising safety concerns. To prevent problems caused by reactive metallic lithium, battery makers modified their designs to keep the lithium in its ionic state. In this state, they were able to reap the electrochemical benefits of lithium-based cells without the safety issues associated with the pure metal.

One of today's newest battery technologies is a refinement of lithium chemistry called the lithium solid polymer cell. Conventional lithium ion cells require liquid electrolytes, but solid polymer cells integrate the electrolyte into a polymer plastic separator between the anode and cathode of the cell. As an electrolyte, lithium polymer cells use a polymer composite such as polyacrylonitrile containing a lithium salt. Because there is no liquid, the solid polymer cell does not require the large cylindrical cases of conventional batteries. Instead, the solid polymer cells can be formed into flat sheets to fit the contours of many surfaces. Manufacturers have identified the shape configuration that utilizes all of the space within the cell, providing it with an approximate 22% greater energy-carrying capacity. Solid polymer batteries are environmentally friendly, lighter because they have no metal shell, and safer because they contain no flammable solvent.

Possibly, the power cell of the future may be the zinc-air battery. This battery offers the most dense energy storage capacity because one component of its chemical reaction is external to the battery, namely atmospheric oxygen. Air is its cathode reactant. Small holes in the battery casing admit air to react with a powered zinc anode through a highly conductive potassium hydroxide electrolyte. This may complicate prosthetic design. Zinc-air batteries have long stable storage life, at least when kept sealed from the air and thus inactive. A sealed zinc-air cell loses only 2% of its capacity after 1 year of storage. Once air infiltrates the cell, zinc-air non-rechargeable cells last only for a few months, whether under discharge or not. Some battery makers have adapted zinc-air technology to be rechargeable. The cells work best when frequently or continuously used in low-drain situations. The primary drawback of zinc-air batteries is their high internal resistance. The prosthesis would need a large battery to overcome the internal resistance, making it unrealistic at the present time.

Ideally, manufacturers would be able to provide consumers with a lightweight, inexpensive, flexible, rechargeable, high energy, safe, and reliable battery solution. As the history has shown, the solution may not be initially designed for prostheses.

MATERIALS

Regardless of whether the prosthesis is externally or body-powered, it is made of several materials selected for their strength, durability, appearance, and ease of fabrication. Some of the most promising developments are in the realm of materials science. Laymen may recall a high-profile patient they saw on television wearing a new type of prosthesis. The prosthesis is usually described as futuristic with space-age materials and technology. In fact, most materials have been used in prostheses for years, although the prosthetic community is still investigating new ways to use familiar materials as well as seeking unconventional ones. Of course, we want the public to notice our patients who run and jump with their prostheses. We should also take pride in patients who go unnoticed during their everyday lives. New materials permit both scenarios.

Wood, metal, and leather have been supplanted or complemented by the use of composite materials, carbon fibers, and plastics.

Biomaterials are a subgroup of materials that interface with the body, usually as internal prostheses. Both internal and external prosthetic devices are regulated by the Food and Drug Administration (FDA). The FDA requires strict testing and design qualifications for each product before it is given approval for interaction with the American consumer. Materials for internal devices must be nontoxic, biologically and chemically stable, and have the mechanical integrity to withstand physiological loads.[19] Ceramics, metals, polymers, glasses, composites, and natural materials, such as lipids, enzymes, and proteins, all must collectively maintain the safe and stable properties of internal prostheses.

Composite materials are a new class of biomaterials.[19] Various materials can be combined to create a structural matrix so the prosthesis can be stronger and lighter. Decreased weight contributes to decrease the amount of shear on the skin inside the socket. Theoretically, the primary benefit of using newer materials would be decreased energy costs during activities. Energy consumption is often the limiting factor determining the patient's overall lifestyle. An untapped area for research is relating prosthetic weight to energy consumption.

Nature provides a blueprint for success. The goal of a composite material is to maintain a high strength-to-weight ratio, similar to bone. Bony tissue is a composite of compact and spongy constituents. Compact bone consists of closely packed osteons. The osteon consists of a central canal called the osteonic (Haversian) canal, surrounded by concentric rings (lamellae) of matrix. Between the rings of matrix, the bone cells (osteocytes) are located in spaces called lacunae. Small channels (canaliculi) radiate from the lacunae to the osteonic (Haversian) canal to provide passageways through the hard matrix. Compact bone has Haversian systems packed tightly to form a solid mass. The osteonic canals contain blood vessels that are parallel to the long axis of the bone. Vessels interconnect, by way of perforating canals, with vessels on the surface of the bone.

Spongy (cancellous) bone is lighter and less dense. It consists of plates (trabeculae) and bars of bone adjacent to small, irregular cavities that contain red bone marrow. The canaliculi connect to the adjacent cavities, instead of a central Haversian canal, to receive blood supply. Trabeculae are arranged to provide maximum strength by following the lines of stress and can realign if the direction of stress changes.

Composites consist of fibrous materials that form a matrix similar to bone. The matrix allows the fibers to function collectively throughout the material, so that force can be distributed throughout the material. Polymers, ceramics, and metals are common matrix materials. They achieve their mechanical properties according to the manner in which they are placed within the material they are reinforcing. Reinforced fabrics demonstrate how weave patterns of the reinforcement affect the overall function of the material. Reinforcing fibers are chosen according to the intended function of the composite material. They are available in woven, chopped, and continuous strand forms. Glass fiber is the most frequently used reinforcing agent in prosthetics. Carbon fibers possess the best combination of high strength and stiffness, and aramid fibers demonstrate lightweight properties and stiffness.[19]

Biomaterials are generally classified according to the tissue response they induce,[20] namely inert, bioresorbable, or bioactive. Inert materials, such as titanium, are almost chemically inert inside the body and have minimal chemical interaction with surrounding tissue. Inert implants are fixated via bone cement, surface irregularities, or press fitting into a defect. These fixation methods are not ideal for long-term durability, and thus are usually considered a temporary solution.

Implant fixation remains one of the largest hurdles for surgeons and researchers. In 2003, Thomas Webster and a postdoctoral researcher from Purdue University presented research that could change the field of internal prosthetic devices and biomaterials. They proved that bone cells attach better to metals with nanometer-scale surface features called nanobumps.[21] The surface of conventional titanium alloys used for internal prostheses possesses irregularities that can be measured in microns, or millionths of a meter. Natural bone has a much rougher surface with bumps approximately 100 nanometers wide. Osteoblast cell production increased 60% when exposed to nanobumps versus the same alloy with micron-sized bumps.

Inert implants demonstrate relatively poor long-term success, whereas bioresorbable materials provide a possible alternative. They are designed to be slowly replaced by biological tissue, such as bone. Gradual replacement allows the body to heal gradually until the entire fixation area is biological tissue. Also, they seem to offer greater strength of bond, with fewer revision surgeries. The future may see the process of replacing biological tissues with biomaterials and eventually replacing biomaterials with bionic limbs.

Bioactive materials are synthetic implants, which can connect to the body directly and elicit a reaction from human tissue. These materials form a chemical bond with tissues, primarily bone, thus creating a strong bond. Certain glasses, ceramics, and glass-ceramics that contain oxides of silicone, sodium, calcium, and phosphorus form a chemical bone with bone.[20] These materials may be the link to wider use of osseointegration, as described in Chapter 19. Several problems must be solved prior to widespread use of ceramics and glass bioactive materials, which have a relatively low load-carrying capacity. Ceramics that are crystalline in structure add strength to bioactive materials, but decrease the bioactivity of the implant.

As bionics and biointegrated materials develop, new prosthetic components will be needed to make best use of them. Product development received a tremendous boost from a process called 3-D nonlinear finite element analysis, which models material stresses and predicts failure throughout complex multi-planar applications. This process, also known as Computerized Prosthetic Modeling, was developed at the Lawrence Livermore National Laboratory.[22] In the past, finite element analysis of prosthetic implants was performed in 2-D (linear) relationships, which eliminated the ability to test such implant materials as polyethylene, which has nonlinear stress-strain properties. Common reasons for failure of the implant include material failure below the articular surfaces, aseptic loosening at the bone-implant interface, and periprosthetic fractures.[22] Each problem happens below the articulating surface of the implant, and is inadequately modeled in 2-D analysis. Three-dimensional computerized prosthetic modeling can predict far more accurately than 2-D analysis.

Internal prostheses are designed to complement joint kinematics to prevent implant wear, bone fractures, and soft tissue deformation.[22] Computer analysis of the joint is necessary to understand the wear pattern of the natural tissues and biomaterials. An internal prosthesis presents several factors that must be considered, including the material properties of the implant, arthrokinematics and neuromuscular control of the joint and limb, and implant design. All factors are necessary for accurate computer modeling.

A new class of organic composites has begun to ignite interest from researchers at Pennsylvania State University. Electroactive polymers have traditionally required a large amount of energy to function, but a new polymer reduces that value by 90%.[23] One organic composite possesses a high dielectric constant dispersed in an electrostrictive polymer matrix. The composite demonstrates much improved properties for manufacturers of actuators.[23] Current applications, such as artificial muscle, tendons, and flexible skin," make the electroactive polymer an attractive material for future studies. The flexibility of the material and its low-voltage operating capacity make it a potential material for prostheses.

Another promising innovation is compliant mechanisms technology, which consists primarily of a series of braided stainless steel cables. Materials properties are based on cable size, length, and configuration, which determine the stiffness and control of rotation about a specific axis.[24] The technology was initiated at the NASA Goddard Space and Flight Center in Greenbelt, Maryland, and has been applied to robotics and prosthetics. The technology is based on the smooth transference of forces between bodies, similar to the function of a tendon. Compliant cable mechanisms are flexible, lightweight, structurally sound, and cost effective, and offer vibration dampening and shock absorption throughout the entire cable.[24] The technology allows structural stiffness during primary planar motion and subtle transitory movements such as twisting.[25] The combination of stability and mobility offered by this technology might lend itself to prosthetic joint design.

Smart memory alloys (SMAs) are being explored for their potential benefits to the field of prosthetics. They are a class of metals demonstrating the abilities of pseudoelasticity and a shape memory effect.[26] Initially observed by Arne Olander in 1938, SMAs made limited progress until the 1960s. Smart metal alloys reemerged on the research front in aeronautics, surgery, and robotics. Smart metal alloys can be deformed and then returned to their initial configuration with the aid of a stimulus. The stimulus may be a temperature change, mechanical traction, or electrical shock. When the SMA is activated by temperature changes, patterns of shape are predictable. The initial shape of the object is changed by heating the alloy, and then it returns to the initial shape when cooled. The stable state when the alloy is at its low temperature phase is called martensite, and it is called austenite when it is at its high temperature stable state.[27] Manufacturing an SMA product begins at its low temperature or martensite form. When it is heated, the atoms become compact and assume a regular pattern. Finally, when the material is cooled it reverts to its former shape. The alloy object can have separate shapes depending on its temperature.

Smart metal alloys have many medical applications. The most popular SMA is nickel-titanium, also known as Nitinol, which has significant biocapability.[27] The Simon Nitinol filter has been used since the 1970s. The cooled device is inserted into the vena cava. Body heat causes the filter to expand into an umbrella-shaped filter, which traps blood clots.[28]

Smart metal alloys demonstrate elasticity. Nitinol returns to its initial shape after having a force applied to it. Materials lacking this ability, such as stainless steel, deform and could be hazardous depending on the intended function of the device. Maintaining temperature of a Nitinol device allows it to demonstrate its elastic property. Load may be applied to the device to cause deformation, but when the load is removed the device returns to its initial shape without changing the structure at the atomic level.

Another medical application of SMAs is the Mitek suture, an anchor used to attach tendons, ligaments, and other soft tissues to bone.[27] The anchor is inserted into the bone and then, as the temperature rises, it expands to form a tight bond with the surrounding bone. Smart metal alloys contribute to fracture management via contraction of a Nitinol plate. The plate is fixated around the fracture site with bone screws. As the plate increases temperature, it contracts to compress the fracture site. Smart metal alloys may be able to benefit people with amputation by managing heterotopic ossification and facilitating osseointegration fixation.

Fabrics

Fabric science is a fast growing aspect of materials, with new fabrics being adapted for prostheses. Coolmax fabrics wick moisture from the body. The moisture crosses to the outside surface where it is carried away by the air by convection, reducing the possibility of skin maceration. This is the same process the body uses to dissipate heat into the environment for cooling.[29] Coolmax (Invista, Wichita, Kan) fabrics use proprietary polyester fibers with microchannel cross sections or two-sided, gradient fabrics, or both. The comfort of Coolmax fabrics can be enhanced by using elasterell-p or introducing Lycra (Invista) elastane. Coolmax is fast drying and resists fading, shrinking, and wrinkling.

Winston Churchill said, "Those that fail to learn from history are doomed to repeat it." One "new" product, which has tremendous therapeutic value, is silver. The precious metal has been used for its medicinal value since ancient Rome. It is widely used for its antibacterial properties in medication, water purification, and wound dressings.[30] A small Pennsylvania company, Noble Fiber Technologies (Summit, Pa), has introduced a product that incorporates silver into textiles. Noble developed a process to permanently adhere pure silver to a basic textile, which allows the fabric to take on the chemical properties of silver. The fabric, X-Static, is used in athletics and by the Department of Defense. Its antimicrobial qualities reduce odor-causing bacteria. Products made with X-Static fibers are nontoxic and have all of the therapeutic benefits of silver. X-Static is used in prosthetic socks and shrinkers, as well as in ordinary socks and undergarments.

Traditionally, fabrics have been used for their flexibility and comfort. Strength has now become another major factor in the selection of fabrics. Materials with a higher strength-to-weight ratio are particularly prized in prosthetics. Kevlar (DuPont, Wilmington, Del), fiberglass, and carbon in woven form allow clinicians to reinforce laminations while maintaining the shape of the socket. The resulting prosthesis is lighter and stronger than its predecessors.

Research and development of biomaterials continues despite lawsuits against manufacturers, health care reform, and FDA guidelines. Several materials suppliers and implant manufacturers have refused to allow their products to be used for medical applications because of such suits.[19] Manufacturers of external prosthetic products also must comply with FDA regulations, which are different from those pertaining to internal devices and biomaterials. Regulations are intended to protect patients from the initial stages of design through the release of the product to the market. The FDA will either continue to apply existing regulations or promulgate new regulations for future developments such as neuro-controlled prostheses and biointegrated materials.

Historically, prosthetists have relied on nature for wooden prostheses. Today most prosthetic suppliers have discontinued wood-based components. Continued developments in materials technology should allow prosthetists to bring new materials to their patients. Although the prosthetic design will always be based on nature, the delivery of the design is increasingly reliant on material science.

LOWER-LIMB PROSTHETICS

Of all the components of lower-limb prostheses, the future for knee units looks especially bright. Since ancient times the primary role of the prosthetic knee has been based on function of the human knee. Even with newer materials, replicating the function of the knee joint is formidable. The anatomical knee joint is a double condyloid joint with two degrees of freedom. The motions of flexion and extension occur in the sagittal plane whereas internal and external rotation occur in the transverse plane.[31] The multiplanar motion of the knee contributes to the difficulties designing a prosthetic knee. Virtually all current prosthetic knee designs maximize the flexion and extension aspects of motion and minimize or eliminate the translation and rotational components.

The predominant knee designs are based on function, except for a purely cosmetic prosthesis. The knee must balance the mix of stability and mobility appropriate to the individual wearer. Stability and mobility have traditionally worked on a continuum with respect to mechanical design. An increase of mobility correlates to a decrease of mechanical stability. Therefore, stability comes from the patient's voluntary control of the prosthesis, from alignment stability added to the design by the prosthetist, and from the attributes of the knee unit. Understanding how the patient's muscular coordination interacts with the knee unit allows the prosthetist to customize stability and mobility.

Stability and mobility of the prosthetic knee reflect the static and dynamic principles of functional activity. Throughout the gait cycle the human knee provides the lower limb with periods of functional shortening and lengthening. During closed kinetic chain activities in stance phase, the ankle, knee, and hip maintain the lower limb in a functionally lengthened position to keep the body in a stable, upright position. The opposite effect is demonstrated during open chain activities in swing phase when lower-limb joints facilitate mobility by functionally shortening the limb. Shortening allows the body to transfer weight efficiently and conserve energy during walking. The combination of tasks demonstrates the difficulty of replicating the human knee.

Recognition of a deficiency in design is the first step towards the development of an alternative solution. Using modern technology, several manufacturers claim to offer the "knee of tomorrow." These units address problems associated with traditional knee units. The mechanical knee was combined with fluid dynamic mechanisms and microprocessor control to bring the "first wave" of microprocessor-controlled knee units to the United States.

Although microprocessor technology was not invented to improve gait, it has been adapted to do so. The technology allows manufacturers to address problems that occur during walking at variable cadences. Traditional knee units, especially those that incorporate sliding friction, respond to one variable, usually the knee extension moment. Microprocessor-controlled knees can monitor and adjust multiple variables depending on the programming of the knee unit.[32] A microprocessor in the knee unit provides the opportunity to attempt to duplicate the hundreds of adjustments the human body makes every step.

Manufacturers have created a competitive marketplace for the microprocessor-controlled knee. Competition drives product research and development to improve products and explore new alternatives. This benefits patients and clinicians by providing advanced technology that may simulate the function of the human knee more closely. Industry and manufacturers evolve science fiction into science fact. The basic principle that continues to surface is the desire to mimic the natural operating system. Just as cavemen used animal skins for protection from the elements and warmth and Leonardo Da Vinci modeled the first "helicopter" from the wing motion of insects, researchers are attempting to pattern their products toward biological design, also known as bionics. The founding principle of bionics is the understanding of biological design to imitate natural models. Human bionics integrates a mechatronic apparatus within the human body, using electronic, informatic, and mechanical technologies to compensate for various physiological or anatomical dysfunctions.[33] Melding bionics and prosthetics should facilitate advances in patient care and enhance patient functional levels.

Manufacturers of new knee units share several characteristics. Each company offers additional training for their product; one even requires certification training before the clinician can order their product, thus maximizing the likelihood of success with the knee unit. Another shared quality is continued product development. Constant feedback from clinicians, positive and negative, reinforces existing designs or fuels change in the structure of the unit. Product development is based on practitioner feedback combined with ongoing company research, maintaining a "checks and balances" approach between practitioners and manufacturers to increase the chance that patients' needs will be met.

Otto Bock Health Care (Minneapolis, Minn) was the first company to introduce microprocessor technology to the United States in 1999 with the C-Leg (Figure 18-1). The company's vision was to provide patients with the closest approximation of natural movement. Otto Bock combined a microprocessor-controlled knee, sensor pylon, dynamic foot, and a servo motor. The system continuously monitors the patient's movements and automatically makes adjustments based on the information.

The microprocessor control of the C-Leg is based on gait analysis and other biomechanical research. The electronic system monitors movements at a rate of 50 times per second. Electronic sensors collect real-time data for immediate adjustment of the prosthesis to changes in walking speed. Real-time gait analysis control is the process of sampling sensory input from knee flexion angle sensors, processing the data through the software algorithm, and creating an output or control signal to adjust resistance through an actuator mechanism or control device. The unit controls swing phase angle and velocity and the direction of the moment created at the knee.

Stance phase stability is managed by data from force sensors in the shin. Heel, toe, and axial loading data determine stance stability adjustments that affect the prosthesis when the wearer ambulates on level and uneven terrain, ramps, and stairs. The C-Leg adjusts automatically to varying walking speeds via the hydraulic valves inside the knee unit. A flexion valve is fully opened at pre-swing for easier control even at slow speeds. Rapid walking causes the valve to be almost completely closed, which increases the dampening force. Flexion and extension valves control stance phase stability and swing phase mobility, together with a high-speed servo-motor, advanced software, and precise sensors. The motor is powered by a lithium-ion battery that functions between 25 and 30 hours before needing to be recharged. The microprocessor provides increased stance stability at initial contact. Suppression of unwanted knee flexion enhances patient confidence in the prosthesis, thus optimizing function.[33]

Magnetic sensors collect knee angle data and pressure sensors report the rate of heel strikes. The sensors provide feedback so the patient can vary walking speed, navigate uneven terrain, and compensate for slopes without actively manipulating the knee unit or altering gait. All adjustments of the system are controlled from the software algorithms used to determine the phase of gait or motion detected by the sensors.

Otto Bock claims that the C-Leg is appropriate for a wide range of patients. The "ideal" candidate for the C-Leg weighs less than 225 pounds and has a K2 or higher functional level. This includes people who are extremely active, as well as those who require additional stance control.

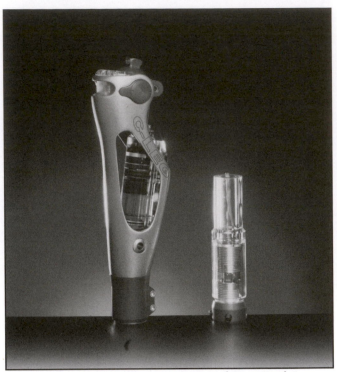

Figure 18-1. C-Leg. (Photo courtesy of Otto Bock.)

Endolite (Blatchford, Hampshire, UK) has also established itself as a leader in microprocessor-controlled knees. The Intelligent Prosthesis (IP), introduced in the European market, was the first microprocessor-controlled knee to be commercially released. Endolite now offers the IP Plus to the North American market. The IP Plus is designed to adjust automatically to the rate of swing of the prosthetic knee to match the user's walking speed. Changes to the knee settings are accomplished by a cordless handheld remote control with audio feedback. The remote control can adjust to slow, normal, and fast walking speeds. The three measured speeds automatically produce five settings for a smooth transition across the full range of walking speeds. The IP Plus has pneumatically controlled swing phase, which provides constant data input to the microprocessor to accommodate to the patient's cadence. Terminal swing phase is controlled by the microprocessor and a knee extension dampener. The dampener is automatically adjusted according to the information provided from a proximity switch to accommodate walking speed.[34] The knee unit also has a weight-activated brake mechanism for stance control and a stance-flex feature to reduce shock at heel strike.

The third generation of microprocessor-controlled Endolite knees, the Adaptive knee (Figure 18-2), incorporates many design principles of the IP Plus, such as the microprocessor, pneumatics, stance-flex, and a wireless remote programmer. The microprocessor on the Adaptive knee interprets feedback from the envi-

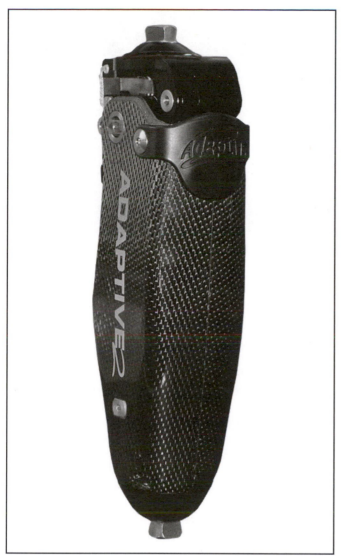

Figure 18-2. Adaptive2 Knee by Endolite. (Courtesy of Endolite.)

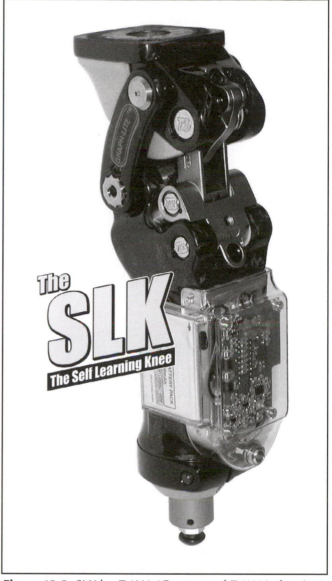

Figure 18-3. SLK by DAW. (Courtesy of DAW Industries.)

ronment, and has additional programs to make stairs, slopes, and uneven terrain more manageable. Sensors provide real-time feedback about time, force, and swing to the microprocessor at a rate of 62.5 times per second.[35] Stance phase stability is adjusted hydraulically.

Wireless programming allows the prosthetist to customize Adaptive knee features, such as variable cadence, ramps, stairs, and stumble recovery. The microprocessor can record information about the patient's walking habits, including level terrain, ramps, stairs, and stumbles.

The Self Learning Knee (SLK) (Figure 18-3) is DAW Industries' (San Diego, Calif) microprocessor-controlled knee unit that uses "blank slate technology." The unit is programmed with normal parameters of gait as its baseline. The microprocessor gathers data to modify the basic gait pattern to accommodate to the patient's unique walking style, thus the self-learning feature.

Data are collected via sensors reading the position of a magnet embedded in the knee cap. This is technology's simulation of proprioception by positional awareness of the magnet. Initially, the knee learns the fastest and slowest gait patterns of the patient, and then formulates 11 gait categories. The categories allow a smooth transition between walking speeds and continuously adjusts as the wearer changes cadence.

The SLK has a stance flexion feature to automatically adjust slight knee flexion between heel strike and mid stance. This attribute helps imitate the natural flexion of a sound knee during early stance phase. The variable cadence feature of the SLK has both pneumatic and hydraulic controls, which are adjusted by the microprocessor throughout swing phase.

The Rheo knee (Figure 18-4) is Ossur's entry into the microprocessor-controlled knee market. This

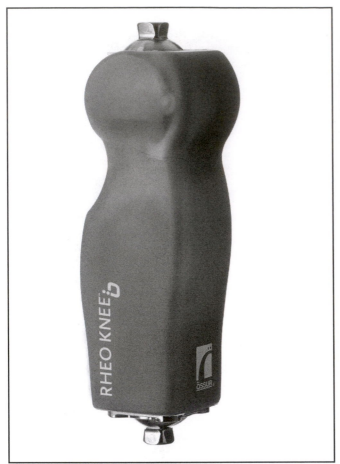

Figure 18-4. Rheo knee. (Photo courtesy of Ossur.)

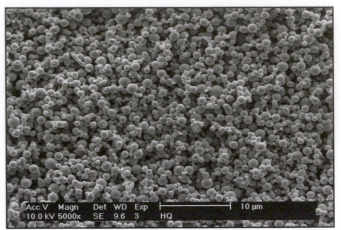

Figure 18-5. MR fluid. (Photo courtesy of Ossur.)

knee resulted from collaboration of Ossur and Hugh Herr from the Artificial Intelligence Laboratory at the Massachusetts Institute of Technology. They developed "mechatronix," which is the combination of mechanical engineering with electronics and intelligent computer controls. Their goals were to enhance dynamic appearance, decrease the metabolic cost of gait, and provide shock absorption.[36] They produced a knee system with intelligent swing and stance control that provides appropriate resistance to flexion and extension through the use of a microprocessor, computer software, integrated sensors, and a magnetorheologic (MR) fluid actuator.

The Rheo knee's microprocessor-controlled swing phase adjusts to the user's velocity at a rate of 1000 times per second by sampling speed and position of the knee. This allows automatic identification of any walking speed changes and updates flexion and extension values throughout swing phase. Stance phase is controlled by the microprocessor, but can also be adjusted manually with the use of the Hewlett Packard (HP) iPAQ PDA (Paolo Alto, Calif). The microprocessor adjusts stance flexion and extension resistance based on the position, load, and velocity of the knee, so that the

wearer can be secure on a variety of surfaces including ramps and uneven terrain. Stability is also maintained automatically by the stumble recovery feature if the wearer has a sudden unwanted change in position or load.

Adjustable stance flexion resistance accommodates to the ground reaction forces placed on the prosthesis. These forces vary according to the walking speed and weight of the wearer. This feature is active during the loading response phase of gait. The stance flexion feature differs from the adjustable stance extension feature, which is active during both loading response and mid-stance phases. The stance extension dampens the ground reaction forces and also allows the wearer to use a step-over-step pattern to ascend stairs.

Smooth operation of this knee unit comes from the MR actuator. Inside the unit, magnetized fluid (Figure 18-5) provides frictional resistance to flexion and extension according to the data provided to the microprocessor. A distinct advantage of the magnetic fluid is its zero pressure actuator, which has a long unit lifespan and decreased maintenance compared to pressurized microprocessor units. A proximal position of the moment of inertia for the MR actuator provides the wearer with more control of the unit when compared to a distal position. Regardless of the length of the amputation limb, a shorter lever arm decreases the perception of weight of the knee unit and the prosthesis.

The Rheo knee incorporates its sensors into the knee frame to decrease the risk of receiving faulty data if the pylon were to become misaligned or from setup errors. Four force and angle sensors are integrated anteriorly and posteriorly into the aluminum knee frame. The sensors detect the load applied to the prosthesis and the distribution of the load to determine torque values, which allow the microprocessor to determine appropriate swing and stance resistance values. The integrated sensor system also accommodates a wide variety of foot options including the high-profile J-shaped foot designs. The combination of Ossur's technology sensing at a rate of 1000 cycles per second, and the MR actuator acting at a rate of 1000 times per second, results in smooth gait dynamics and decreased energy costs.[37] The Rheo samples approximately 1200 times during a normal 1.2 second gait cycle. This allows for optimal coordination between swing and stance controls throughout the gait cycle.

The overall function of the Rheo knee is controlled by Ossur's control software, known as the Dynamic Learning Matrix Algorithm (DLMA). It is the real-time, on-board, continuous gait feature that allows the knee to detect and automatically accommodate to the wearer's gait characteristics without additional external programming.[37] The control software provides the Rheo knee with the ability to self-program initial swing and stance control parameters through "floating" parameters of gait established within a conventional linear control system. These parameters are maintained in a matrix that is unique to each patient. The system continually monitors kinematic and kinetic parameters and adjusts the dampening values within the matrix. The software results in faster accommodation between the user and the knee unit. The established matrix can also be modified at any time by the prosthetist for fine tuning of the knee unit.

Manual adjustments and monitoring of the Rheo can be accomplished with the HP iPAQ PDA. It offers manual and automatic programming features for determining the swing and stance controls. The initial programming is completed in the "Setup" mode. The unit self-calibrates during this mode to establish baseline data for operation. The "Manual" mode allows the prosthetist to fine tune swing and stance control parameters. The PDA can also monitor the state of the lithium-ion battery. With a 5400 mAh capacity, the battery can hold a charge for up to 48 hours depending on the wearer's activity. The battery requires 3 to 4 hours of charging time using home and automobile charging accessories.

Building on their successful partnership with Hugh Herr and the Artificial Intelligence Laboratory, Ossur joined with the Canadian company Victhom to delve into the field of bionics. Victhom (Saint Augustin de-Desmaures, Quebec, Canada) and Ossur presented their prototype bionic knee based on the vision of Stephane Bedard. Following the biological model of control systems, Bedard recognized that to truly meet the needs of people with amputations he would have to develop bidirectional interaction between patient and prosthesis. His work created an active autonomous system, instead of a passive mechanism, that provides active flexion and extension for the patient. The decreased energy costs should allow the patient to walk more smoothly for a longer time.[38] The Victhom system

uses sensors in the shoes to provide feedback to the microprocessor to generate the appropriate values for the patient's activity. The constant stream of information dictates the amount of power generated by a small motor in the "Power Knee" to replace the function of amputated muscles.[39]

The use of motors to replace amputated muscles has been successful for decades to treat people who wear upper-limb prostheses. Now it appears possible that this technology will be able to help people with lower limb amputations. Victhom also continues its research and development on a motorized ankle, artificial muscles, and a neuro implant to replace the bionic leg's external sensors.[40]

The Prolite Smart Magnetic knee also uses MR technology. This knee was created through the combined efforts of German-based Biedermann OT Vertrieb and the Lord Corporation located in Cary, North Carolina. Civil engineers explored the possibility of controlling undesirable motion with the use of a semi-active vibration control device.[41] Magnetorheologic fluid dampers are semi-active control systems due to their high force capacity, low power requirements, minimal cost, and mechanical simplicity.[42] Following successful use of MR technology to limit unwanted movements with bridges, researchers concluded that MR fluid dampers can be miniaturized for prostheses. The Lord Corporation applied the technology to other products such as real-time vibration control seating systems, adjustable MR fluid shock absorbers and braking systems, as well as the Prolite Smart Magnetix knee unit.[43-45]

The Prolite system uses an MR fluid damper to control knee flexion and extension resistance. Similar to other microprocessor-controlled knee units, the Prolite knee offers a smoother gait at less energy cost than traditional knee units. A powerful 2-day battery derived from cell phone battery technology powers the knee.[35] The sensors and control systems, developed by Biedermann, adjust to movement within a millisecond, enhancing the patient's ability to perform many activities. The Lord Corporation is exploring other prosthetic applications for MR technology, such as ankle joints, elbow joints, and rehabilitation equipment.[35]

Another cooperative effort to develop a "smart" leg is taking place between the Department of Energy's Sandia National Laboratories (Albuquerque, NM), Seattle Orthopaedic Group (Poulsbo, Wash), and Chelyabinsk 70 (Russia). Each organization brings a high level of expertise from their field to the project. A project of this size demonstrates how government agencies and independent companies can work together for the betterment of mankind. The final result of their efforts will result in the Smart Integrated Lower Limb (SILL). The sensors and microchip technology for the SILL will be supplied from Sandia National Laboratories. The sensors will provide information from the socket, knee, ankle, and foot to the microprocessor for processing and coordination of the components.[35] Technical requirements and prosthetic expertise are contributed by the Seattle Orthopedic Group. The final component of the development team is Chelyabinsk 70, a Russian nuclear weapons laboratory and peacetime partners of Sandia. They will be responsible for the material work and testing of the SILL. When the SILL is released, it will be the first digitally controlled prosthetic limb system on the market. It is intended to simulate normal gait, regardless of slopes or terrain.[42] To accomplish this, a microprocessor-controlled module implanted in the leg will respond to sensor input from multiple sources. The microprocessor will modulate hydraulic joints and piezoelectric motors that power the ankle, knee, and socket.[42]

A unique feature of the SILL prosthesis is its socket. The socket can change its shape to accommodate to the patient's limb changes throughout the day. It accomplishes this from the feedback the microprocessor receives from the sensors incorporated into the socket to measure volumetric changes of the limb. Automatic adjustment to the thigh will produce a better fitting socket throughout the day and reduce skin disorders caused by excessive pressure or shear. The design team will place sensors in the foot-ankle complex of the prosthesis to gain feedback from each dynamic point throughout the system. The team continues to develop a power source light enough for the patient to carry comfortably to ensure the energy conservation from the prosthesis is not lost to the energy cost of carrying the battery.

This survey of new and future developments in lower-limb prosthetic technology suggests that microprocessors could become the key to a bi-directional neurologically controlled prosthesis. Research involving larger numbers of pilot wearers will help provide the scientific evidence demanded by insurance companies and patients to justify the added cost of current and prospective microprocessor-controlled prostheses.

UPPER-LIMB PROSTHETICS

The upper-limb prosthesis is the most visible artificial limb. History records many attempts to create a device that resembles the human hand both in appearance and function. The first upper-limb prostheses were designed primarily to recreate the appearance of an intact limb. The earliest record concerns a Roman general, Marcus Sergius, who sustained traumatic arm amputation in the Second Punic War, 218-201 BC. He wore an iron fist fashioned by armor makers. He did not want his adversaries to see any sign of weakness as he wielded his shield in battle. No major advancements occurred until the 19th century when Peter Ballif, a dentist from Berlin, designed a harness that could open and close a prosthetic hand. Although the hand had little

functional use, the harness is still the basis for contemporary figure-of-eight and figure-of-nine harnesses. In 1912, D.W. Dorrance invented the split hook, marking a shift in emphasis from appearance to function. Later, Dorrance designed task-specific devices for farming or other trades. The idea for a device that was both cosmetic and functional resulted in cable-controlled hands introduced in the 1950s. Subsequent hands were made with pneumatic and electrical switch controls, the first externally powered prosthetic components. In the early 1960s, clinicians and the public were astounded by the Russian myoelectrically controlled arm, which used electromyographic signals to open and close an electric terminal device (TD). Future development seeks to improve the socket interface, control systems, and power sources, as well as TDs.

Upper-limb prostheses, unlike lower-limb ones, do not require substantial weight bearing through the appliance. The design of the upper-limb prosthesis must still cope with the effects of the socket on the limb. The socket interface must provide a comfortable, stable way to attach the prosthesis to the body and support the loads placed on it.

MYOELECTRIC CONTROL

Socket design is influenced by the type of surgery, as well as the physical characteristics of the amputation limb. Osseointegration, described in Chapter 19, has been more successful with patients who have upper-limb amputation than lower-limb amputation. Most of the socket fitting issues of suspension, volume fluctuations, skin contact pressure, and stabilization can be reduced or eliminated when the prosthesis is attached directly to the bone. Patients with compromised healing or fragile bone are not candidates for osseointegration, and thus need to be fitted with an external socket. Materials technology is resulting in cooler, lighter, more flexible sockets.

Powered prostheses use a control system to operate various components on the wearer's command. Traditionally, surface-mounted electrodes mediate signals between the patient and the prosthesis. Such electrodes present several problems. The subcutaneous layer of adipose tissue surrounding muscles insulates the signal and disrupts the transmission of electrical signals through the skin. The system can only monitor large muscle groups rather than individual muscles, as is possible with needle electrodes. Typical control muscles in the transradial level are wrist extensors and wrist flexors. Even if a prosthetic hand which had independent finger motion, were invented, it could not function because only two muscle groups are currently used to control the device.

Other problems include inconsistent donning of the prosthesis; external forces exerted when the wearer lifts heavy objects can move the electrode contacts or change the amount of pressure applied to the skin. A great deal of information is lost when microvoltage signals at the motor neuron are amplified. Perspiration alters the conductive properties of the skin, causing inconsistent electrical signals throughout the day. Without consistent and predictable monitoring of muscle activity, the user cannot reliably control grip strength or speed, and must rely on visual cues.

In the near future, electrodes may be implanted in the muscle or attached directly to nerves. Previously, implanted electrodes have failed because of power and biocompatibility problems. Inductive technology could allow the internal electrodes to be recharged through the skin. A charging plate or wire ring would be placed around the limb and the batteries could be recharged without a wired connection. First generation implants used rigid tips to connect to nerves, which caused fibrosis. Newer electrode implants use flexible silicone, which should lead to more durability. Internal electrodes should produce predictable monitoring of electrical activity within specific muscles without being affected by the external environment. Internal electrodes might lead to individual finger control or pattern recognition for multiple degrees of movement. Pattern recognition examines the electrical activity of multiple electrodes while the user mimics a specific task. For example, the microprocessor could record the user while mimicking forearm pronation, then associate the pattern with a specific task and send power to an electric wrist rotator. For higher levels of amputation, this technology could be used to control an elbow unit, wrist unit, and hand simultaneously.

Eventually we should see activity-specific secondary and tertiary modes for upper-limb prostheses, similar to the C-leg knee unit. The user could select a preprogrammed series of movements. For example, someone with a shoulder disarticulation could wear a prosthesis programmed for eating; the hand would hold a fork, the wrist would rotate, and the elbow would flex to bring food to the mouth with only one signal to initiate the series of complex movements. Movements of prostheses tend to look artificial, because the motions are typically performed with one motor at a time. Self-leveling wrists with tilt sensors could keep the fork level while the elbow is flexed, making the movement look more natural.

TERMINAL DEVICES

Probably the most fascinating aspect of upper-limb prostheses is the TD. External power combined proportional grip strength with an anthropomorphic device. Controlling the hand with only two muscle groups prevents independent finger motions in commercial hands. As control technology advances, manufacturers will be able to design TDs that can produce multiple grasp patterns and wrist motions.

Servo motors can operate the motor-driven TDs. A servo motor is a small device that has an output shaft ,which can be placed at a specific angle by sending the servo a coded signal. As long as the coded signal exists on the input line, the servo will maintain the angular position of the shaft. The motors are relatively small including the control circuitry, but are extremely powerful. The motor draws power proportional to the mechanical load. A lightly loaded servo, therefore, does not consume much energy. The amount of power applied to the motor is also proportional to the distance it needs to travel. If the shaft needs to turn a large distance, the motor will run at full speed. If it needs to turn only a small amount, the motor will run at a slower speed. This is called proportional control.

Engineers are working to build smaller, lighter, faster, and quieter motors for many applications. Thermoplastics, ceramics, and carbon fiber composites reduce the weight of the TD, but these materials are not widely used due to manufacturing cost. Piezoelectric motors would also reduce weight. They do not require a gearbox, unlike current motors. When a current is applied to the ceramic material it vibrates. Vibrations can be transferred to linear motion to operate a prosthetic hand. When the current is stopped, the motion stops, eliminating the need for a braking system.

Future TDs will incorporate sensory feedback. The long-term goal is to integrate the prosthesis directly into the body's sensory nervous system. Currently, grip strength is monitored primarily by visual cues and secondarily via proprioception through the harness, especially with a voluntary-closing TD or through the power and duration of muscle contraction in a myoelectric system. Until technology allows direct integration, input can be transferred to the body through vibration or pressure within the socket. As the TD makes contact with an object, the current draw for the motor increases. The microprocessor can monitor any increase in current and send a signal to a vibratory device in the prosthesis to vibrate at varying frequency as grip strength increases.

Some systems have expandable bladders that increase pressure against the amputation limb with increase in grip pressure. Auto-grasp or "slip detection" is used in current prosthetic TDs to make control self-monitoring. The Sensor hand from Otto Bock uses force-sensing resistors in the thumb and a sensor in the linkage to monitor grasp and automatically adjust without patient input.

As technology progresses, a hierarchy of control may range from direct patient input to self-monitoring functions to allow seamless prosthetic usage. Shape memory alloys, osseointegration, and artificial muscles are especially promising.

Continued research will always be needed. The beauty of science is the way that it continues to develop.

New inventions and discoveries will be made during the printing of this book, which will always be the case when discussing futuristic concepts. Clinicians must maintain familiarity with new technology to provide their patients with the best care. New materials, components, and techniques are bringing the field of prosthetics to an exciting time.

REFERENCES

1. Cerny FJ, Burton HW. *Exercise Physiology for Health Care Professionals*. Champaign, Ill: Human Kinetics; 2001:82-83.

2. Stark G. *The future of O&P (or at least our best guess!)* Fillauer Inc. Available at: http://www.fillauer.com/education/ED_future.html. Accessed June 19, 2004.

3. Boone DA, Burgess EM. Automated fabrication of mobility aids: clinical demonstration of the UCLA computer aided socket design system. *Journal of Prosthetics and Orthotics*. 1989;1:187-190.

4. Smith DG, Burgess EM. The use of CAD/CAM technology in prosthetics and orthotics—current clinical models and a view to the future. *J Rehabil Res Dev*. 2001;38:327-334.

5. Dalton-Taggart R. Creator: Ivan Sutherland. *Desktop Engineering*. 2004;10.

6. Murdoch G. Editorial. *Prosthet Orthot Int*. 1985;9:1-2.

7. Houston VL, Burgess EM, Childress D, et al Automated fabrication of mobility aids (AFMA): below-knee CASD/CAM testing and evaluation program results. *J Rehabil Res Dev*. 1992;29:78-124.

8. Saunders CG. State-of-the-art in CAD/CAM for orthotic applications. In: *International Society for Prosthetics and Orthotics 11th World Congress; Hong Kong*. 2004:245.

9. Reynolds D. CAD/CAM development in the field of prosthetics. In: *International Society for Prosthetists and Orthotists 11th World Congress; Hong Kong*. 2004:243.

10. Kristinsson O. The ICEROSS concept: a discussion of a philosophy. *Prosthet Orthot Int*. 1993;17:49-55.

11. Lilja M, Oberg T. Volumetric determinations with CAD/CAM in prosthetics and orthotics: errors of measurement. *J Rehabil Res Dev*. 1995;32:141-148.

12. Johnson S, Oberg T. Accuracy and precision of volumetric determinations using two commercial CAD systems for prosthetics: a technical note. *J Rehabil Res Dev*. 1998;35:27-33.

13. Smith DG, Boone DA, Harlan JS, et al. Automated prosthetics fabrication in the developing world: the experimental prosthetics center in Hanoi, Vietnam. *Loyola Univ Orthop J*. 1993;2:49-60.

14. Monash. Rapid 3D prototyping in prosthetics. *REHAB Tech*; 1998.

15. Lokhande M, Crawford RH. Testing of compliance in a prosthetic socket fabricated using selective laser sintering. In: *Proceedings of the 2001 Solid Freeform Fabrication Symposium Austin, Tex*. 2001:513-526.

16. Rovick S, Childress DS, Chan R. An additive fabrication technique for the CAM of prosthetic sockets. *Dept Veterans Affairs, Rehabilitation Research and Development Progress Reports*. 1997:33.

17. Goh JC, Lee PV, Ng P. Structural integrity of polypropylene prosthetic sockets manufactured using the polymer deposition technique. *Proc Inst Mech Eng [H]*. 2002;216:359-368.

18. Batteries. Massachusetts Institute of Technology. Available at: http://web.mit.edu/solar-cars/www/generalinfo/batteries.html. Accessed December 3, 2004.

19. Mittal A, Srikanth G, Biswas S. Composite materials for orthopaedic aids. TIFAC. Available at: http://www.tifac.org.in/news/isc.htm. Accessed July 29, 2004.

20. Blanchard C. Biomaterials: Body parts of the future. *SWRI Technology Today*. Available at: http://www.swri.org/3pubs/ttoday/fall95/implant.htm. Accessed August 1, 2004.

21. Nanobumps: New hope for implant success, 2003. Available at: https://engineering.purdue.edu/BME/News/2003/november_18_html?pp=1. Accessed August 1, 2004.

22. Hollerbach K, Hollister A. O&P: Computerized Prosthetic Modeling. *Biomechanics*. September 1996. Available at: http://www.biomech.com/db_area/archives/1996/9609oandp.bio.html. Accessed June 15, 2004.

23. Space Daily. New organic composites could add muscle to artificial body parts. *Space Daily*. Available at: http://www.spacedaily.com/news/spacemedicine-02m.html. Accessed November 3, 2004.

24. Kelley R. Technology and the future of O&P. *O&P World*. 202, 29-33.

25. Ibrahim A. Compliant Cable Mechanism. NASA Goddard Space Flight Center. Available at: http://techtransfer.gsfc.nasa.gov/compliantcable/benifits.cfm. Accessed September 4, 2004.

26. SMA/MEMS Research Group. Shape Memory Alloys. Available at: http://www.cs.ualberta.ca/~database/MEMS/sma_mems/sma.html. Accessed October 31, 2004.

27. Freiherr G. Shape-memory alloys offer untapped potential. 1998. Available at: http://www.devicelink.com/mddi/archive/98/03/005.html. Accessed October 31, 2004.

28. Bard CR. Simon Nitinol Filter. Available at: http://www.bardpv.com/prod-simon.php. Accessed October 31, 2004.

29. Michlovitz SL. *Thermal Agents in Rehabilitation*. 3rd ed. Philadelphia, Pa: FA Davis Company; 1996:115-116.

30. New and innovative materials and fabrics in O&P. *O&P Business News*. 2004;27-32.

31. Levangie PK Norkin CC. *Joint Structure and Function: A Comprehensive Analysis*. 4th ed. Philadelphia, Pa: FA Davis Company; 2005.

32. Michael J. O&P: Prosthetic knee mechanisms: centuries of progress. Available at: http://biomech.com/db_area/archives/1997/9708op.bio.html. Accessed August 10, 2004.

33. Buckley JG, Spence WD, Solomonidis SE. Energy cost of walking: comparison of "Intelligent Prosthesis" with conventional mechanism. *Arch Phys Med Rehabil*. 1997;78:330-333.

34. Michael JW. Modern prosthetic knee mechanisms. *Clin Orthop*. 1999;361:39-47.

35. Otto J. Prosthetic knees: what's currently new and impressive? *O&P Edge*. 2003;2:29-31.

36. Wilkenfeld A, Herr H. An auto-adaptive external knee prosthesis. Artificial Intelligence Laboratory at Massachusetts Institute of Technology. Available at: http://www.ai.mit.edu/research/ abstracts/ abstracts2000/ps/z-Herr1.ps. Accessed June 19, 2004.

37. *RHEO KNEE™ Product Profile*. Aliso Viejo, Calif: Ossur; 2004.

38. Otto J. Prosthetic knees: what's on the way? *O&P Edge*. 2003;2:22-28.

39. Keegan P. The new bionic man. *Business 2.0*. 2004;104-108.

40. Calleja D. Victhom develops a souped-up bionic leg. June 2003, CanadianBusiness.com. Available at: http://www.canadianbusiness.com/article.jsp?content=20030609_54224_54224. Accessed July 9, 2004.

41. Carlson JD. *Magnetorheological Fluids—Ready for Real-Time Motion Control*. Cary, NC: Lord Corporation, Materials Division; 2002.

42. Prosthetic limb to be controlled by microchip. Sandia National Laboratories, 2000. Available at: http://www.sandia.gov/media/NewsRel/NR2000/smartleg.htm. Accessed August 3, 2004.

43. Carlson JD. Commercial magneto-rheological fluid devices. In: Bullough WA, ed. *Proceedings of 5th International Conference on ER Fluids, MR Fluids and Associated Techniques*. Singapore: World Scientific; 1996:20-28.

44. Design Engineering. A smoother ride for vehicle seats. *Design Engineering*. 1999;54-55.

45. Mehri D. Economical actuator provides simple precise motion control. *Design News*. 2000;55:63-65.

Chapter 19

In the Future: Surgical and Educational Advances and Challenges

Matthew A. Parente, PT, CPO and Mark Geil, PhD

OBJECTIVES

1. Explore principles of osseointegration and its prosthetic implications
2. List the contributions of robotics and microsurgery to the replacement of body parts
3. Relate pneumatic artificial muscles and reimplantation to future prostheses
4. Describe the present and future status of entry-level and continuing prosthetics education

---

INTRODUCTION

Will osseointegration become the standard for amputation surgery? Will technology eventually create a robot to do the job of a practitioner? How should clinicians and the public balance the desire for substantial practitioner education with the need to meet the immediate needs for patient service? Clinicians must take the initiative to improve the way they practice. New concepts will accelerate improvement, only if the clinician uses education as the catalyst to incorporate innovations into practice. Prosthetists incorporate ideas from many fields into a prosthetic design. This is why they keep a close eye on research and inventions in a wide range of scientific disciplines.

OSSEOINTEGRATION

Innovations do not always arise by improving existing practices. New ideas may represent radical departures from the norm. With all of the research and development devoted to components, exemplified by modern materials and computer-controlled actuators in knee units and hands, as described in Chapter 18, the performance of any component is secondary to proper fit of the prosthesis. It must be securely attached to the amputation limb. Faulty sockets are too tight or too loose, or they can distribute too much force to tender

areas, or because the residual limb is dynamic, they might fit well one day and not the next. If the socket is uncomfortable, the prosthesis, even with the most modern components, is a hindrance rather than an enabler. For the appropriate candidate, an innovative surgical procedure called osseointegration avoids the socket altogether.

Osseointegration is the direct attachment of the prosthesis to the amputation limb. An osseointegrated prosthesis is a conventional prosthesis that connects to an abutment that has been surgically attached to the weight-bearing bone of the amputation limb. The abutment breaches the skin to protrude from the distal end of the limb (Figure 19-1). The surgery to attach the abutment occurs in multiple stages and involves a lengthy recovery period. Once healed and functional, the prosthetic pylon is bolted onto the abutment to obtain a secure attachment. The technique is appropriate for a select group of patients. It provides many advantages as compared with traditional socket attachment, and it has its enthusiastic proponents. The technique, however, may introduce medicosurgical complications and involves several other disadvantages. As with any procedure in its relative infancy, one can hope the procedure improves to the point where many more people with amputations are eligible and complications are minimized.

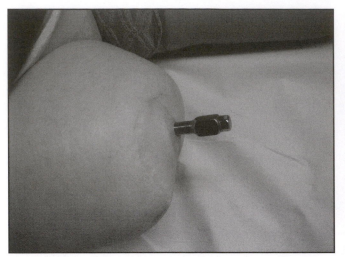

Figure 19-1. Osseointegration abutment.

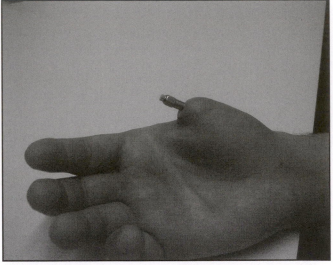

Figure 19-2. Finger osseointegration.

History of Osseointegration

Although the direct attachment of a prosthetic limb to the appendicular skeleton is a relatively new idea, the penetration of the skeleton in other anatomical areas is not. In 1843, Joseph Malgaigne pioneered securing fractures with metal. Metal implants have held dental prostheses in place since the 1960s, and craniomaxillofacial osseointegration is well established. Finger prostheses have been successfully implanted (Figure 19-2). Since World War II physicians have experimented with direct attachment of prosthetic limbs.[1] However, mainstream application to leg prostheses did not appear until the early 1990s, through the work of Swedish orthopedic surgeon Per-Ingvar Brånemark. His son, Rickard Brånemark, continues his work. Because the procedure originated in Göteborg, Sweden, most of the procedures and research have been performed there. The first prosthetic osseointegration surgery performed in the United Kingdom occurred in 1997, and a trial continues at Queen Mary's Hospital in Roehampton, London. Procedures have also been performed at Alfred Hospital in Melbourne, Australia. Some work has also been done in Germany,[2] and in the United States, a few clinicians are working toward a clinical trial. The total number of procedures performed worldwide is under 100.

Surgical Procedure

Current practice entails surgeries in two stages. Stage I involves placement of an implant into the distal end of the weight-bearing bone of the amputation limb. In stage II, the abutment is permanently attached to the implant through the skin.

Stage I

The implant is usually a threaded titanium tube meant to eventually receive the abutment. Implantation engages the inner cortex of the distal end of the larger bone in the amputation limb and is expected to be held firmly in place by subsequent bone modeling. This stage of surgery also involves significant repositioning of soft tissue to produce a distal amputation limb most suitable for prosthesis attachment. Following the surgery, the amputation limb is closed. Healing and establishing bony integration take 6 months (Figure 19-3).

Stage II

In stage II, the amputation limb is reopened, and a metal abutment is attached to the implant. Most abutments are threaded on the proximal end and contain a distal end shaped for prosthesis attachment with a simple hexagonal key. Soft tissue and skin are closed around the abutment to create a healthy interface of metal and skin, which can be maintained without infection or injury.

Recovery

The process of enabling a useful abutment following surgery must take into account soft tissue healing, infection control, and, for lower-limb prostheses, the development of a mechanical structure capable of bearing loads greater than body weight. The last consideration results in a lengthy process of gradual load bearing on the abutment while it becomes integrated with the skeleton. Including surgeries and recovery, the entire process required to integrate a useable abutment can take 2 years. Reducing this long and sometimes painful process is a primary consideration among orthopedic surgeons investigating possible improvements.

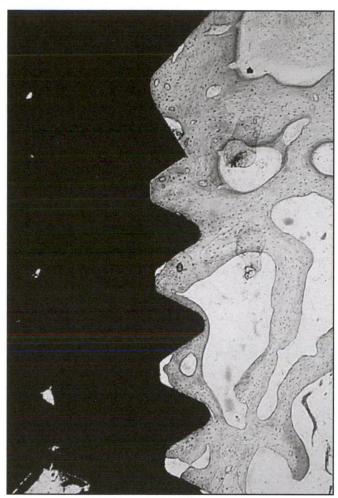

Figure 19-3. Microscopic healing of osseointegration.

Advantages

An osseointegrated prosthesis eliminates a socket. The fact that the prosthesis is directly anchored to the bone preserves sensation. "Osseoperception" describes awareness of the prosthesis. In 2004, osseointegration patient Eric Ax reported the unusual perception of stepping on a pebble. In a conventional prosthesis, such an event creates a force that is distributed through the socket, possibly altering the bending moment applied to the amputation limb. With an osseointegrated prosthesis, the altered force is transferred directly to bone to be perceived by sensory nerves. Discomfort sometimes associated with a socket is avoided. The encumbrance a socket imposes, particularly when sitting on a short stool, is also avoided.[3] Inside a socket, both amputation limb soft tissue and bone can move, with amputation limb motion being limited by the moment it can apply to the socket walls. In contrast, direct skeletal attachment markedly improves control of prosthetic motion and enables the patient to have significantly more hip excursion than with a socket.[3] Absence of a socket, with

its flares and trim lines, also improves the silhouette under clothing. Finally, donning and doffing of the prosthesis is much simpler, especially as compared with complex suspension systems used in many modern sockets.

Disadvantages

Although osseointegration completely avoids many problems associated with sockets, the procedure introduces its own difficulties. In current practice, direct skeletal attachment limits some activity because high impact forces could damage the bone. Of the complications associated with the procedure, infection is potentially the most hazardous. Infections around the attachment site sometimes occur, and far more serious systemic infections have produced some cases of osseointegration failure. Mechanical failure can affect the abutment, with loosening, bending, or fracturing. When a socket breaks, a new one can be made fairly easily, but fracture of an abutment may require much more involved treatment. Finally, a major disadvantage is the duration of the procedure. The two-stage surgery process takes 6 months, and the second surgery is then followed by a lengthy and, at times, painful process of gradual weight bearing during bone healing and modeling.

Indications

Certain patients are candidates for osseointegration, namely those for whom the benefits are likely to outweigh the risks. Those with very short amputation limbs, tissue problems, or a scarred residual limb are usually suitable. Robust, active people are ideal, as long as they are aware of the activity limitations imposed by the procedure. Individuals with long amputation limbs who are good candidates for conventional sockets do not gain much from osseointegration

Contraindications

The procedure is not intended for people older than 70 years, or those with vascular disease, diabetes, osteoporosis, infection, weight exceeding 100 kg, or skeletal immaturity.

Research

Peer-reviewed research on osseointegrated limb prostheses is confined to reports by the developers. In 2001, the elder and younger Brånemarks described the procedure but note an emphasis in the literature on applications in dentistry, facial prosthetics, hearing aids, and finger prostheses.[4] Bone remodeling surrounding an intermedullary implant and osseoperception have been studied in animal models.[5] The significantly larger body of literature regarding dental applications may guide investigators concerned with limb prosthetics.

Summary

Osseointegration in lower-limb prosthetics represents a complete departure from traditional thinking regarding prosthetic attachment. The process is innovative and avoids the many problems associated with the traditional socket. Widespread application of osseointegration is limited by the contraindications and by the daunting length of the medical procedures and recovery. Future research is directed towards improving the medicosurgical procedure and the rehabilitation process and treatment for more levels of amputation.

REPLACING BODY PARTS AND FUNCTIONS

The field of prosthetics is based on the ability of an artificial device to replace an absent or dysfunctional body part. The expectations of prostheses range from restoring the appearance of the missing body part to reproducing the motor and sensory capabilities of the absent segment. The most important factor is the overall function the patient desires from the prosthesis.

Theoretically, the design aspect of product development is not difficult, because engineers and designers already have the blueprints for the desired finished product. The human body has been studied for centuries. Areas of specialization that most directly lend themselves to prosthetic applications are kinesiology, biomechanics, and arthrokinematics. These fields dictate the effectiveness of devices fabricated to benefit the patient. Each prosthesis is evaluated on many variables, always compared to the original natural design.

A prosthesis, internal or external, must reflect the merit of every aspect of the design. The inventor should consider how limiting factors affect the final product. These factors act along a continuum with respect to their properties. For example, using stainless steel instead of titanium decreases the overall cost, but increases the weight of the device. Other considerations include biocapability and durability of the materials. Researchers are developing new ways to replace body parts and replicate human movement. Several research projects are underway, bringing us closer to these objectives.

A device that produces limb movement must satisfy several functional and mechanical principles. Mechanically, it should have high torque-to-weight and power-to-weight ratios, shock absorbing qualities, energy storage capabilities, and a simple actuator located near the joint.[6] Functionally, an upper-limb prosthesis would provide variable grip forces to manipulate objects, tactile sensation, finite movement control, and fluid movement patterns.[7] Rather than having one prehension pattern, the ideal prosthetic hand would offer many grasp patterns with hand span comparable to the human model.

Using nature as the compass, a logical starting point was to create an artificial muscle to provide movement to an artificial limb. This involves simulating neuromuscular physiology, biomechanics, and musculoskeletal stabilizers by using sensors, actuators, microprocessors, and control systems. One approach focused on one component of the complex system, the actuator.

An original and popular actuator was initially developed as a power assist for orthoses for patients with poliomyelitis. The device was the design of J.L. McKibben and is powered by compressed gas.[8] The actuator consists of an inflatable inner bladder covered with a braided woven shell, which contracts lengthwise when the bladder expands radially.[9] Performance characteristics of the McKibben actuator are a direct function of the weave characteristics of the braided shell, material properties of the elastic bladder, actuation pressure, and length of the "muscle." The McKibben actuator is an actuator whose performance is most similar to biological muscle.[10] The primary difference has been the limited amount of natural dampening, a velocity-dependent component. As noted in 1999, a possible improvement to the McKibben actuator could be made by adding dampening to create an actuator whose properties more closely resembled muscle with respect to both length and velocity.[9]

Pneumatic Artificial Muscles (PAMs), such as the McKibben actuator, have been used primarily in robotics. Continued research into PAMs may be beneficial to people who wear prostheses. A promising variation of the PAM is the Pleated Pneumatic Artificial Muscle (PPAM). PPAMs have unidirectional motion that provides adjustable compliance due to gas compressibility, varying force-displacement relation, absence of friction and hysteresis, and the ability to operate at a wide range of gas pressures. Most notable may be their ability to connect directly to a robotic joint; because of their high force output at all speeds.[11] They are safe because their materials cause no fire, explosions, or pollution. These contractile devices controlled by pressurized gas may make a pivotal contribution toward bridging robotics and prosthetics.

Several attempts, aside from PAMs and PPAMs, have been made to replicate motion with artificial muscles. One experiment employed Shape Memory Alloys (SMAs), which can mimic the tissue characteristics of human muscles and tendons. Typically used in robotics because of their strength and ability to be formed into large groups, SMAs are able to create fluid motion.[7] Movements are achieved by initial bias of the SMA to a static position. Then an electric current is passed through the "muscle" that needs to contract. When the SMA wire shortens it simulates movement of the intended joint. After the current is removed the joint returns to its resting or extended position. The timing and magnitude of the current can be controlled to simulate graded contraction of muscle tissue. Studies at the University of Alberta have generated a functional hand to demonstrate the properties of SMAs and how they relate to joint motion.

Yobotics (Cincinnati, Ohio), a consulting, research, and design company, is working on an orthotic project that has tremendous potential in the prosthetic community. The company specializes in robots, force-controllable actuators, and powered leg orthoses. Their product, known as the Robowalker, is an exoskeletal device designed to help patients with lower-limb weakness achieve more ambulatory mobility.[12] The Robowalker responds to the wearer via strategically placed electrodes. They detect trace neurological impulses. The signals are converted to provide the patient with the corresponding motion, produced by the Robowalker. This project relates directly to neurologically controlled prosthetic devices. The development of powered exoskeletal technology has fueled inquiry into powered endoskeletal prostheses.

Prostheses with direct connection to the body, both skeletally and neurologically, are often referred to as bionic. The cochlear implant is a most successful bionic prosthesis.[13] It causes direct stimulation of the auditory nerves. Patients with the implants report a high return of functional hearing.[13] The success of the cochlear implant, as well as the cardiac pacemaker, provide valuable information about microelectronics and biointegrated devices.

Surgery to implant a wide variety of devices appears to be a trend, although not always a viable option. One tool that has facilitated implantation is the operating microscope, which can magnify structures forty times their original size.[14] The operating microscope, in turn, has driven the development of ultra sensitive tools for operating on microscopic structures.

Advances in microsurgical procedures have made replantation of a body part a reality. Replantation refers to surgical reattachment of a finger, hand, or limb that has been completely detached from a person's body. The goal is to revive maximum function of the reattached body part. In many cases, replantation is not an option due to the extent of damage of the severed limb or the potential attachment site. The Mangled Extremity Severity Score (MESS) (Table 19-1) established by Johansen et al in 1990 is an accurate predictor of the viability of replantation. In both prospective and retrospective studies, according to the MESS scale, a score >7 had a 100% predictive value for reimplantation.[15]

A sequential inspection of the surgical procedure demonstrates the intricacies of the operation. First, the area must be debrided and prepared for the operation. Then the bone must be shortened and prepared for reattachment. Next the tendons are reattached to their appropriate fixation point. Then the surgeon repairs the nerve, prior to releasing the tourniquet. Afterward, the arteries, then veins are repaired. The final step is skin closure.[15]

Replantation is not an option if the patient has a low MESS score, or if the limb is unlikely to regain at least as much function as if the patient were to use a prosthesis. The physical and occupational therapy associated with replantation does not always restore the function that the patient anticipates.

Hand transplantation is a dramatic procedure, resulting from advances in microsurgical techniques. Several transplantation procedures have been successful, although long-term success is still vague. Warren C. Breidenbach, MD, a member of the surgical team that performed the first hand transplantation, tells his patients to expect a 10-year survival rate of the transplanted segment of <50%.[16] The body's rejection of the hand is often controlled by medication, which depresses the immune system.

Although the human body is an amazing organism, it cannot regenerate a severed part. Urodele amphibians are the only group of vertebrates that possess this ability. Specifically, the axolotls (*Ambystoma mexicanum*) have been used to study this unique quality. Their limb cells dedifferentiate and then reinitiate growth.[17] The limb then regenerates to form a fully functional adult limb.[18] Better understanding of tissue regeneration could bring a drastic change in the field of rehabilitating people with amputations.

The premise that the future of prosthetics is only limited by our imagination may be a lot closer to the truth than anyone thought. The brain is the key to the future of thought-controlled prostheses. Using a microchip implanted onto the brain, researchers at Brown University have enabled monkeys to operate a video game by thought alone.[19] Neural impulses were recorded on the monkeys' motor cortex while they played the game. The signals were then mathematically translated into a computer program. The program then translated new information during real-time activities to control the cursor on the screen. Conceivably, mapping the motor cortex could lead to a wireless thought-controlled prosthesis.

EDUCATION

One of the largest hurdles that prosthetists face is justification to insurance companies and the entire medical community about the work they perform. No longer is the prosthetist just a "leg maker" or "limb fitter." Increased levels of professional and post professional education for prosthetists mirror that of other health professions. Research has accelerated the transition from craft to science, enabling prosthetists to gain greater collegial respect.

Prosthetists are expected to have more knowledge than at any other time in history. They need to master anatomy, biomechanics, physiology, pathology, psychology, physics, computer science, mechanics, and material science as well as have substantial technical skill in evaluating patients and fabricating prostheses. Until the mid 20th century, prosthetics education was limited, in part, by the paucity of materials and components and relatively basic scientific knowledge. Practitioners relied primarily on clinical and technical skills to treat their patients. Today, the constant influx of new technology has increased the expectations of health care providers and patients who insist that prosthetists have up-to-date knowledge of new products and techniques. If prosthetists are to work successfully with the rest of the rehabilitation team, they must have comprehensive knowledge from many sciences and research-based evidence to support their recommendations.[20]

Baccalaureate prosthetics and orthotics education begun at New York University in the early 1960s and has evolved into the current four entry-level curricula at the baccalaureate or master's degree level, in addition to three post baccalaureate certificate programs for entry-level students. Representatives from the collegiate programs focus on the didactic aspect of a student's education through the North American Prosthetic and Orthotic Educators (NAPOE). Residencies, at a minimum of 12 months, are overseen by the National Commission of Orthotic and Prosthetic Education (NCOPE). A student who has completed the requirements of both organizations is eligible to take the examination administered by the American Board for Certification in Orthotics and Prosthetics (ABC). Upon successful completion of all components of the ABC examination, the candidate is now an ABC certified prosthetist.

Prosthetists must adapt as the field continues to change. Several states now license them. Licensure requires that practitioners complete a minimum number of continuing education hours over a 5-year period. Professional excellence, however, demands that prosthetists exceed the minimum continuing education. Academic institutions, manufacturers, and other organizations recognize the need to present continuing education.

Distance learning is one means of providing continuing education. In September 2002, the Newington Certificate Program in Orthotics and Prosthetics, Newington, Connecticut, became the first to enroll students for a practitioner distance learning program (DLP). The DLP was modeled on traditional programs and NCOPE requirements. Candidates have a baccalaureate degree and have completed one discipline, either orthotics or prosthetics, at a college accredited by the Commission on Accreditation of Allied Health Education Programs (CAAHEP). DLP students receive a digital videodisc (DVD) of every lecture from the core courses—transtibial, transfemoral, and upper-limb prosthetics. Students have several days to view

Table 19-1	
MANGLED EXTREMITY SEVERITY SCORE (MESS)	
Skeletal/Soft-Tissue Injury	
• Low energy (stab, simple fracture, pistol gun shot wound)	1
• Medium energy (open or multiple fractures, dislocation)	2
• High energy (high speed RTA or rifle GSW)	3
• Very high energy (high speed trauma + gross contamination)	4
Limb Ischemia	
• Pulse reduced or absent but perfusion normal	1*
• Pulseless, paraesthesias, diminished capillary refill	2*
• Cool, paralyzed, insensate, numb	3*
Shock	
• Systolic BP always >90 mm	0
• Hypotensive transiently	1
• Persistent hypotension	2
Age (Years)	
• <30	0
• 30 to 50	1
• >50	2
*Score doubled for ischemic period longer than 6 hours	

the DVD and prepare for a conference call with the instructor. During this call, the students question the instructor to clarify the material. They take their written examinations through an online examination service. With regard to practical education, Newington students negotiate with a sponsoring facility to permit them to see patients. Students send digital pictures of class projects to the course instructors at Newington. At the end of each semester, students come to Newington for a multi-day comprehensive practical examination graded with the same criteria as for traditional students.

DLP is an innovative response to the need to educate prosthetists. Not being in a classroom environment on a daily basis, the student has to have the dedication to succeed. Newington's DLP students have achieved higher grade point averages compared to traditional students.

Educational institutions are responsible for integrating new technology into their curricula. Advanced technology is a great lure for prospective students and should help increase the applicant pool. As the number of applicants increases, so does the potential to accept more able students. A relative "snowball" effect would then lead to more knowledgeable graduates to take their skills into the field.

The American Academy of Orthotists and Prosthetists (AAOP) has expanded its educational programming via distance learning. For a small fee, members and non-members can access courses and take quizzes to confirm acquisition of knowledge. A passing grade qualifies the registrant for continuing education units (CEUs). AAOP offers other options for obtaining CEUs. NetED allows one to view video and audio programs on the computer.[21] Audio Conference Educational Series enables participants to listen to a presentation and ask questions of the presenter. Professional Audio Web Educational Series features a computer-driven presentation accompanied by a telephone connection to the presenter.[22]

Many manufacturers offer continuing education based on their product lines. Some require prosthetists to complete product coursework before being allowed to purchase the specific component. The practitioner receives product-specific training and CEUs. The manufacturer insures that prosthetists use their product according to its intended design to maximize its performance for the patient. Ossur has established a combination of seminars and online education through the Ossur Academy, an Internet-based educational series that offers programs primarily based on its products. Ossur also offers a professional presentation series to educate groups of clinicians at local facilities.

Hanger Orthopedic Group's program, E-versity, is a company-wide effort devoted to continuing education. E-versity is a combination of academic presentations on clinical, technical, and office management subjects delivered electronically. DVD will soon augment Internet presentations.

Computer aided learning can supplement hands-on training. A notable educational application is the teaching of anatomy. Historically, practical anatomical learning was done with the aid of cadavers, and many institutions retain this practice. Virtual anatomy dissection can now be performed via computer software. Three-dimensional images can be manipulated to be viewed at infinite angles. Computer tomography accompanies many images, so the student can correlate the anatomical image to the diagnostic image. Most of these programs are limited to normal, rather than pathological, anatomy.[22]

Computer technology is changing the future of surgery from an educational and practical perspective. Computer imaging has an increasing number of surgical applications, such as surgical planning and rehearsal. A unique aspect of this process is a technique known as deformable modeling, the combination of computerized models of anatomy, tissue behavior, joint motions, real-time deformation of bones and tissues, all of which result in a visual interactive environment. Deformable

modeling helps the surgeon plan and simulate the potential consequences of a proposed procedure.

Image-guided surgery, a minimally invasive procedure, allows surgeons to view video images on a monitor that are projected from an endoscopic camera. This procedure decreases recovery time and has proven to be an invaluable tool for neurosurgeons, although it leaves little room for error, and allows only a limited field of view.[22]

The success of image-guided surgery has led to the development of robotically assisted surgery, which melds image-guided surgery with robotics. Telesurgery could allow surgeons to operate with the assistance of robotically controlled instrumentation and real-time computer feedback. The surgeon would wear a virtual reality interface glove to provide the robots with the appropriate degree of motion and receive feedback to their hands as if they were standing in the operating room. Telesurgery requires additional surgeons to be on standby in case of complications. Surgeons could operate on a patient in a robotically controlled operating room almost anywhere in the world from a remote computerized surgical center in their home town. Numerous obstacles must be overcome. Applied technology must make a procedure easier than is the case without the use of technology. Cost is another hurdle. The best way to quantify the cost is through a cost-to-benefit ratio, calculated by relating the cost of implementing technology to the clinical benefit of the treatment. This ratio must be favorable before a specific technology will be accepted.

The Internet is arguably the most significant technological advancement in the past decade. It enables individuals all over the world to access almost any piece of information within seconds. Patients have gained from the Internet. Rather than going to the library or relying solely on medical advice, the patient seeks answers from the privacy of their home through the use of online search. A more informed patient is likely to be a more active participant in treatment. Patient compliance is often increased with greater understanding and less confusion. Compliance is paramount, for the best prosthesis in the world is meaningless if the patient does not wear it.

The Internet can contribute to patient care by giving clinicians instant access to the patient's treatment history, pathologies, and medications. Documentation is more accurate and efficient with the use of a wireless dictation device that automatically entered notes into the patient's electronic chart. The system has direct links to physicians' offices for patient care concerns and legible prescriptions.

Online information security is a great concern regarding Internet-based patient information.[23] Unauthorized access to patient information violates the patient's right to maintain all of his/her medical treatments under strict confidentiality. Communication between patient and clinician via e-mail is speedy if communications are brief. The simple telephone call is still more efficient with lengthy communications.[23]

Although computers have revolutionized communication, education, and technology, some older clinicians are reluctant to use computers. In contrast, newer practitioners will tend to be more technologically savvy and will act as a catalyst to integrate technology into clinics.[23]

Many clinicians, facilities, and companies recognize an international need for high quality prosthetic care. Some needs are met via the donation of components and services. Patients in developing countries should receive excellent, realistic prosthetic care. The continuum of prosthetic care should be explored so that clinicians can extract the most important factors. The goal is to produce an inexpensive, lightweight, well functioning, biomechanically sound, durable, easily repaired prosthesis that is cosmetically acceptable and can adapt to varying climates. Materials and components for the prosthesis must be locally available, manually fabricated, and reproducible by trained personnel.[24]

Although each factor is necessary for long-term prosthetic success, arguably the most important is educating local practitioners. The need to have trained personnel as a part of the local community has been acknowledged since the 6th century BC when Lao Tzu, the father of Taoism, recognized the societal value associated with educating those in need. "Give a man a fish and you feed him for a day. Teach him how to fish and you feed him for a lifetime."

Education drives the field of prosthetics. As products, materials, and techniques are developed it is imperative for clinicians to have the education to maximize the potential of the products. Entry-level education, whether traditional or distance learning, must be extended by continuing education. Although computerized instruction is an excellent teaching tool, it cannot replace hands-on experience and interpersonal treatment skills gained from human interactions. The combination of skills and expanded knowledge enables clinicians to bring patients the benefit of future advances.

CONCLUSION

The inherent problem with a "futuristic concept" is that it is relatively short-lived before it is reassigned to a different category. The concept may become "common practice" or a "crazy idea." Wherever it ends, the important aspect of the concept is the research that was associated with it. Inspirational writer Dale Turner said, "Some of the best lessons we ever learn are learned from past mistakes. The error of the past is the wisdom and success of the future." The field must learn from previous successes and failures in order to move into the future.

REFERENCES

1. Hayes E. Osseointegration: where man meets machine. *BioMechanics*. 2002;9:17-24.
2. Staubach KH, Grundei H. The first osseointegrated percutaneous prosthesis anchor for above-knee amputees [German]. *Biomed Tech (Berl)*. 2001;46:355-361.
3. Hagberg K, Haggstrom E, Uden M, Brånemark R. Socket versus bone-anchored trans-femoral prostheses: hip range of motion and sitting comfort. *Prosthet Orthot Int*. 2005;29:153-163.
4. Brånemark R, Brånemark P-I, Rydevik B, Myers RR. Osseointegration in skeletal reconstruction and rehabilitation: a review. *J Rehabil Res Dev*. 2001;38:175-181.
5. Ysander M, Brånemark R, Olmarker K, Myers RR. Intramedullary osseointegration: development of a rodent model and study of histology and neuropeptide changes around titanium implants. *J Rehabil Res Dev*. 2001;38:183-190.
6. Pneumatic artificial muscles (PAMs). Brussels University, Department of Engineering. Available at: http://lucy.vub.ac.be/gendes/actuators/muscles.htm. Accessed December 4, 2004.
7. SMA/MEMS Research Group. (2001) Robotic Muscles. University of Alberta. Available at: http://www.cs.ualberta.ca/~database/MEMS/sma_mems/muscle.html. Accessed October 31, 2004.
8. Nickel VL, Perry J, Garrett AL. Development of useful function in the severely paralyzed hand. *J Bone Joint Surg Am*. 1963;45:933-952.
9. Klute GK, Czerniecki JM, Hannaford B. McKibben Artificial Muscles: Pneumatic actuators with biomechanical intelligence. IEEE/ASME International Conference on Advanced Intelligent Mechatronics; September 19-22, 1999; Atlanta, Ga.
10. Chou CP, Hannaford B. Measurement and modeling of artificial muscles. *IEEE Transactions on Robotics and Automation*. 1996;12:90-102.
11. Daerden F, Lefeber D, Verrelst B, Van Ham R. Pleated Pneumatic Artificial Muscles: Compliant Robotic Actuators. University of Brussels, Department of Mechanical Engineering/Multibody Mechanics Group; 2001.
12. Otto J. What O&P technology has gained from robotics. *O&P Business News*. 2002; 47-67.
13. Pescovitz D. Reality Check: The future of Bionics. Wired Magazine, 1997. Available at: http://www.wired.com/wired/5.02/reality_check.html. Accessed August 1, 2004.
14. Showalter JF. Hand and upper extremity surgery. Available at: http://www.orthodupage.com/handsurgery2.htm. Accessed August 3, 2004.
15. Hand replantation. 2002. Available at: http://www.orthoteers.co.uk/Nrujp~ij33lm/Orthmess.htm. Accessed November 3, 2004.
16. Holliman K. Ethics of hand transplants. *O&P Business News*. 2002; 27-30.

17. Bryant SV. Molecular basis of limb development and regeneration. Available at: http://Darwin.bio.uci.edu/%7emrjc/bryants.html. Accessed August 27, 2004.

18. Brant I. Axolotol Limb Regeneration. University of California, Irvine. Available at: http://Darwin.bio.uci.edu/%7emrjc/regen.html. Accessed August 27, 2004.

19. Kelley R. Technology and the future of O&P. *O&P World.* 2002; 29-33.

20. Conn D. The evolution of the O&P practitioner. *O&P Almanac.* 2004; 61-63.

21. Otto J. Distance learning: No longer a remote possibility. *O&P Business News.* 2002; 24-34.

22. Oakman A. The future of medicine? Available at: http://www.doc.ic.ac.uk/~nd/surprise_96/journal/vol1/ao2/article1.html. Accessed July 30, 2004.

23. Roniger LR. Practitioners and the Internet: the future comes into focus. Biomechanics, 2002. Available at: http://www.biomech.com/db_area/archives/2002/0205.cover.bio.shtml. Accessed June 15, 2004.

24. Michael JW, Bowker JH. Prosthetics/Orthotics Research for the Twenty-first Century: Summary 1992 Conference proceedings. *Journal of Prosthetics and Orthotics.* Available at: http://www.oandp.org/jpo/library/printArticle.asp?printArticleId=1994_40_100. Accessed August 6, 2004.

Physical Therapy Intake

Melissa Wolff-Burke, PT, EdD, MS, ATC; Elizabeth Smith Cole, PT; Mary Witt, PT

Please complete this form before your physical therapy appointment on (date)_____ at (time) _____.
Please bring the completed form with you to your appointment or fax it to us: Fax #: _____

Adapted from Boissonnault, WG. Koopmeiners MB. Medical history profile: orthopedic physical therapy outpatients. *JOSPT.* 1994;20:2-10.

Patient Name: _____ **Date:**_____

1. What side is your amputation(s)/ what level? _____

2. What was/were the date(s) of your amputation(s)? _____

3. What was the cause/reason for the amputation(s)? _____
_____

4. Have you recently noticed: (Check all that apply)
❏ Unexplained weight loss   ❏ Fever/chills/sweats   ❏ Fatigue
❏ Nausea/vomiting   ❏ Weakness   ❏ Numbness or tingling

5. Current Care: (Check all that apply)
❏ Medical Doctor (MD)   ❏ Psychiatrist/Psychologist   ❏ Massage Therapist
❏ Osteopath (DO)   ❏ Physical Therapist   ❏ Prosthetist
❏ Dentist   ❏ Chiropractor   ❏ Other_____
For what reason have you seen this/these provider(s) in the past 3 months:_____
Name and phone number of primary care physician: _____

6. Have you declared an Advanced Directive (Living Will, Durable Power of Attorney for Health Care or DNR)?
    ❏ Yes   ❏ No (If yes, please bring a copy of this document with you to your first appointment)

7. Have you been hospitalized for other surgeries or conditions?

DATE	REASON FOR SURGERY/HOSPITALIZATION
(1) _____	_____
(2) _____	_____
(3) _____	_____
(4) _____	_____
(5) _____	_____

8. OVER-THE-COUNTER medications you have taken in the past week. (Check all that apply)
❏ Aspirin ❏ Antihistamines ❏ Decongestants ❏ Laxatives
❏ Acetamenophen ❏ Antacid ❏ Vitamins/mineral supplements
❏ Ibuprofen ❏ Homeopathic remedies ❏ Other _____

9. PRESCRIPTION medications are you currently taking (including pills, injected medications, skin patches, creams or ointments). (Use back of page if necessary.)
(1) _____ (2) _____ (3) _____ (4) _____
(5) _____ (6) _____ (7) _____ (8) _____

10. Allergies: List any medications your are allergic to: _____
    Are you sensitive to Latex? ❏ Yes ❏ No
    List any other allergies we should know about: _____

11. Have you EVER been diagnosed as having any of the following conditions?
❏ Cancer ❏ Heart problems ❏ High blood pressure
❏ Circulation problems ❏ Asthma ❏ Emphysema/bronchitis
❏ Chemical dependency ❏ Thyroid problems ❏ Diabetes
❏ Multiple sclerosis ❏ Rheumatoid arthritis ❏ Other arthritic conditions
❏ Depression ❏ Hepatitis ❏ Tuberculosis
❏ Stroke ❏ Kidney disease ❏ Anemia
❏ Epilepsy ❏ HIV ❏ Other _____

12. Do you smoke cigarettes or chew tobacco? ❏Yes ____packs/day ❏ No

13. Are you currently wearing a prosthesis? ❏Yes ❏No
    If yes, how many hours/day do you have it on? _____ hours/day
    What percent of that time are you up/walking? _____%
    How many days/week do you wear your prosthesis? _____ days/week
    Are you having any problems with your prosthesis? ❏Yes ❏No
    If yes, what are they? _____

14. Do you need assistance of another person to walk? ❏Yes ❏No
    How far can you walk? _____
    What is the reason you stop walking? _____

15. Are you having problems with your prosthesis? ❏Yes ❏No
    If yes, what are they? _____

16. Do you have any concerns regarding your skin? ❏Yes ❏No
    If yes, what are your concerns? _____

17. Are you experiencing pain? ❏Yes ❏No (If yes, complete pain questionnaire if provided)

18. Do you use a wheelchair? ❏All the time ❏Some of the time ❏Rarely ❏Never

19. Do you use an crutches, walker, or a cane? ❏Yes (Circle device) ❏No ❏All the time
    ❏Some of the time ❏Rarely ❏Never

20. Do you live alone? ❏Yes ❏No
    If you are living with others, how much do they help you, and to do what? _____

21. Do you have stairs at home? ❏Yes ❏No ❏ Ramp
    If yes, how many to get into the home? _____ With railing? ❏Yes ❏No
    How many to reach your bedroom? _____ With railing? ❏Yes ❏No

22. Are you currently working/volunteering outside your home? ❑Yes　❑No
　　If yes, what do you do? How many hours/day? _____　How many hours/week? _____

23. What do you like to do for fun/recreation/relaxation? _____

24. Do you see any limitations in returning to your previous activity due to your amputation? ❑Yes　❑No
　　Describe: _____

25. What are your goals for physical therapy? What do you expect be able to do after physical therapy is finished?
(Be specific: For example, Be able to walk 2 blocks to my friend's house without a walker.) _____
_____
_____

LOWER EXTREMITY FUNCTIONAL SCALE (LEFS)

Today, do you or would you have any difficulty at all with the following activities?
(Circle a number for each activity)

Activity	Extreme Difficulty or Unable to Perform	Quite a Bit of Difficulty	Moderate Difficulty	A Little Bit of Difficulty	No Difficulty
Usual work, housework, schoolwork	0	1	2	3	4
Performing light tasks at home	0	1	2	3	4
Performing heavy tasks at home	0	1	2	3	4
Usual sports, hobbies, recreation	0	1	2	3	4
Getting into or out of the bathtub	0	1	2	3	4
Walking between rooms	0	1	2	3	4
Putting on your shoe and sock	0	1	2	3	4
Lifting an object like a bag of groceries from the floor	0	1	2	3	4
Squatting	0	1	2	3	4
Getting into and out of your car	0	1	2	3	4

continued

Walking 2 blocks	0	1	2	3	4
Walking a mile	0	1	2	3	4
Going up and down 10 stairs	0	1	2	3	4
Sitting for 1 hour	0	1	2	3	4
Standing for 1 hour	0	1	2	3	4
Running	0	1	2	3	4
Hopping	0	1	2	3	4
Roll over in bed	0	1	2	3	4
SCORE					

Adapted from: Binkley M. The Lower Extremity Functional Scale (LEFS): Scale development, measurement properties, and clinical application. *Phys Ther*. 1999;79:371-383.

If you have diabetes, remember to eat a regular meal 1 ½ to 2 hours prior to PT. Do not skip a meal. Check your blood sugar. If it is over 240, please contact the physical therapist to reschedule your appointment.

What to bring and wear to your physical therapy appointment:
1. Loose, comfortable shorts
2. The shoes that were worn when the prosthesis was aligned
3. Extra stump socks
4. An elastic skrinker
5. Crutches or a wheelchair

Please continue to work on your home exercise program.

Thank you for taking the time to complete this questionnaire.

Facility name: _____
Facility address:_____
Contact number: _____

Pain Questionnaire

Melissa Wolff-Burke, PT, EdD, MS, ATC; Elizabeth Smith Cole, PT; Mary Witt, PT

NAME: _____ DATE: _____

Amputation site(s):_____ ❐ Left   ❐ Right

I. Residual Limb (Stump) Pain

If you have pain in your residual limb(s), please continue with this section, if you do **NOT** have pain in your residual limb, you may continue to Section II.

1. Is your pain: ❐ Constant   ❐ Comes and goes

2. Where is this pain? _____

3. Please circle the words below that best describe this pain (circle all that apply):

Dull	Sore	Hurting	Aching	Heavy
Tender	Taught	Tiring	Splitting	Other _____

4. On a scale of 0-10 (0 = no pain, 10 = worst pain imaginable), what was your WORST pain level each day of the past week?

Monday	Tuesday	Wednesday	Thursday	Friday	Saturday	Sunday

5. What helps to relieve the pain? (Please circle all that apply)

Rest	Massage	Ice	Music	Acupuncture
Heat	Medications	Other _____		

6. What makes it worse? _____

7. Does the pain affect: (Please circle all that apply)

Appetite	Concentration	Relationships	Physical activity	Sleep
Emotions	Nothing	Other _____		

8. What pain level, from 0 to 10, is acceptable/tolerable to you? _____

II. Phantom Pain

If you have **PAIN** in the part of your leg(s) that is/are no longer there (NOT just feelings), please continue with this section. If you do **NOT** have phantom pain in this/these area(s), you may continue to Section III.

1. Is your pain: ❑ Constant   ❑ Comes and goes

2. Where is this pain? _____

3. Please circle the words below that best describe this pain (circle all that apply):
   Dull   Sharp   Aching   Throbbing   Hot   Cold
   Piercing   Other _____

4. On a scale of 0-10 (0 = no pain, 10 = worst pain imaginable), what was your WORST pain level each day of the past week?

Monday	Tuesday	Wednesday	Thursday	Friday	Saturday	Sunday

5. What helps to relieve the pain? (Please circle all that apply)
   Rest   Massage   Ice   Music   Acupuncture   Heat
   Medications   Other _____

6. What makes it worse? _____

7. Does the pain affect: (Please circle all that apply)
   Appetite   Concentration   Relationships   Physical activity   Sleep
   Emotions   Nothing   Other _____

8. What pain level, from 0 to 10, is acceptable/tolerable for you? _____

III. Phantom Feeling

If you have FEELING, BUT NOT PAIN, in the part of your leg(s) that is/are no longer there, please continue with this section. If you do not have this feeling, you may continue to Section IV.

1. Is this feeling: ❑ Constant   ❑ Comes and goes

2. Where is this feeling? _____

3. Please describe the feeling: _____

4. Does this feeling bother you?   ❑ Yes   ❑ No

5. What helps to relieve the feeling? (Please circle all that apply)   ❑ N/A
   Rest   Massage   Ice   Music   Acupuncture
   Heat   Medications   Other _____

6. Does the phantom feeling affect: (Please circle all that apply)
   Appetite   Concentration   Relationships   Physical activity   Sleep
   Emotions   Nothing   Other _____

IV. Previous Pain

If you had pain before your amputation, please continue with this section.

1. What areas of your body were painful and why? _____

_____

_____

Physical Therapy Evaluation for Prosthetic Candidate

Melissa Wolff-Burke, PT, EdD, MS, ATC; Elizabeth Smith Cole, PT; Mary Witt, PT

Date: _____

Name: _____   **DOB**: _____   **Height**: _____   **Weight**: _____

BMI: _____   (Weight in pounds) X 700/(height inches) squared

Dates of Amputation: _____   **Amputation(s) sides**: _____   **Level(s)**: _____

Mental status: ❑ Intact x 4   **Impaired orientation to**: ❑ Person   ❑ Place   ❑ Time   ❑ Condition

Patient Concerns: _____

_____

Vital signs: ❑ N/T

HR at rest: _____	After exercise: _____	After 5 min rest: _____
BP at rest: _____	After exercise: _____	After 5 min rest: _____
RR at rest: _____	After exercise: _____	After 5 min rest: _____
RPE at rest: _____	After exercise: _____	After 5 min rest: _____

Balance:

	Unsteady	Steady with Support	Independent
Sitting – Eyes open			
Sitting – Eyes closed			
Sitting reach			
Sitting nudge			
Standing – Eyes open			
Standing – Eyes closed			
Standing reach			
Standing nudge			

Assistive Devices Used:
❏ Tub seat   ❏ Tub transfer bench   ❏ Gab bars   ❏ Wheelchair

Transfers	Independent	Min Assist	Mod assist	Max assist
Supine-to-sit				
Sit-to-supine				
Sit-to-stand				
Stand-to-sit				
Stand-to-floor				
Floor-to-stand				

Ambulation: ❏ With prosthesis   ❏ Without prosthesis   ❏ Nonambulatory/WC
                    ❏ Walker   ❏ Wheeled walker   ❏ Quad cane
                    ❏ Cane(s)   ❏ Crutches   ❏ No assistive device
                    ❏ Other

Gait assessment: _____

_____

_____

RESIDUAL LIMB: ❏ Right   ❏ Left

Shape: ❏ Cylindrical   ❏ Conical   ❏ Bulbous   ❏ Other: _____

Redundant Tissue: ❏ None   ❏ Present: _____

Incision: ❏ Healed   ❏ Sutures   ❏ Staples   ❏ Steristrips   ❏ Other: _____

Scar: ❏ Mobile   ❏ Adherent   ❏ Invaginated   ❏ Flat   ❏ Keloid   ❏ Other: _____

Wound: Eschar: ❏ None   ❏ _____ %   Slough: ❏ Mobile   ❏ _____ %
            Granulated: ❏ None   ❏ _____ %

Drainage: ❏ None   ❏ Scant   ❏ Minimal   ❏ Moderate   ❏ Severe   ❏ Serous   ❏ Serosanguinous
               ❏ Bloody   ❏ Purulent   ❏ Other: _____

Odor: ❏ None   ❏ Present: _____

Callus: ❏ None   ❏ Present: _____

Skin Temperature: ❏ Normal   ❏ Warm   ❏ Cold

Skin Color: ❏ Normal   ❏ Red   ❏ Blue   ❏ Pale   ❏ Ashen   ❏ Jaundiced   ❏ Other: _____

Turgor: ❏ Normal   ❏ Fair   ❏ Poor

Moisture: ❏ Normal   ❏ Dry   ❏ Moist   ❏ Sweaty

Edema: ❏ None   ❏ Mild   ❏ Moderate   ❏ Severe   ❏ Pitting   ❏ 1+   ❏ 2+   ❏ 3+

Girth: Point of Reference: _____

At reference point: _____cm		Contralat: _____cm	
5 cm below: _____cm		_____cm	
10 cm below: _____cm		_____cm	
20 cm below: _____cm		_____cm	

Sensation:

Light Touch: ❑ normal ❑ decreased ❑ increased
Pin Prick: ❑ normal ❑ decreased ❑ increased
Smallest Semmes-Weinstein Monofilament perceived: _____ (5.07 Normal)

Vascular Status: ❑ N/A (HP or HD) ❑ N/T

Pulse	0 (absent)	1+ (diminished)	2+ (normal)	3+ (increased)

Knee: ❑ N/A ❑ N/T

Extension   *Flexion*

MMT	A/PROM	MMT	A/PROM

Hyper/hypomobility noted: ❑ none ❑ M/L ❑ A/P
Standing position: ❑ genu recurvatum ❑ genu valgum ❑ genu varum
Other: ❑ crepitus ❑ c/o pain _____

Hip: ❑ N/A ❑ N/T

Flexion   *Extension*   *Abduction*   *Adduction*

MMT	A/PROM	MMT	A/PROM	MMT	A/PROM	MMT	A/PROM

Internal rotation   *External rotation*

MMT	A/PROM	MMT	A/PROM

❑ c/o pain _____

Comments: _____

CONTRALATERAL LIMB: ❑ right ❑ left ❑ N/T

Skin Temperature: ❑ normal ❑ warm ❑ cold

Skin Color: ❑ normal ❑ red ❑ blue ❑ pale ❑ ashen ❑ jaundiced ❑ other _____

Turgor: ❑ normal ❑ fair ❑ poor

Moisture: ❑ normal ❑ dry ❑ moist ❑ sweaty

Edema: ❑ none ❑ mild ❑ moderate ❑ severe ❑ pitting ❑ 1+ ❑ 2+ ❑ 3+ ❑ 4+

Sensation:

Light Touch: ❑ normal ❑ decreased ❑ increased
Pin Prick: ❑ normal ❑ decreased ❑ increased
Smallest Semmes-Weinstein Monofilament perceived: _____ (5.07 Normal)

Vascular Status: ❑ N/A (HP or HD) ❑ N/T

Pulse	0 (absent)	1+ (diminished)	2+ (normal)	3+ (increased)

Ankle: ❑ N/A ❑ N/T

Dorsiflexion		Plantarflexion		Inversion		Eversion	
MMT	A/PROM	MMT	A/PROM	MMT	A/PROM	MMT	A/PROM

❑ c/o pain _____

Knee: ❑ N/A ❑ N/T

Extension		Flexion	
MMT	A/PROM	MMT	A/PROM

Hyper/hypomobility noted: ❑ none ❑ M/L ❑ A/P
Standing position: ❑ genu recurvatum ❑ genu valgus ❑ genu varus
Other: ❑ crepitus ❑ c/o pain _____

Hip: ❑ N/A ❑ N/T

Flexion		Extension		Abduction		Adduction	
MMT	A/PROM	MMT	A/PROM	MMT	A/PROM	MMT	A/PROM

Internal rotation		External rotation	
MMT	A/PROM	MMT	A/PROM

❑ c/o pain _____

Comments: _____

_____

Prosthesis:

Socket style: ❑ suction ❑ nonsuction ❑ auxiliary suspension
# of socks: am _____ pm _____
Knee unit: _____ Foot: _____ Other: _____

Previous prostheses usage and components (if different from current prosthesis): _____

_____

Upper Extremities: ❏ AROM/PROM WFL   ❏ MMT at least 4/5 throughout

_____

_____

LEFS Score: _____   **2-minute walk distance**: _____

PT Diagnosis: _____

Problem List
1.
2.
3.
4.

Equipment needs: _____

Referrals/Contacts: _____

Goals: (with time frame)
1.
2.
3.
4.

Patient goals: _____

Prognosis: _____

Plan of Care:
      Interventions: _____
      Frequency and duration: _____
      Discharge plans: _____

Precautions: _____

Contraindications: _____

Signature/Title: _____

Case Study for a Person With a Transfemoral Amputation

Melissa Wolff-Burke, PT, EdD, MS, ATC; Elizabeth Smith Cole, PT; Mary Witt, PT

HISTORY

The patient is a 55-year-old white male, who was in an excellent state of health prior to his amputation. He had no significant health history, was not taking any medications and was working full time as a ferrier. He smoked two packs of cigarettes/day, and drank alcohol moderately. He was independent in all self-care and lived with his wife in a two-story home. An undiagnosed aneurysm in his right popliteal region ruptured ten weeks prior resulting in an emergency bypass which failed. A transtibial amputation was unsuccessful and a subsequent revision to the transfemoral level was done 8 weeks later. He was referred to physical therapy 2 weeks post-transfemoral amputation for rehabilitation.

The first 4 weeks of rehabilitation were nonprosthetic and focused on core strength, trunk and limb flexibility, and pelvic control. The patient was unable to drive during this time as he had not been tested for driving with the left leg, nor had any adjustments been made to his truck. At 6 weeks postamputation, he received his current prosthesis; an ischial containment suction socket with a swing control knee, a single axis foot, and auxiliary suspension from a Silesian belt.

INTAKE EXAMINATION

The patient is independent in self-care without the prosthesis and is using the crutches in and around his home, except on stairs. His incision is well healed, the residual limb is cylindrical, edematous (1+) with significant redundant tissue. The distal 3 inches are indurated and the shrinker is not fitting properly, nor applying enough compression at the distal end of the residual limb. His femoral pulse is normal (2+) on the right. He is using pain medications prn. He reports phantom sensation of the right foot. His vitals are stable at rest and after crutch ambulation in the clinic using the prosthesis. His 2-minute walk distance, using crutches and prosthesis, is 100 feet. His LEFS score at intake is 13/80. There are no problems or concerns on the left lower extremity, except for the patient report of osteoarthritis of the left knee. There are no functional limitations of his upper extremities. His lumbar backward bending demonstrates marked hypomobility with no reversal of the lumbar curve. The patient's goal is to quickly return to work.

EVALUATION

The examination identifies a physical therapy diagnosis of impaired mobility due to the right transfemoral amputation. The evaluation determines the following problem areas. The patient is: unable to don the prosthesis with the pull sock; is not fully seated in the socket; is unable to weightbear on the right; is unable to stand without an assistive device; is unable to resist challenges to his standing balance; is unable to maintain knee extension at midstance; is unable to ambulate using the prosthesis and bilateral axillary over any surface without pain in the residual limb.

No additional equipment is needed at this time. A referral is made to the driver retraining program, and contact with the prosthetist is necessary due to concerns about fit, alignment, and comfort. Physical therapy long term goals are: pain free, independent ambulation without an assistive device over level and uneven ground; ambulation distance sufficient to meet personal and work needs; return to previous employment.

PROGNOSIS

The prognosis for ambulation is excellent as the patient is not debilitated by other health problems and is motivated. The prognosis for return to work as a ferrier is guarded due to limitations in the capabilities of a prosthesis to allow for the necessary speed and agility to safely work around horses.

The next section describes physical therapy interventions used to achieve the patient and physical therapy goals over a 12 week period. The LEFS at discharge –48/80 and the patient had started a consultation practice as a ferrier.

PATIENT/CAREGIVER EDUCATION

A. *Prosthetic care and function*: Explained components of prosthesis, how they function, care and cleaning of prosthesis.
B. *Skin checks*: Discussed frequency and procedure for skin checks post ambulation, using a mirror and palpation. Frequent skin checks with the physical therapist during early weeks of ambulation training. Explained hygiene for residual limb.
C. *Edema management*: Patient is given well-fitting shrinker and instructed in elastic bandage wrap, over or under shrinker, to improve compression at distal residual limb.
D. *Wearing schedule*: Given wearing schedule and parameters for walking and wearing time.
E. *General education*: Given local and national support group information. Offered magazines, videos and books related to amputations, prosthetics, prosthetists, and living with an amputation.
F. *Care of remaining limb*: Discouraged hopping due to OA and increased stress on remaining limb. Patient is not diabetic.
G. *Fitness*: Reviewed previous independent fitness program of weight lifting, Yoga and Pilates. Modified program for safety and feasibility with one limb. Developed HEP for right residual limb, lumbar strengthening and flexibility.

PROSTHESIS CHECK

A. *Donning*: Experimented with pullsock, elastic bandage wrap, lotion to determine easiest entry into socket with best contact. Selected lotion.
B. *Sock management*: None. Suction fit.

C. *Fit*: No contact at distal socket, adductor role evident. Patient reports pain at distal, lateral femur and in groin. Prosthetist contacted and follow-up appointment scheduled. Adjustments made to socket resulted in improved contact and comfort.
D. *Alignment*: Observed knee axis anterior of weight line on initial contact, resulting in unstable knee at loading response. Lateral whip noted. Prosthetist contacted and alignment changes made resulted in improved knee stability and patient confidence during stance.

STANDING BALANCE AND WEIGHTBEARING

A. Stable and soft surfaces used to practice maintaining upright posture with and without perturbations.
B. Balloon toss and reach.
C. Balance board for finding midline and moving away from midline in lateral, diagonal, and a/p directions.
D. Weighted ball toss.
E. Step-up on 2- to 8-inch step, using hands for support → hands free.
F. Hip hiking from a 2-inch step with full weight bearing on amputated side.

SOCKET CONTROL

A. Visualization for position of residual limb in socket.
B. Placement of prosthetic foot without visual cues.
C. Active contraction of the residual limb in socket against resistance.
D. Sidestepping, crossover and inline stepping in parallel bars.
E. Single limb stance not tolerated until socket and alignment adjustments made.

AMBULATION

A. Components of swing and stride practiced in parallel bars. Begin with two hands and sequentially progressed to amputated side hand, sound side hand, no hands.
B. Full strides using parallel bars → One crutch and one side of parallel bar → Outside of bars two crutches used in reciprocating pattern → one crutch and PT for stabilization on amputated side → cane and PT → cane at discharge. Likelihood of ambulation without an assistive device is good.

C. Manual and elastic cord resistance to pelvis and shoulders during ambulation to encourage forward rotation of pelvis on amputated side and trunk stability.

D. Stair training using crutches, rail.

E. Practiced inclines and declines using various methods depending on terrain, condition of surface and patient confidence.

ENDURANCE

A. Upper body ergometer.

B. Recumbent bike with sound limb and arms. Bike used when prosthesis fit is comfortable.

C. Pool therapy for endurance.

D. Treadmill, full body weight, using rails for stability. Emphasized full use of prosthetic foot through terminal stance.

ACTIVITIES OF DAILY LIVING

A. Encouraged community ambulation with and without prosthesis; shops, restaurants.

B. Scheduled and passed driver safety test. Adaptive gas pedal installed allowing patient to drive.

C. Modified seat of truck for ease of entry and comfort while driving.

RETURN TO WORK

A. Squat, with and without a weight, between knees to simulate shoeing a horse.

B. Ambulate over uneven ground, across street, inclines, ramps.

C. Ambulate with cane and object in sound side hand to simulate carrying equipment for shoeing horses.

Index

WAIT
...There's More!

SLACK Incorporated's Health Care Books and Journals offers a wide selection of products in the field of Prosthetics and Orthotics. We are dedicated to providing important works that educate, inform and improve the knowledge of our customers. Don't miss out on our other informative titles that will enhance your collection.

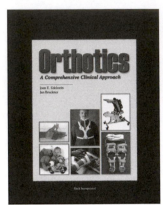

Orthotics: A Comprehensive Clinical Approach

Joan Edelstein, MA, PT, FISPO and Jan Bruckner, PhD, PT
192 pp., Hard Cover, 2002,
ISBN 1-55642-416-7,
Order #44167, **$46.95**

Orthotics: A Comprehensive Clinical Approach is an innovative and comprehensive text that provides essential information about contemporary orthoses to guide the student and clinician in prescribing and utilizing these appliances in neuromuscular, musculoskeletal, and integumentary rehabilitation.

Individual chapters cover orthoses for the foot, ankle, knee, hip, trunk, neck, shoulder, elbow, wrist, and hand. Orthoses for patients with paraplegia, burns, and soft tissue contractures are detailed and illustrated. Prescription guidelines, evaluation techniques, goal setting, and training procedures are presented. Each chapter also includes interesting "thought" questions and case studies to promote clinical reasoning and problem-solving skills.

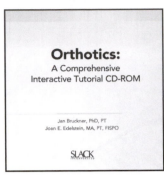

Orthotics: A Comprehensive Interactive Tutorial

Jan Bruckner, PhD, PT and Joan Edelstein, MD, PT, FISPO
CD-ROM, 2003,
ISBN 1-55642-744-1,
Order #47441, **$49.95**

Orthotics: A Comprehensive Interactive Tutorial provides a dynamic presentation of orthotic management for patients with lower-limb, spinal, cervical, and upper-limb disorders. This user-friendly CD-ROM utilizes an interactive format to exhibit a wide range of orthoses in use and on display.

Jan Bruckner, PhD, PT and Joan E. Edelstein, MA, PT, FISPO present a library of lower-limb, spinal, cervical, and upper-limb orthoses, evaluations of orthoses on and off patients, six case studies, and a self-assessment quiz written in the format of the physical therapy licensure examination. Componentry is demonstrated as well as multiple aspects of the appliances and donning procedures.

Please visit
www.slackbooks.com
to order any of these titles!
24 Hours a Day...7 Days a Week!

Attention Industry Partners!
Whether you are interested in buying multiple copies of a book, chapter reprints, or looking for something new and different — we are able to accommodate your needs.

Multiple Copies
At attractive discounts starting for purchases as low as 25 copies for a single title, SLACK Incorporated will be able to meet all your of your needs.

Chapter Reprints
SLACK Incorporated is able to offer the chapters you want in a format that will lead to success. Bound with an attractive cover, use the chapters that are a fit specifically for your company. Available for quantities of 100 or more.

Customize
SLACK Incorporated is able to create a specialized custom version of any of our products specifically for your company.

Please contact the Marketing Manager of the Health Care Books and Journals for further details on multiple copy purchases, chapter reprints or custom printing at 1-800-257-8290 or 1-856-848-1000.

*Please note all conditions are subject to change.

CODE: 328

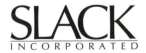

SLACK Incorporated • Health Care Books and Journals
6900 Grove Road • Thorofare, NJ 08086

1-800-257-8290 or 1-856-848-1000
Fax: 1-856-853-5991 • E-mail: orders@slackinc.com • Visit www.slackbooks.com